# Palliative Care

*Guest Editor*

SERIFE ETI, MD

# PRIMARY CARE:
# CLINICS IN OFFICE PRACTICE

www.primarycare.theclinics.com

*Consulting Editor*
JOEL J. HEIDELBAUGH, MD

June 2011 • Volume 38 • Number 2

SAUNDERS an imprint of ELSEVIER, Inc.

**W.B. SAUNDERS COMPANY**
*A Division of Elsevier Inc.*

1600 John F. Kennedy Boulevard, Suite 1800 • Philadelphia, PA 19103-2899

http://www.theclinics.com

**PRIMARY CARE: CLINICS IN OFFICE PRACTICE Volume 38, Number 2**
**June 2011 ISSN 0095-4543, ISBN-13: 978-1-4557-0497-2**

Editor: Yonah Korngold

*Primary Care: Clinics in Office Practice* (ISSN: 0095–4543) is published quarterly by Elsevier Inc., 360 Park Avenue South, New York, NY 10010-1710. Months of issue are March, June, September, and December. Periodicals postage paid at New York, NY and additional mailing offices. Subscription prices are $203.00 per year (US individuals), $336.00 (US institutions), $101.00 (US students), $248.00 (Canadian individuals), $395.00 (Canadian institutions), $159.00 (Canadian students), $309.00 (international individuals), $395.00 (international institutions), and $159.00 (international students). Foreign air speed delivery is included in all *Clinics* subscription prices. All prices are subject to change without notice. POSTMASTER: Send address changes to *Primary Care: Clinics in Office Practice*, Elsevier Periodicals Customer Service, 11830 Westline Industrial Drive, St. Louis, MO 63146. Customer Service Health Sciences Division, Subscription Customer Service, 3251 Riverport Lane, Maryland Heights, MO 63043. **Customer Service: 1-800-654-2452 (U.S. and Canada); 314-447-8871 (outside U.S. and Canada). Fax: 314-447-8029. E-mail: journalscustomerservice-usa@elsevier.com (for print support); journalsonlinesupport-usa@elsevier.com (for online support).**

*Reprints.* For copies of 100 or more, of articles in this publication, please contact the Commercial Reprints Department, Elsevier Inc., 360 Park Avenue South, New York, NY 10010-1710. Tel. (212) 633-3812; Fax: (212) 482-1935; E-mail: reprints@elsevier.com.

*Primary Care: Clinics in Office Practice* is covered in *MEDLINE/PubMed (Index Medicus)* and *EMBASE/ Excerpta Medica, Current Contents/Clinical Medicine, and ISI/BIOMED.*

Printed and bound by CPI Group (UK) Ltd, Croydon, CR0 4YY

Transferred to Digital Print 2011

# Contributors

## CONSULTING EDITOR

**JOEL J. HEIDELBAUGH, MD**
Clinical Assistant Professor and Clerkship Director, Department of Family Medicine;
Clinical Assistant Professor, Department of Urology, University of Michigan Medical
School, Ann Arbor, Michigan

## GUEST EDITOR

**SERIFE ETI, MD**
Director of Fellowship Program in Hospice and Palliative Medicine, Department of Pain
Medicine and Palliative Care, Beth Israel Medical Center, New York; Assistant Professor,
Department of Family and Social Medicine, Albert Einstein College of Medicine, Bronx,
New York

## AUTHORS

**ANDREW R. BERMAN, MD**
Associate Professor of Clinical Medicine, Division of Pulmonary Medicine, Department
of Medicine, Albert Einstein College of Medicine; Montefiore Medical Center,
Bronx, New York

**CRAIG D. BLINDERMAN, MD, MA**
Division Chief, Adult Palliative Medicine, Assistant Professor of Palliative Care
(Anesthesiology and Medicine), Department of Anesthesiology, Columbia University,
New York, New York

**EDUARDO BRUERA, MD**
Department of Palliative Care and Rehabilitation Medicine, The University of Texas MD
Anderson Cancer Center, Houston, Texas

**MARIE-ANDRÉE BRUNEAU, MD**
Institut Universitaire de Gériatrie de Montréal; Assistant Professor, Department of
Psychiatry, University of Montreal, Montreal, Quebec, Canada

**RABBI MOLLIE CANTOR, BCC**
Center for Pastoral Education, Jewish Theological Seminar, New York, New York

**LESLIE CUNNINGHAM, PhD**
Licensed Clinical Psychologist and Instructor, Division of Pediatric Hematology/Oncology,
Albert Einstein College of Medicine, Children's Hospital at Montefiore, Bronx, New York

**SHALINI DALAL, MD**
Assistant Professor, Department of Palliative Care and Rehabilitation Medicine, The
University of Texas MD Anderson Cancer Center, Houston, Texas

## SERIFE ETI, MD
Director of Fellowship Program in Hospice and Palliative Medicine, Department of Pain Medicine and Palliative Care, Beth Israel Medical Center, New York; Assistant Professor, Department of Family and Social Medicine, Albert Einstein College of Medicine, Bronx, New York

## JAMES A. FAUSTO Jr, MD
Assistant Professor, Palliative Care Program, Department of Family and Social Medicine, Montefiore Medical Center, Albert Einstein College of Medicine, Bronx, New York

## ALLEN HUTCHESON, MD
Regional Medical Director, Visiting Nurse Service of New York Hospice Care, Bronx, New York

## DANIELLE N. KO, MBBS, LLB
Palliative Care Fellow, Division of General Internal Medicine; Palliative Care Service, Massachusetts General Hospital; Medical Ethics Fellow, Division of Medical Ethics, Harvard Medical School, Boston, Massachusetts

## HANNAH I. LIPMAN, MD, MS
Assistant Professor of Medicine, Divisions of Cardiology and Geriatrics; Chief, Bioethics Consultation Service; Associate Director, Montefiore-Einstein Center for Bioethics, Montefiore Medical Center, Albert Einstein College of Medicine, Bronx, New York

## DAVID LUSSIER, MD
Institut Universitaire de Gériatrie de Montréal; Assistant Professor, Department of Medicine, University of Montreal; Adjunct Professor, Division of Geriatric Medicine, Alan-Edwards Centre for Research on Pain, McGill University, Montreal, Quebec, Canada

## MARLENE E. MCHUGH, DNP, FNP-BC, RN
Assistant Professor of Clinical Nursing, Columbia University, School of Nursing, New York; Associate Director, Palliative Care Service, Department of Family Medicine, Montefiore Medical Center, Bronx, New York

## DEBBIE MILLER-SAULTZ, DNP, FNP-BC, RN
Assistant Professor of Clinical Nursing, Columbia University Nurse Practitioner; Department of Anesthesiology, Divison of Pain Medicine and Palliative Care, New York Presbyterian Medical Center, New York, New York

## KAREN MOODY, MD, MS
Assistant Professor, Division of Pediatric Hematology/Oncology, Albert Einstein College of Medicine, Children's Hospital at Montefiore, Bronx, New York

## SANDHYA MURTHY, MD
Cardiology Fellow, Division of Cardiology, Montefiore Medical Center, Albert Einstein College of Medicine, Bronx, New York

## PEDRO PEREZ-CRUZ, MD
Palliative Care Fellow, Division of General Internal Medicine, Massachusetts General Hospital, Boston, Massachusetts; Instructor, Department of Internal Medicine, School of Medicine, Pontifical Catholic University of Chile, Santiago, Chile; Palliative Care Service, Massachusetts General Hospital, Boston, Massachusetts

## KATHRYN SCHARBACH, MD
Assistant Professor, Division of Social Pediatrics, Albert Einstein College of Medicine, Children's Hospital at Montefiore, Bronx, New York

**PETER A. SELWYN, MD, MPH**
Professor and Chairman, Department of Family and Social Medicine, Montefiore Medical Center, Albert Einstein College of Medicine, Bronx, New York

**LINDA SIEGEL, MD, FAAP**
Assistant Professor, Division of Pediatric Critical Care, Albert Einstein College of Medicine, Children's Hospital at Montefiore, Bronx, New York

**JUAN MANUEL VILLALPANDO, MD**
Institut Universitaire de Gériatrie de Montréal, Assistant Professor, University of Montreal, Montreal, Quebec, Canada

**RONALD WERB, MB, ChB, MRCP(UK), FRCP(C)**
Clinical Professor of Medicine, Division of Nephrology, Department of Medicine, University of British Columbia; Staff Nephrologist, Providence Health Care, Vancouver, British Columbia, Canada

# Contents

Foreword: "Dying with Dignity"                                                    xi

Joel J. Heidelbaugh

Preface                                                                           xiii

Serife Eti

Palliative Care: An Evolving Field in Medicine                                    159

Serife Eti

Palliative care is an approach that improves the quality of life of patients and their families facing the problems associated with life-threatening illness, through the prevention and relief of suffering by means of early identification and impeccable assessment and treatment of pain and other problems: physical, psychosocial, and spiritual. This article discusses illness trajectories and prognostic estimates, prognostic tools, educating physicians and nurses in palliative care, research in palliative medicine, and palliative care in hospitals and the community.

Hospice Care in the United States                                                 173

Allen Hutcheson

Hospice affirms the concept of palliative care as an intensive program that enhances comfort and promotes quality of life for individuals and their families. When cure is no longer possible, hospice recognizes that a peaceful and comfortable death is an essential goal of health care. Hospice believes that death is an integral part of the life cycle and that intensive palliative care focuses on pain relief, comfort, and enhanced quality of life for the terminally ill. Hospice also recognizes the potential for growth that exists within the dying experience for individuals and their families and seeks to protect and nurture this potential.

Ethical Issues in Palliative Care                                                 183

Danielle N. Ko, Pedro Perez-Cruz, and Craig D. Blinderman

Ethical problems in medicine are common, especially when caring for patients at the end of life. However, many of these issues are not adequately identified in the outpatient setting. Primary care providers are in a unique and privileged position to identify ethical issues, prevent future conflicts, and help patients make medical decisions that are consistent with their individual values and preferences. This article describes some of the more common ethical issues faced by primary care physicians caring for patients with life-limiting illness.

Assessment and Management of Pain in the Terminally Ill                           195

Shalini Dalal and Eduardo Bruera

Regular assessment for the presence of pain and response to pain management strategies should be high priority in terminally ill patients. Pain management interventions are most effective when treatments are individualized based on the various physical and nonphysical components of pain at the end of life, and patients and family are educated and involved in the decision making. Opioids remain the cornerstone of pain management, and adjuvant analgesics and nonpharmacologic options are usually considered after relative stabilization of pain. This article describes the various issues that are pertinent to the assessment and treatment of pain in terminally ill patients.

**Assessment and Management of Gastrointestinal Symptoms in Advanced Illness**    225

Marlene E. McHugh and Debbie Miller-Saultz

Primary care clinicians increasingly encounter patients with advanced illness, many suffering from symptoms other than pain. Key principles that guide palliative care must be incorporated into a plan of care for each patient and family. Although medical management continues to be the mainstay of treatment, the generalist in palliative care needs to be familiar with the patient's preferences and goals of care. This article provides an overview of gastrointestinal symptoms including anorexia, cachexia, nausea, vomiting, and constipation. Advanced progressive illnesses are defined here as incurable conditions that have significant morbidity in the later stages of illness.

**Management of End-Stage Dementia**    247

David Lussier, Marie-Andrée Bruneau, and Juan Manuel Villalpando

Dementia is a progressive and noncurable illness, and its management in late stages should follow a palliative care approach. However, many patients with advanced dementia sustain aggressive interventions that do not improve their survival and might hinder their comfort and quality of life. This is likely explained by a lack of research on this population; a lack of knowledge from health care providers, patients, and family members; and lack of communication between those caring for these patients. There is therefore an urgent need for research and education on this topic, as well as palliative care services devoted to this population.

**Management of End-Stage Heart Failure**    265

Sandhya Murthy and Hannah I. Lipman

The prevalence of heart failure (HF) is increasing and morbidity and mortality remain high. There is a clear need for palliative care for the growing population of chronically ill patients with HF. Because HF-specific therapy modifies disease and palliates symptoms, recommended treatments for chronic and acute decompensated HF are reviewed. This article discusses symptom burden in advanced HF and specific considerations for patients with HF regarding advance care planning and symptom-directed therapy. Options for care at the end of life, including hospice, chronic inotropic support, and deactivation of an internal cardiac defibrillator, are also discussed.

**Management of Patients with End-Stage Chronic Obstructive Pulmonary Disease**    277

Andrew R. Berman

Patients with end-stage chronic obstructive pulmonary disease (COPD) have poor quality of life, with limited activity, breathlessness, dependence on others, and recurrent needs for medical evaluation and treatment. Such patients demonstrate significant and progressive impairments in physical, mental, and social functioning. Because the rate of decline is variable, however, it is difficult to predict prognosis of survival. Currently available treatments only partially relieve symptoms, and patients become increasingly more disabled. This article reviews quality of life issues, proposed prognostic indicators, and pharmacologic and nonpharmacologic treatments in advanced COPD. Palliative measures to address breathlessness and unmet needs among patients with end-stage COPD are discussed.

**Palliative Care in the Treatment of End-Stage Renal Failure**    299

Ronald Werb

Palliative care begins with establishing goals of care based on estimated prognosis in end-stage renal disease (ESRD). Patients with ESRD are increasingly characterized by older age and multiple comorbid illnesses, and have a mortality rate 8 times higher than the general Medicare population. Dialysis patients are appropriate for palliative care because of their high mortality rate and high symptom burden. More patients and families are choosing not to start or withdraw dialysis for multiple reasons, particularly in patients older than 60 years. Advance directives and resuscitation directives are important in ensuring compassionate and goal-directed palliative care of ESRD patients. Drug toxicities are avoidable by using appropriate drugs at the correct doses and dosing intervals.

**Palliative Care in the Management of Advanced HIV/AIDS**    311

James A. Fausto Jr and Peter A. Selwyn

The basic elements of palliative care can be translated into practice for patients with HIV/AIDS. More than half of clinical events and deaths occurring among patients on highly active antiretroviral therapy are classified as non-AIDS illnesses. Thus, end-of-life care for patients with late-stage AIDS needs to include any palliative measures that are used for patients without AIDS. This article reviews the epidemiology of HIV/AIDS, prognostic indicators, opportunistic infections, specific AIDS-defining and non–AIDS-defining malignancies, substance abuse/liver disease, and highly active antiretroviral therapy and comfort measures for late-stage AIDS patients.

**Pediatric Palliative Care**    327

Karen Moody, Linda Siegel, Kathryn Scharbach, Leslie Cunningham, and Rabbi Mollie Cantor

Progress in pediatric palliative care has gained momentum, but there remain significant barriers to the appropriate provision of palliative care to ill and dying children, including the lack of properly trained health care professionals, resources to finance such care, and scientific research, as well as a continued cultural denial of death in children. This article reviews the epidemiology of pediatric palliative care, special communication concerns, decision making, ethical and legal considerations, symptom assessment and management, psychosocial issues, provision of care across settings, end-of-life care, and bereavement. Educational and supportive resources for health care practitioners and families, respectively, are included.

Index    363

## FORTHCOMING ISSUES

*September 2011*
Gastrointestinal Disease
James Winger, MD, and
Aaron Michelfelder, MD, FAAFP,
*Guest Editors*

*December 2011*
Immunizations
Marc Altshuler, MD, and
Edward Buchanan, MD,
*Guest Editors*

## RECENT ISSUES

*March 2011*
Substance Abuse in Office-Based Practice
Robert Mallin, MD,
*Guest Editor*

*December 2010*
Rheumatology-A Survival Guide for the
Primary Care Physician
Allen Perkins, MD, MPH,
*Guest Editor*

*September 2010*
Primary Care Urology
Karl T. Rew, MD and
Masahito Jimbo, MD, PhD, MPH,
*Guest Editors*

## VISIT THE CLINICS ONLINE!

Access your subscription at:
www.theclinics.com

# Foreword

# "Dying with Dignity"

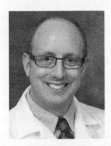

Joel J. Heidelbaugh, MD
 *Consulting Editor*

> *"Death is not the greatest of evils; it is worse to want to die… and not [to] be able to with dignity…"*
>
> —Sophocles

The role of the primary care clinician in caring for our patients with devastating and terminal illnesses cannot be understated, given the complex and often long-standing relationship many of us have with our patients. Unfortunately in many cases, once a patient is diagnosed with a chronic condition that progresses to a terminal condition, the role of the primary care clinician becomes minimized, as the specialist(s) may assume the majority of their health care needs toward the end of life.

Current LCME (Liason Committee on Medical Education) and ACGME (Accreditation Council for Graduate Medical Education) guidelines for US medical school and residency education, respectively, are sparse relative to teaching the concepts of palliative/hospice/end-of-life care. However, this rapidly expanding field of medicine is fast becoming deemed as necessary for all clinicians to embrace, understand, and implement into practice on the level of a multidisciplinary and team-based approach. Current and future research will prove this concept increasingly beneficial on many levels, demonstrating improved qualitative and quantitative outcome measures.

A recent study published in *Health Affairs*[1] found that patients with Medicaid at four hospitals in New York who received comprehensive palliative care services incurred $6,900 less in hospital costs compared to matched controls who didn't receive these services. Consistent with the goals of most patients and their families, this study proved that recipients of palliative care services spent fewer days in intensive care units, were less likely to die there, and were more likely to receive hospice referrals than matched patients who did not receive such services. The authors of this study estimated an impressive potential future annual reduction in Medicaid hospital spending from $84 million to $252 million if hospitals created and offered multidisciplinary palliative care consultation team services to patients with terminal conditions.

Prim Care Clin Office Pract 38 (2011) xi–xii
doi:10.1016/j.pop.2011.03.012
0095-4543/11/$ – see front matter © 2011 Elsevier Inc. All rights reserved.

Future medical education initiatives will see enhanced curricula to teach medical students and residents necessary provisions of end-of-life care, pain management in terminal illness, and strategies to develop the inherent compassionate care that such patients deserve. While palliative and hospice care fellowships currently exist, more will be needed in the future as demand for these services expands greatly.

This volume of the *Primary Care Clinics* serves as an outstanding primer for clinicians to use as a daily reference when called upon to assist patients and their families in the management of end-of-life conditions, from both a medical and a humanitarian standpoint. Introductory articles create a framework for clinicians to understand key terms and statistics relative to palliative and hospice care, as well a conceptual basis of the ethical considerations of such care. This volume also provides excellent detail from the current literature on palliative care options for patients with chronic diseases including dementia, congestive heart failure, chronic obstructive pulmonary disease (COPD), renal disease, and acquired immunodeficiency syndrome (AIDS). Last, an article dedicated to palliative care practices in pediatric patients offers significant guidance in this area.

I sincerely thank Dr Serife Eti, the director of the fellowship program Pain Medicine and Palliative Care at the Albert Einstein College of Medicine, as well as her dedicated authors, for compiling this much needed compendium of information. It is with this knowledge that we will become better stewards of care for our patients at the end of their lives, to maximize their care, to minimize the suffering of our patients and their loved ones, and to help our patients die with respect and dignity.

Joel J. Heidelbaugh, MD
Departments of Family Medicine and Urology
University of Michigan Medical School
Ann Arbor, MI 48109, USA

Ypsilanti Health Center
200 Arnet Street, Suite 200
Ypsilanti, MI 48198, USA
E-mail address:
jheidel@umich.edu

**REFERENCE**

1. Morrison RS, Dietrich J, Ladwig S, et al. Palliative care consultation teams cut hospital costs for Medicaid beneficiaries. Health Affairs 2011;30(3):454–63.

# Preface

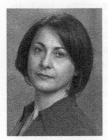

Serife Eti, MD
*Guest Editor*

For more than 25 years, palliative care has been an evolving medical discipline in the United States and many other countries. It is now viewed as a therapeutic approach. It is essential in the comprehensive care of patients with serious or life-threatening illnesses, including those receiving aggressive treatments. Specialist-level palliative care can be delivered through many models, the most common of which in the United States are institution-based palliative care programs and hospice programs. Multiple studies have shown that specialist palliative care is beneficial for patients in reducing pain and other symptom burden, addressing other factors that may contribute to the suffering of the patient and family, increasing satisfaction with care, and reducing cost. It has been accepted as a specialty by the American Board of Medical Specialties, and completion of an Accreditation Council for the Graduate Medical Education (ACGME)-accredited hospice and palliative medicine fellowship will be necessary for certification after 2012.

Specialist-level palliative care often focuses on far advanced illness or end-of-life care because the complexity of problems during this time necessitates the involvement of a specialist team. This volume focuses on understanding final stages of chronic illness, reducing the severity of symptoms in order to prevent and relieve suffering, and improving the quality of life for adults and children facing serious, complex illness. It reviews the current status of delivery systems for palliative care, including hospice. Important topics in palliative care, such as disease trajectories, management of several end-stage diseases, and management of pain and nonpain symptoms, pediatric palliative care, and ethics, are included.

The evidence base supporting therapies central to the delivery of palliative care is very limited. Most treatments are based on expert consensus and some empirical basis. Despite having established practice guidelines, growing in scope and sophistication, palliative care needs far more research to guide practice and create the strongest service delivery models.

Primary care providers are often the coordinators of medical care in inpatient and outpatient settings and need to be well versed in all aspects of providing palliative care for the terminally ill. Tomorrow's primary care physicians will require skills in palliative care as demographics change in the country. An aging population, the growing prevalence of chronic illnesses with functional disability, and the potential for palliative

Prim Care Clin Office Pract 38 (2011) xiii–xiv
doi:10.1016/j.pop.2011.03.013
0095-4543/11/$ – see front matter © 2011 Elsevier Inc. All rights reserved.
**primarycare.theclinics.com**

care to reduce health care costs will increase the importance of palliative care in health care system reform. Primary care physicians can provide guidance for patients and families, support palliative care interventions, and, when appropriate, refer to specialist-level care. This is critical in all settings: community, nursing homes, and hospitals.

The education and training of primary care physicians in the precepts and principles of palliative care will expand patients' access to necessary care when it is needed. This volume hopefully will expand the knowledge and skills of the primary care physician caring for those with advanced illnesses.

Serife Eti, MD
Department of Pain Medicine and Palliative Care
Beth Israel Medical Center
First Avenue at 16th Street
New York, NY 10003, USA

Department of Family and Social Medicine
Albert Einstein College of Medicine
1300 Morris Park Avenue, Bronx, NY 10461, USA

E-mail address:
seti@chpnet.org

# Palliative Care: An Evolving Field in Medicine

Serife Eti, MD[a,b,]*

**KEYWORDS**

• Palliative care • End-of-life care • Prognostic tools

The first use of the word "palliative" as applied to the field was in early 1975 when the first Palliative Care Service of the Royal Victoria Hospital in Montreal was established. The hospice movement was started and spread rapidly in the late 1960s. The pioneering work of Cicely Saunders in London and Florence Wald in New Haven established the foundations of the modern hospice and palliative care movement and highlighted the end-of-life care needs of patients with advanced malignant disease. The Medicare hospice benefit was designed to limit access to patients who were dying of terminal illness, which led to late hospice referrals and reduced access for hospice care for patients with advanced chronic illnesses (**Fig. 1**).

Palliative care began to be defined as a care model for the terminally ill in the 1970s and came to be synonymous with the physical, social, psychological, and spiritual support of patients with life-limiting illness, delivered by a multidisciplinary team. The transition period from curative care to palliative care can be one of the most difficult phases of caring for patients with advanced chronic illnesses. The treatment goals change from life-prolonging treatment to symptom control and quality of life. Palliative care originally referred to the care of patients with terminal illnesses, but now it refers to the care of patients with advanced chronic illnesses (**Fig. 2**). The stark redirection of goals may fit only a few patients' expectations from health care providers. Most patients want palliation of symptoms; and most are well served by some preparations for dying, even while there is substantial hope to prolong life with "aggressive" treatment.[1,2] In fact, most patients are probably best served with a model that mixes treatments to correct physiology (or to extend life) with treatments aimed at symptom control and alleviation of disability. Studies of the use of palliative care have found that

The author has nothing to disclose.
[a] Department of Pain Medicine and Palliative Care, Beth Israel Medical Center, First Avenue at 16th Street, New York, NY 10003, USA
[b] Department of Family and Social Medicine, Albert Einstein College of Medicine, 1300 Morris Park, Bronx, NY 10461, USA
* Department of Pain Medicine and Palliative Care, Beth Israel Medical Center, First Avenue at 16th Street, New York, NY 10003.
*E-mail address:* seti@chpnet.org

Prim Care Clin Office Pract 38 (2011) 159–171
doi:10.1016/j.pop.2011.03.001

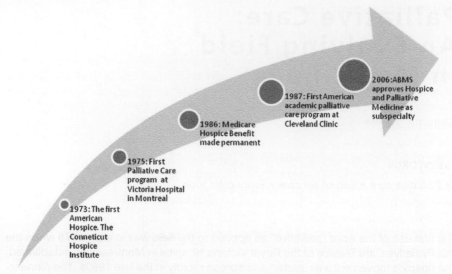

**Fig. 1.** Cornerstones of the hospice and palliative care movement in the United States.

patients with chronic, incurable conditions generally report a much better quality of life when they receive palliative care than patients who do not. In the past 2 decades, we have tried to improve end-of-life care, have granted patients the "right to refuse treatment," have introduced advance directives, and have supported physicians' claims that a treatment would be futile.

The groundbreaking randomized clinical trial by Temel and her colleagues[3] evaluated the impact of early palliative care on the care of patients with metastatic cancer. The study showed that specialty-based palliative care improved quality of life (QOL) and reduced the use of aggressive end-of-life care. Patients who received palliative care rated their quality of life as being significantly higher than those who did not receive palliative care (98.0 vs 91.5 on the Functional Assessment of Cancer Therapy-Lung scale, $P = .03$).[3]

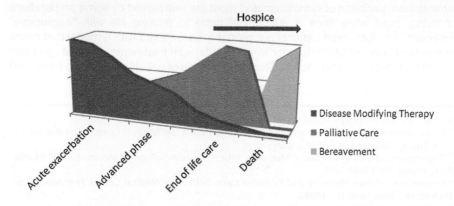

Chronic life-limiting illness

**Fig. 2.** Palliative care and hospice care in the management of chronic life-limiting illness: integrative model of care.

## DEFINITION OF PALLIATIVE CARE

In 2002, the World Health Organization (WHO) revised and described palliative care in a broader definition.[4]

Palliative care is an approach that improves the quality of life of patients and their families facing the problems associated with life-threatening illness, through the prevention and relief of suffering by means of early identification and impeccable assessment and treatment of pain and other problems, physical, psychosocial, and spiritual. Palliative care:

- Provides relief from pain and other distressing symptoms
- Affirms life and regards dying as a normal process
- Intends neither to hasten nor postpone death
- Integrates the psychosocial and spiritual aspects of patient care
- Offers a support system to help the family cope during the patient's illness and in their own bereavement
- Uses a team approach to address the needs of patients and their families, including bereavement counseling, if indicated
- Enhances quality of life and may also positively influence the course of illness
- Is applicable early in the course of illness, in conjunction with other therapies that are intended to prolong life, such as chemotherapy or radiation therapy, and includes those investigations needed to better understand and manage distressing clinical complications.

## WHY DO WE NEED PALLIATIVE CARE?

Modern medicine has helped in the growth of the number of older adults with chronic illness. Although the current generation of older people is less disabled than its predecessors, the probability of functional dependency, cognitive impairment, and living with advanced chronic illness increases with age. According to the Federal Interagency Forum on Aging-Related Statistics, between 1981 and 2008, age-adjusted death rates for all causes of death among people age 65 and older declined by 21%. Heart disease and cancer are the top 2 leading causes of death among all people age 65 and older, irrespective of sex, race, or origin. Americans are living longer than ever before. Life expectancies at both age 65 and age 85 have increased. Under current mortality conditions, people who survive to age 65 can expect to live an average of 18.5 more years, about 4 years longer than people age 65 in 1960.[5] In 2007, 42% of people age 65 and older reported a functional limitation. Individuals with 5 or more diseases are the largest consumers of health care and account for two-thirds of all Medicare spending.[5]

Overall, hospitalization rate was 336 per 1000 Medicare enrollees in 2007. Skilled nursing facility stays increased significantly from 28 per 1000 Medicare enrollees in 1992 to 81 per 1000 in 2007. The number of home health care visits increased to 3409 per 1000 enrollees in 2007. After adjusting for inflation, health care costs increased significantly among older Americans from 1992 to 2006.[5] In the United States, the health care system is structured around easy access to hospital care and does not have a good support system for community-based organized care for chronically ill patients. Despite being one of the highest spenders for per-capita expenditures, recipients of health care services are not satisfied with the care system in the United States.[6]

Hospice providers grew by more than 30% between 1997 and 2007 in the United States. The reasons for the growth in hospice use include increased hospice services in nursing homes, growth in the aging population living with advanced chronic illness, and greater recognition of hospice benefit.[7]

As the population continues to age in the United States, we will be faced with greater number of patients with advanced life-limiting illnesses. Health care providers will be needed to provide optimal care for these patients. The Institute of Medicine has made several recommendations regarding end-of-life care.[8] Some of these recommendations include the following: (1) People with advanced potentially fatal illnesses and those close to them should be able to expect and receive reliable, skillful, and supportive care. (2) Health care professionals must commit themselves to improving care for dying patients and to using existing knowledge effectively to prevent and relieve pain and other symptoms. (3) Educators and other health professionals should initiate changes in undergraduate, graduate, and continuing education to ensure that practitioners have relevant attitudes, knowledge, and skills to provide appropriate care for dying patients. Today, in New York State, physicians and nurse practitioners are required to offer to provide terminally ill patients with information and counseling concerning palliative care and end-of-life care options.

## ILLNESS TRAJECTORIES AND PROGNOSTIC ESTIMATES

Excellent palliative care begins with an understanding of disease processes and trajectories, end-stage disease indicators, and the clinician prediction skills needed at each stage of the dying process.

Lunney and colleagues[9] studied 4 types of illness trajectories and described different patterns of dying: sudden death, cancer death, death from organ failure, and frailty. The study included 14,456 participants from 4 US regions and was called the Established Populations for Epidemiologic Studies of the Elderly (EPESE) study. The trajectories of functional decline for the 4 categories differed markedly. Only short-term expected deaths are likely to have a predictable terminal period. Patients with cancer do not usually suffer severe functional disability until the final stages. The illness trajectory therefore is of a slow overall decline until a relatively rapid decline in function toward the end of life (**Fig. 3**). Patients with far-advanced noncancer illnesses

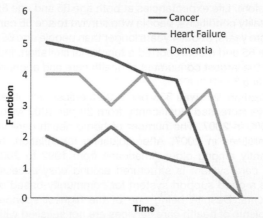

**Fig. 3.** Model of common trajectory in cancer, organ failure (heart failure), and dementia. (*Data from* Murtagh FE, Preston M, Higginson I. Patterns of dying: palliative care for non-malignant disease. Clin Med 2004;4(1):39–44.)

and high risk of death may have slowly declining health and relatively good functional status, such as patients with ischemic heart disease (see **Fig. 3**).[10] Deteriorations may be associated with hospitalizations and intensive care unit (ICU) admissions. This pattern also applies to those dying from chronic lung disease, with a similar pattern of acute relapse, active treatment, and improvement, but underlying steady decline and sudden death is always a possibility. In fact, the risk of sudden death for patients with advanced heart failure is 6 to 9 times that of the general population.[10] This trajectory may not be true for all patients with organ failure. The high levels of comorbidity with renal disease (especially cardiovascular and cerebrovascular disease) make this trajectory particularly difficult to predict. Those with dementia or general frailty have a much lower baseline level of functioning, with a declining but variable downward course toward death (see **Fig. 3**). In patients with an "entry–reentry" pattern, such as heart failure and chronic lung disease, decisions about *when* palliative care is appropriate are particularly difficult.

Studies assessing the accuracy of the physician's clinical prediction are conflicting and contradictory; however, some investigators consider that it tends to overestimate survival by a factor of 3 to 5[11–13] and is overly pessimistic in only 20% of cases. Clinical predictions of survival seem more accurate for short-term than long-term survival. Therefore, for greater accuracy, survival estimates must be considered in conjunction with more widely used criteria, such as biochemical findings and comorbidities. Physicians, patients, and families can all become accustomed to periods of severe illness, with subsequent improvement, which may detract the provider from awareness of the overall decline. Patients may be well known to their general practitioner or specialist over a long period, a factor known to contribute to a more optimistic prognostic assessment by the clinicians.[11]

There are more and more patients dying of acute complications rather than underlying chronic illness without the discreet terminal phase.[14] Palliative medicine is facing the need for finding ways to help patients in whom a serious chronic illness presents with unpredictable illness trajectory, ongoing sudden exacerbations, and high risk of sudden death. Palliative care must also include frail elderly patients who have diminishing reserve capacity. What makes the trajectory even more complex is the difficulty in predicting who is at risk for sudden death and the limitation of clinical prediction models to identify the terminal phase of the disease.[15] With the rise in prevalence of advanced chronic diseases in the United States, there is a compelling need to adopt comprehensive models of disease-specific palliative care that are responsive to the ongoing challenges of living with an unpredictable chronic illness that is marked by a high death rate.

The identification of prognostic and predictive factors concerning both life expectancy and quality of life in patients is very important to facilitate ethical, clinical, and organizational decisions, but also to use resources as efficiently as possible. A life expectancy of 6 months or less is required for admission to government-funded hospices. Predictive models in palliative care should mainly concern the prognostication of life expectancy with the following objectives[16]:

- To inform patients, families, and caregivers about the prognosis, in an appropriate culturally sensitive way within the patient-physician relationship, so as to involve them in the decision-making process
- To make clinical decisions concerning withdrawing curative-intent therapies
- To make clinical decisions regarding the use of oncologic therapies, such as chemotherapy/radiotherapy with palliative intent
- To minimize the risks of undertreatment or overtreatment

- To define the "appropriate time" for initiating a certain palliative option
- To establish the most appropriate therapy for symptom control in each individual patient
- To select the most appropriate setting of care (hospital, hospice, home care)
- To answer the patient's question: "How long do I have to live?" with the aim of helping patients, families, and caregivers to make personal decisions and plans.

## PROGNOSTIC TOOLS IN PALLIATIVE CARE

There have been several studies of prognostic indicators of survival for advanced cancer patients and less attention has been paid to noncancer but equally life-threatening illnesses. Data derived from prospective studies are scant. Four systematic reviews on survival prediction in terminally ill patients have identified a set of prognostic factors that are found to be predictive of survival time. These studies have taken the following into consideration: clinical prediction of survival, performance status, some physical symptoms, some biologic markers, some psychosocial and economic variables, and tumor type and cancer stage.[17–20] Although prognostic tools have been shown to improve survival prediction accuracy, only a few have undergone independent validation. Two of non–disease-specific prognostic tools, the Palliative Prognostic (PaP) score and the Palliative Prognostic Index (PPI), have been validated in different settings, countries, and in terminally ill cancer patients.[21–24]

The PaP score and the PPI are the most validated and used prognostic tools in palliative care.[25] The PaP score was developed in the 1990s as the end result of a series of prospective, multicenter Italian studies that aimed to identify clinical and biologic factors relevant to the prognosis of patients with advanced cancer referred to hospice, and then to produce a composite of those factors as a prognostic index. Survival times were measured from the date of study enrollment, and the outcome was death from all causes. The score includes the following clinical and biologic variables: (1) symptoms such as dyspnea and anorexia (presence or absence); (2) Karnofsky Performance Score (KPS) (**Table 1**); (3) clinical prediction of survival, ranging from 1 to 2 weeks up to 12 weeks; (4) total white blood cell count; and (5) lymphocyte counts (classified as normal, high, or very high). A numerical partial score is given to each variable, based on the relative weight of the independent prognostic significance shown by each single category in the multivariate analysis. The sum of the single scores gives the total, which can range from 0 to 17.5. The higher the score, the lower the likelihood of survival at 30 days.

The prognostic variables of the PPI are the following: KPS, amount of oral intake, presence/absence of edema, dyspnea at rest, and delirium. A numeric partial score was given to each variable, and the sum of the single scores gives the total, which ranges from 0 to 15. Patients were stratified into 3 groups depending on their score (Group A: PPI ≤2; Group B: PPI of 2 to ≤4; and Group C: PPI >4). When a PPI greater than 6 was adopted as a cutoff, 3-week survival was predicted with 80% sensitivity and 85% specificity. When a PPI greater than 4 was used as a cutoff, 6-week survival was predicted with 80% sensitivity and 77% specificity. The PPI can acceptably predict whether a patient will survive for longer than 3 or 6 weeks.

Clinical prediction estimates, palliative scores, dyspnea, anorexia, dysphagia, delirium, leukocytosis, and lymphocytopenia are all considered factors of primary importance in survival prognosis in patients with advanced solid cancers. However, further research is still needed to better identify the prognostic factors for survival in palliative care patients at any stage of a wide spectrum of diseases. On the other hand, we should keep in mind that PaP scores and the PPI are like other survival estimate tools and predicted results are only a number that acts as a guide.[26]

| Table 1 | |
|---|---|
| The Karnofsky performance scale | |
| **Karnofsky Performance Scale (%)** | |
| 100 | Normal no complaints; no evidence of disease |
| 90 | Able to carry on normal activity; minor signs or symptoms of disease |
| 80 | Normal activity with effort; some signs or symptoms of disease |
| 70 | Cares for self; unable to carry on normal activity or to do active work |
| 60 | Requires occasional assistance, but is able to care for most of his personal needs |
| 50 | Requires considerable assistance and frequent medical care |
| 40 | Disabled; requires special care and assistance |
| 30 | Severely disabled; hospital admission is indicated although death not imminent |
| 20 | Very sick; hospital admission necessary; active supportive treatment necessary |
| 10 | Moribund |
| 0 | Dead |

Available at: http://www.hospicepatients.org/karnofsky.html.

Estimating survival remains an inexact science, but prognostic uncertainty should not prevent us from talking with our patients when the question arises. Over the past decade, we learned to ask, "Is this patient sick enough that you would not be surprised to find that he or she had died 6 months (or a year) from now?" The patients who are "sick enough to die" are usually appropriate targets for the care that recognizes the eventuality of dying, even if any particular patient may live for many months.

## EDUCATING PHYSICIANS IN PALLIATIVE CARE

Despite increased societal concern about end-of-life care issues, there is no clear indication that care for most patients with advanced life-limiting illnesses in the United States has dramatically improved. Most physicians, residents, and medical students have received sporadic and nonstandardized training in the principles and practice of palliative care.

Between 1989 and 1994, the Robert Wood Johnson Foundation funded a large study called SUPPORT, the Study to Understand Prognoses and Preference for Outcomes and Risks of Treatment, to improve the care given to seriously ill hospitalized patients by having patients and their families discuss their treatment options with trained nurses. The study has shown that most patients were receiving aggressive life-prolonging treatments and had heavy symptom burden.[27] The results of the study were conveyed to treating clinicians, but did not have a big impact on the care of terminally ill patients. Thus, the Robert Wood Johnson Foundation has started a multi-year, multidisciplinary effort in collaboration with the Open Society Institute's Project on Death in America to improve the care given to patients with serious, life-threatening illnesses. As palliative care enters mainstream medicine, we are now witnessing major efforts to improve the care of patients with advanced chronic diseases as they approach the terminal phase.

Previous studies showed that palliative care content in general medical and subspecialty books was very vague.[28] We now have textbooks for palliative care,[1,2] multiple journals, and multiple research projects.[3] The Project on Death in America has supported 50 academician-leaders who are transforming medical education.[7]

In 2000, the Liaison Committee on Medical Education added a requirement in end-of-life care and doctor-patient communication. The American Board of Medical

Specialties (ABMS) approved subspecialty status for palliative medicine in 2006 and the first official ABMS-certified board examination for physicians was given in 2008 (see **Fig. 1**). Teaching palliative care for both undergraduate and graduate levels has been improved in past 10 years.[7] More than 80% of teaching hospitals reported having a palliative care program.[29] However, finding the resources to pay the faculty to teach palliative care has been challenging for most teaching hospitals.

## NURSING EDUCATION IN PALLIATIVE CARE

Expertise in symptom assessment, communication, and advocating well-communicated care are core competencies for nurses. Nurses hold a very important position in delivery of palliative care and home hospice care. The End-of-Life Nursing Education Consortium (ELNEC), administered by the American Association of Colleges of Nursing, has prepared and disseminated palliative care resources for undergraduate and graduate levels.[30] Nurses have developed formal accreditation requirements and certification examinations for nurse practitioners and registered nurses. The National Board of Hospice and Palliative Care Nurses has been offering certification examinations for advanced practice nurses and registered nurses.

## RESEARCH IN PALLIATIVE MEDICINE

Research, professional education, and clinical practice are convening to provide substantial improvement in care for people with serious chronic diseases. In a systemic review, researchers found that strong to moderate evidence supports interventions to improve important aspects of end-of-life care and many critical issues still lack high-quality evidence.[31] Existing evidence does not support palliative care delivery interventions. Lorenz and colleagues[31] found weak evidence for the effectiveness of specific palliative service delivery innovations for managing pain and dyspnea, no evidence addressing pain management in advanced noncancer conditions, and insufficient evidence addressing dyspnea in cancer and heart failure. They identified research priorities about short-acting antidepressants and caregiving challenges in populations other than patients with dementia and reported important research gaps in the field. In 2008, the article "Putting evidence into practice: palliative care" was released as a valuable source. http://clinicalevidence.bmj.com/downloads/end-of-life.pdf.[32]

Hospice programs have been established in many countries, often showing that good care for the end of life is within reach for a wide array of patients and cultures. The American Academy of Hospice and Palliative Medicine and the National Institutes of Health have called for investments in palliative care research because of the lack of evidence base in the field, and because models of care delivery need to be improved. But federal funding for palliative care research remains inadequate.[33] The National Palliative Care Research Center was established in 2005 to develop a new generation of researchers in palliative care. From July 1997 through July 1998, the Center to Improve Care of the Dying and the Institute for Healthcare Improvement sponsored a collaborative quality improvement endeavor for 48 teams from as many health care programs.[7] All aimed to improve care for persons facing the end of life. They formed goals, devised measurements, and tried innovations. The Institute of Medicine has released 2 more reports: "Improving palliative care for cancer" and "When children die: improving palliative care and end-of-life care for children and their families."[34,35]

For more than 20 years, the Dartmouth Atlas Project has documented variations in how medical resources are distributed and used in the United States. The project uses Medicare data to provide information and analysis about national, regional, and local markets, as well as hospitals and their affiliated physicians. Researchers have shown wide regional variation in health care resource use, and care effectiveness during chronic illness.[36] The data suggest that extra spending on doctors' visits, consultations, tests, and frequency of hospitalizations in the high-use regions do not necessarily buy longer and better life for Medicare beneficiaries. According to the Dartmouth Atlas Project's first-ever report on cancer care at the end of life released in November 2010, whether Medicare patients with advanced cancer will die while receiving hospice care or in the hospital varies markedly depending on where they live and receive care. The researchers found no consistent pattern of care or evidence that treatment patterns follow patient preferences, even among the nation's leading academic medical centers. Across the United States, about 29% of patients with advanced cancer died in a hospital between 2003 and 2007. A link to the full study can be found at www.dartmouthatlas.org.

## PALLIATIVE CARE IN HOSPITALS

The number of palliative care teams has been increased over the past decade and teams are available at most US hospitals, including more than 75% of large hospitals and all Department of Veterans Affairs medical centers.[29] The National Consensus Project for Quality Palliative Care (www.nationalconsensusproject.org) has developed Clinical Practice Guidelines for Quality Palliative Care. Palliative care teams including a physician and/or advanced practice nurse, nurse, social worker, and/or chaplain have demonstrated dramatic improvement in quality of care in symptom management,[37] advance care planning,[38] family and patient satisfaction and use of inpatient services,[39] and cost. Patients receiving inpatient palliative care consultation are more likely to receive follow-up services, such as home care services, hospice care, and nursing home placement when compared with usual care patients matched on age, mortality risk, and disease severity.[40]

The palliative care team acts as a consulting service within a hospital. The team should ideally be available 24 hours a day, 7 days a week. Generally, a palliative care team is invited by the patient's attending physician to provide the following services[41]:

- Provide treatment of pain and other symptoms
- Communicate with patient/family regarding goals of care
- Assess for hospice eligibility and discharge planning
- Provide emotional support
- Arrange transfer of patient to a palliative inpatient unit.

Palliative care professionals provide consultative services not only to medical and surgical wards and emergency rooms, but also to adult and pediatric ICUs. Because rates of mortality and other unfavorable outcomes are relatively high in ICUs, many critically ill patients and their families have palliative care needs. Today, many critical care physicians are supporting educational efforts targeted to physicians, nurses, and other staff members of the critical care team. Several studies have shown that integrating palliative care services to improve quality of care in the ICU were associated with reductions in use of nonbeneficial ICU interventions, length of ICU stay, and conflict over goals of care.[42]

## PALLIATIVE CARE IN THE COMMUNITY

Most patients with life-limiting illness are trying to manage complex chronic illness at home with minimal support from the insurance system. Moderate evidence supports the ability of multidisciplinary interventions that target continuity to affect outcomes of use in advanced illness. Strong evidence derived from many high-quality randomized clinical trials shows that reducing readmissions and other inappropriate use in advanced heart failure is possible, and the evidence is more consistent among more comprehensive and multidisciplinary approaches.[31]

### Outpatient Palliative Care Clinics

Meier and Beresford[43] suggest that outpatient palliative care clinics are a "new frontier" for palliative care, but the growth of outpatient clinics has been hampered by poor reimbursement, limited space, and lack of palliative care staff. Many clinics support the patients referred by an inpatient palliative care program. Palliative care outpatient clinics may provide supportive care for patients with cancer; patients with human immunodeficiency virus (HIV); and patients with chronic advanced illnesses, such as end-stage heart disease, lung disease, and neurologic disease.

### Hospice Palliative Care Programs

Hospices are discovering that hospice does not meet the needs of all patients. Terminally ill patients may not meet the stringent criteria of the hospice conditions of participation, and there are patients who refuse to elect the hospice benefit for several other reasons. A few large community hospice programs, such as the Metropolitan Jewish Hospice and Palliative Care Program in New York and the Hospice of the Bluegrass and Palliative Care Center of the Bluegrass in Lexington, Kentucky, are offering palliative care consultation services for patients cared for at home or in nursing homes. These programs can provide a smooth transition from usual care to hospice care for patients whose illnesses progress to the level where they are eligible or willing to receive hospice care. These hospice palliative care programs are model services that heavily depend on philanthropic support. Palliative care services may not be available across the country until financial support is provided for patient-centered services in the community.

### Home Health Palliative Care Programs

Home health care agencies that meet the Medicare guidelines for home health services are beginning to introduce palliative care into their programs in various ways. In one study, patients with a prognosis of approximately 12 months to live were randomized into usual (n = 155) versus palliative in-home care (n = 155). Usual care was services provided through the Medicare home health benefit. Palliative in-home care consisted of an interdisciplinary team providing medical, social, and other palliative services. The study suggested significant improved patient/family satisfaction, fewer emergency department visits, lower medical costs, and increased deaths at home with palliative in-home care.[44]

The Program of All-inclusive Care for the Elderly (PACE) and hospice programs incur a serious discontinuity at entry, but thereafter they are solidly allied with the patient and family. Fee-for-service care has little incentive to ensure continuity, to accept responsibility for patients' experiences across multiple programs, or to ensure prevention of exacerbations. Patients with chronic serious illness could be matched with a special service array that emphasizes symptom control, family support, function, reasonable planning for death, and continuity.

### SUMMARY

Palliative care is an approach that improves the quality of life of patients and their families facing the problems associated with life-threatening illness, through the prevention and relief of suffering by means of early identification and impeccable assessment and treatment of pain and other problems: physical, psychosocial, and spiritual. Palliative care uses a team approach to address the needs of patients and their families. This approach requires the interdisciplinary effort of health care professionals to address the physical, psychological, social, spiritual, and practical supportive needs of patients and their families. Ideally, the continuum of palliative care begins at the time of diagnosis of serious illness and creates a seamless delivery of supportive care. Palliative care complements therapies that aim to cure or modify disease process throughout an advanced illness process. It is an integral part of comprehensive care for adult and pediatric patients with life-limiting illnesses.

During the past 2 decades, palliative medicine has evolved from the hospice movement and has been recognized as a medical subspecialty. There are 3 key competencies that are central to providing general palliative care for any physician:

1. Providing a multidimensional assessment of the patient's situation. "Are there issues related to communication and goal setting? Are they getting medically appropriate care? Are there unmet needs in terms of physical symptoms, psychological issues, social concerns, family difficulties, or spiritual distress? Are they informed about prognosis in a culturally sensitive way?"
2. Therapeutic core competency. This means providing treatment to improve those sources of distress, including skills in pain control and symptom control, as well as the ability to have conversations about tough issues like advanced care planning and choices at the end of life.
3. Knowledge of referral resources and willingness to refer for additional specialist palliative care. An aging population and growing incidence of multiple noncommunicable diseases has brought increased attention on palliative care as a public health issue. As the health care system faces these issues, palliative care presents an opportunity for policy makers, clinicians, and community organizations to immediately provide cost-effective care that will have significant effect on patients and their families.

There is a need to build on successful programs to provide palliative care and a need to enhance the services of long-term care facilities and home care for patients with life-limiting illnesses. Hospital palliative care teams and inpatient units are becoming a standard of high-quality care in American hospitals and ICUs.

## REFERENCES

1. Lynn J. An 88-year-old woman facing the end of life. JAMA 1997;277:1633–40.
2. Lynn J, Harrell FE Jr, Cohn F, et al. Defining the "terminally ill": insights from SUPPORT. Duquesne Law Rev 1996;25:311–36.
3. Temel JS, Greer JA, Muzikansky A, et al. Early palliative care for patients with metastatic non-small-cell lung cancer. N Engl J Med 2010;363:733–42.
4. "WHO definition of palliative care". World Health Organization. Available at: http://www.who.int/cancer/palliative/definition/en/. Accessed December 5, 2010.
5. Federal Interagency Forum on Aging-Related Statistics. Older Americans 2010. Key indicators of well-being. Available at: http://www.agingstats.gov/. Accessed November 23, 2010.
6. Employee Benefit Research Institute. 2006 Health Confidence survey: dissatisfaction with health care system doubles since 1998. 2006. Available at: http://www.ebri.org/publications/notesindex.cfm?fa=notesDisp&content_id=3758. Accessed December 6, 2010.

7. Meier DE, Isaacs SL, Hughes RG. The development, status and future of palliative care. In: Meier DE, Isaacs SL, Hughes RG, editors. Palliative care: transforming the care of serious illness. Princeton (NJ): Jossey-Bass; 2010. p. 3–76.

8. Doyle D, Hanks GWC, MacDonald N, editors. Oxford textbook of palliative medicine. 2nd edition. New York: Oxford University Press; 1998.

9. Lunney JR, Lynn J, Foley DJ, et al. Patterns of functional decline at the end of life. JAMA 2010;289(18):2387–92.

10. Murtagh FE, Preston M, Higginson I. Patterns of dying: palliative care for non-malignant disease. Clin Med 2004;4(1):39–44.

11. Christakis NA, Lamont EB. Extent and determinants of error in doctors' prognoses in terminally ill patients: prospective cohort study. BMJ 2000;320(7233):469–73.

12. Vigano A, Dorgan M, Buera E, et al. The relative accuracy of the clinical estimation of the duration of life for patients with end of life cancer. Cancer 1999;86: 170–6.

13. Bruera E, Miller MJ, Kuehn, et al. Estimate survival of patients admitted to a palliative care unit: a prospective study. J Pain Symptom Manage 1992;7:82–6.

14. Lynn J. Serving patients who may die soon and their families: the role of hospice and other services. JAMA 2001;285:925–32.

15. Levenson JW, McCarthy EP, Lynn J, et al. The last six months of life for patients with congestive heart failure. J Am Geriatr Soc 2000;48(Suppl 5):S101–9.

16. Ripamonti CI, Farina G, Garassino MC. Predictive models in palliative care. Cancer 2009;115(Suppl 13):3128–34.

17. Maltoni M, Caraceni A, Brunelli C, et al. Prognostic factors in advanced cancer patients: evidence-based clinical recommendations. A study by the Steering Committee of the European Association for Palliative Care. J Clin Oncol 2005; 23:6240–8.

18. Vigano A, Bruera E, Jhangri GS, et al. Clinical survival predictors in patients with advanced cancer. Arch Intern Med 2000;160:861–8.

19. Glare P, Virik K. Independent prospective validation of the PaP score in terminally ill patients referred to a hospital-based palliative medicine consultation service. J Pain Symptom Manage 2001;22:891–8.

20. Hauser CA, Stockler MR, Tattersall MHN. Prognostic factors in patients with recently diagnosed incurable cancer: a systematic review. Support Care Cancer 2006;14:999–1011.

21. Harrold J, Rickerson E, Carroll JT, et al. Is the palliative performance scale a useful predictor of mortality in a heterogeneous hospice population? J Palliat Med 2005; 8(3):503–9.

22. Head B, Ritchie C, Smoot TM. Prognostication in hospice care: Can palliative performance score help? J Palliat Med 2005;8(3):492–502.

23. Maltoni M, Nanni O, Pirovano M, et al. Successful validation of the Palliative Prognostic Score in terminally ill cancer patients: Italian Multicenter and Study Group on Palliative Care. J Pain Symptom Manage 1999;17:240–7.

24. Caraceni A, Nanni O, Maltoni M, et al. Impact of delirium on the short term prognosis of advanced cancer patients: Italian Multicenter and Study Group on Palliative Care. Cancer 2000;89:1145–9.

25. Morita T, Tsunoda J, Inoue S, et al. The Palliative Prognostic Index: a scoring system for survival prediction of terminally ill cancer patients. Support Care Cancer 1999;7:128–33.

26. Lau F, Cloutier-Fisher D, Kuziemsky C, et al. A systematic review of prognostic tools for estimating survival time in palliative care. J Palliat Care 2007;23(2): 93–112.

27. A controlled trial to improve care for the seriously ill hospitalized patients. The study to understand prognoses and preferences for outcomes and risks of treatments (SUPPORT). JAMA 1995;274:1591–8.
28. Carron AT, Lynn J, Keaney P. End-of-life care in medical textbooks. Ann Intern Med 1999;130:82–6.
29. Goldsmith B, Dietrich J, Du Q, et al. Variability in access to hospital palliative care in the United States. J Palliat Med 2008;11(8):1094–102.
30. Ferrell BR, Grant M, Virani R. Strengthening nursing education to improve end-of-life care. Nurs Outlook 1999;47:252–6.
31. Lorenz K, Lynn J, Dy MS, et al. Evidence for improving palliative care at the end of life: a systematic review. Ann Intern Med 2008;148:147–59.
32. Brunnhuber K, Nash S, Meier D, et al. Putting evidence into practice: palliative care. London: The BMJ Publishing Group Limited; 2008. Available at: http://clinicalevidence.bmj.com/downloads/end-of-life.pdf. Accessed December 5, 2010.
33. Gelfman LP, Morrison RS. Research funding for palliative medicine. J Palliat Med 2008;11:36–43.
34. Institute of Medicine. Improving palliative care for cancer. Washington, DC: National Academies Press; 2001.
35. Institute of Medicine. When children die: improving palliative care and end-of-life care for children and their families. Washington, DC: National Academies Press; 2002.
36. Fisher ES, Wennberg DE, Stukel TA, et al. The implications of regional variations in Medicare spending. Part 1: the content, quality, and accessibility of care. Ann Intern Med 2003;138(4):273–87.
37. London MR, McSkimming S, Drew N, et al. Evaluation of a comprehensive, adaptable life-affirming, longitudinal (CALL) palliative care project. J Palliat Med 2005; 8:1214–25.
38. Lilly CM, Sonna LA, Haley KJ, et al. Intensive communication: four-year follow-up from a clinical practice study. Crit Care Med 2003;31(Suppl 5):S394–9.
39. Casarett D, Pickard A, Bailey FA, et al. Do palliative care consultations improve patient outcomes? J Am Geriatr Soc 2008;56:593–9.
40. Brody AA, Clemins E, Newman J, et al. The effects of an inpatient palliative care team on discharge disposition. J Palliat Med 2010;13(5):541–8.
41. Weissman DE, Meier DE. Center to Advance Palliative Care palliative care consultation service metrics: consensus recommendations. J Palliat Med 2008; 11:1294–8.
42. Nelson JE, Bassett R, Boss RD, et al. Models for structuring a clinical initiative to enhance palliative care in the intensive care unit: a report from the IPAL-ICU Project (Improving Palliative Care in the ICU). Crit Care Med 2010;38:1765–72.
43. Meier DE, Beresford L. Outpatient clinics are a new frontier for palliative care. J Palliat Med 2008;11:823–8.
44. Brumley R, Enguidanos S, Jamison P, et al. Increased satisfaction with care and lower costs: results of a randomized trial of in-home palliative care. J Am Geriatr Soc 2007;55:993–1000.

# Hospice Care in the United States

Allen Hutcheson, MD

KEYWORDS

• Hospice • Primary care • Prognosis • Medicare hospice benefit

Hospice care is a special way of caring for a patient whose disease cannot be cured. It is available as a benefit under Medicare Part A hospital insurance. Medicare beneficiaries who choose hospice care receive noncurative medical and support services for their terminal illness. To be eligible, they must be certified by a physician as terminally ill with a life expectancy of 6 months or less. Although they no longer receive curative treatment, they require close medical observation and supportive care, which are provided by hospice interdisciplinary team. Hospice care under Medicare includes both home care and inpatient care, when needed, and a variety of services.

This article should help primary care physicians use hospice to deliver effective care for patients in the final stages of life, specifically, to make timely referrals to hospice, counsel patients regarding hospice services, and work effectively with a hospice interdisciplinary team.

## HISTORY OF HOSPICE AND HOSPICE PHILOSOPHY

The modern hospice movement developed as a reaction to deficiencies in a medical system that in the first half of the twentieth century had made marked technologic and pharmacologic advances, leading to a focus on specialization, inpatient care, and interventional techniques. One person in particular, Cicely Saunders,[1] noticed the pain and isolation of dying patients she cared for as a nurse and social worker at a "home for the dying poor." She retrained as a physician and founded St Christopher's Hospice in London as a treatment center for those whose illnesses were beyond curative treatment.[1]

Dame Cicely Saunders (she was knighted by Queen Elizabeth II in 1979 for her pioneering medical work) laid the foundations for the hospice philosophy, which has several central features: the concept of total pain, a focus on interdisciplinary care, and the recognition of dying as a potentially valuable and enriching segment of a person's life.[2]

---

The author has nothing to disclose.
Visiting Nurse Service of New York Hospice Care, 1250 Broadway, 7th floor, Bronx, NY 10001, USA
*E-mail address:* allen.hutcheson@vnsny.org

Prim Care Clin Office Pract 38 (2011) 173–182
doi:10.1016/j.pop.2011.03.002        **primarycare.theclinics.com**

Total pain means that suffering can come from many sources. Many terminal illnesses cause physical pain, but in her writings and lectures, Saunders argued that pain can have psychological, social, spiritual, and practical sources:

*A patient described it: "All of me is wrong." She did not mean merely her many related symptoms but also her feelings of isolation, the family's social problems connected with her illness and her need for a sense of meaning and security. Our treatment should be based on an equally wide approach.*[2]

So an interdisciplinary team was needed to treat total pain, with a nurse, a social worker, a chaplain, a physician, and others, each contributing his or her own expertise.

In 1969, the psychiatrist Elisabeth Kübler-Ross published *On Death and Dying*,[3] a critique of the US medical system's neglect of dying patients, which created a public awareness of the potential for improving the experience of death and dying and prompted introspection and reform in the academic medical system.[4] Kübler-Ross' focus was on grief and bereavement, the intense psychological response to death and dying. Kübler-Ross later turned her attention to bereavement in friends and family members, but her first formulation of the now well-known outline of grief—denial, anger, bargaining, depression, and acceptance—was originally an observation of patients' own reactions to terminal diagnosis and fatal illness—self-bereavement.[3] Addressing bereavement in both patients and families is a core task in hospice care.

In the United States, a few free-standing hospices were founded on the model of Dame Cicely Saunders' St Christopher's Hospice, but most efforts were directed toward home care. Volunteers organized hospice agencies to minister to the dying in their homes, often over the objections or despite the lack of participation of physicians. Today hospice remains focused on home care; 40% of hospice patients died at home in 2008, and approximately 20% in nursing homes or inpatient hospice facilities.[5] The mission of home-based hospice is to provide medical care and support to terminally ill patients and their families, helping people who are dying remain comfortable. Patients and family members are assisted in transitioning from a high-tech medical environment focused on cure to a home-like environment focused on comfort. Even though the number of hospices has grown rapidly in the last 20 years, still fewer than 25% of dying patients in the United States access hospice services. But public awareness of this benefit is growing: in 1992, only 9% of Medicare beneficiaries who died used hospice benefits; by 2000, 23% of them did.

## VALUING DEATH

It is difficult to touch only briefly on the effort to treat death as a valuable life experience, but many investigators have pointed out that dying need not be seen as a horrifying, shameful, avoidable event. For hospice advocates this means "the notion of the good death, the idea that the end of life could be a fulfilling phase of life and an opportunity for personal growth—a time of reflection, of resolving emotional rifts and achieving satisfying farewells, of wrapping up one's life's work, of finding meaning in one's life and legacy, of realizing peace and grace and forgiveness and true comfort as death draws near. This idealized good death might involve writing or videotaping messages for future generations, finishing a major art project, talking to a long-estranged friend or family member, revisiting an old house or favorite natural vista, leaving financial affairs in good order, and just spending quality time with the important people in their lives."[6]

## HOSPICE: A CARING ALTERNATIVE

In the formative years of hospice, one of its primary services to patients was to insulate them from conventional medical treatment. It still can be difficult for a busy primary care physician to shift mindsets in the middle of a day for a call from a hospice nurse. In fact, a visit only to talk and make contact, with no treatment agenda at all, can be an invaluable contribution from the doctor.[1]

Hospice interdisciplinary teams are necessary to assess and treat total pain, provide dignity in the final months of life, and mitigate the trauma of bereavement. Care at home has priority over inpatient or institutional living and dying. Studies indicate that patients receiving hospice compared with conventional care in the end of life have better pain management[7,8] and symptom control and higher perceived quality of care for emotional needs. Hospice can also help families of terminally ill patients, and evidence indicates that benefits include improved family functioning, greater caregiver satisfaction, increased survival, and better bereavement adjustment.[9,10]

## HOSPICE REGULATIONS

In the early 1980s, the lobbying efforts of affiliated hospices coincided with government efforts to reduce health care costs, and Congress enacted the Medicare hospice benefit provisionally in 1982, and then permanently in 1986, creating a new division of Medicare to fund palliative care for the terminally ill. Since that time, Medicare laws have been amended several times, most recently with new regulations (known as Conditions of Participation [COPs]) in 2009.[11] The hospice regulations are complex and require extensive documentation of services provided. For patients who do not qualify for Medicare, most private insurance plans, managed care organizations, and state Medicaid programs generally include a hospice benefit in their insurance plans with features that closely follow the format of the Medicare benefit.

## ELIGIBILITY

Any patient who is terminally ill is eligible for hospice: "*Terminally ill* means that the individual has a medical prognosis that his or her life expectancy is 6 months or less if the illness runs its normal course" (COP 418.3).[12] Under Medicare regulations, a beneficiary is eligible for hospice care coverage only if both a patient's attending physician and the medical director of the hospice certify that the individual's prognosis is for a life expectancy of 6 months or less.

## DETERMINATION OF PROGNOSIS

The best way for a primary care physician to screen for whether a patient is eligible for hospice is to ask, "Would I be surprised if this person died in the next 6 months?"[13] If the answer is no, then in effect the prognosis is 6 months or less, and the next tasks are to consider whether hospice services would be beneficial and discuss the option of hospice with the patient or family if the patient lacks capacity. The predictable final course of cancer with progressive decline at the end of life is well suited to hospice. But for individuals dying of chronic conditions whose courses are difficult to predict, such as chronic obstructive pulmonary disease (COPD), congestive heart failure (CHF), end-stage liver disease (ESLD), Alzheimer's dementia, and end-stage renal disease (ESRD), access to hospice benefit remains limited. It has been shown that for seriously ill hospitalized patients with advanced COPD, CHF, or ESLD, recommended clinical prediction criteria are not effective in identifying a population with a survival prognosis of 6 months or less.[14] The prognosis and symptom burden of patients with advanced COPD, CHF, or ESLD is even worse than the prognosis of many terminal cancer patients. The cause of death is often a relatively sudden and unpredictable event, such as a pulmonary infection or a cardiac arrhythmia that has a substantial per-incident mortality rate. Disease-specific criteria regarding end-stage COPD, CHF, and ESRD and dementia for hospice referral are discussed in related articles elsewhere in this issue.

## CERTIFICATION OF TERMINAL ILLNESS

Initially, based on a review of the medical record, both a patient's attending physician and the hospice medical director sign a certification of terminal illness that specifies a prognosis "of 6 months or less if the terminal illness runs its normal course" (COP 418.22[b][1]).[11]

Criteria for several common hospice diagnoses are laid out in hospice-specific local coverage determinations (LCDs).[15] These checklists were originally formulated as suggested guidelines, and their accuracy in predicting a 6-month prognosis is debatable (discussed previously), but they have become required criteria for hospice eligibility. The intricacies of the LCDs are beyond the scope of this article; they can be obtained through Centers for Medicare & Medicaid Services websites or from a local hospice, and primary physicians should collaborate with hospice personnel regarding eligibility criteria for any particular diagnosis or regarding recertification of patients who are not clearly worsening.

The hospice benefit covers only treatment related to a terminal diagnosis, but comorbidities can be taken into account when judging terminal prognosis. For example, someone might be referred with cirrhosis but not meet the specific criteria in the LCDs. In that case, a prognosis of less than 6 months might be supported by comorbid moderate COPD and coronary artery disease. Once a patient enrolls in hospice, treatments for edema, hepatic encephalopathy, abdominal pain, and hemorrhoids secondary to cirrhosis are covered by the hospice provider, but long-term oxygen therapy related to COPD or nitrates for coronary artery disease continue to be covered through Medicare or private insurance.

For diagnoses that are not included in the LCDs, physicians are to use their own judgment and review of the literature to certify terminal illness. There is a nonspecific category for certifying terminal illness called decline or debility (previously often termed failure to thrive). Patients with poor functional status, multiple comorbidities, and weight loss can be certified under decline or debility; the hospice then generally covers treatments related to one or two of the underlying illnesses.

## REFERRALS TO HOSPICE

Referrals can be made by anyone connected with a patient. Often this is a physician but just as often it is someone else—a social worker, a family member, or sometimes a patient himself or herself—who recognizes that a patient is terminally ill and might benefit from hospice services. The hospice is required to consult with the attending physician before admitting a patient; if that physician objects, the patient has the option of choosing another physician as a primary attending physician (COP 418.25[a]).[11]

Usually a hospice referral requires only one call to the main listed number of a hospice agency. A hospice admissions nurse or social worker takes demographic and medical information and gives some guidance regarding if the person is eligible and what services will be received. The hospice staff contacts the patient's attending physician and other medical providers to get medical details, confirm the prognosis, and begin collaboration.

## ELECTION OF HOSPICE BENEFIT

A hospice staff member meets with the patient or representative for counseling regarding hospice services and signature of enrollment forms. The patient or a representative signs an election statement confirming "that he or she has been given a full understanding of the palliative rather than curative nature of hospice care, as it relates to the individual's terminal illness" (COP 418.24[b]).[11] There is no requirement for a do-not-resuscitate order.

The election statement also technically waives all rights to any Medicare coverage for treatment of a terminal condition except for the services provided under the auspices of the hospice agency (COP 418.24[d]).[11] Subsequently, the patient or representative can revoke the hospice election, for example, to receive nonpalliative treatments related to the terminal condition. Patients can also be discharged from hospice if they move, if they are abusive and disruptive, or if they are no longer considered terminally ill (COP 418.260).[11]

## HOSPICE PAYMENT SYSTEM: CAPITATED PAYMENT

A hospice agency receives a daily payment for each patient enrolled. The amount depends on the area of the country and the setting of a patient's care, but, as an example, the standard rate in 2010 was $142 daily for home care.[16] All treatment related to the hospice diagnosis is paid for through this daily rate, including staff visits, medications, home health aide hours, equipment, and supplies. Treatments not related to the hospice diagnosis are covered through Medicare Part B.

The 4 categories of hospice care based on setting are as follows.

### Routine Home Care

Routine home care includes care in a nursing home, assisted living facility, or hospice residence. Nurses and other staff visit regularly, and a few hours a day of home health aide hours are usually available if needed. Hospice home care usually requires that someone from the family is available to provide the daily care and monitoring of a patient.

### Continuous Home Care

Continuous care means a skilled nurse (a licensed practical nurse or a nurse with a more advanced degree) is at the bedside over a 24-hour period. It is available at times of crisis, such as uncontrolled symptoms or imminent death.

### Inpatient Respite Care

Respite care entails admitting a patient from home into a facility to give respite to the caregivers. Families often use this time to attend functions, such as graduations or weddings, or sometimes to take a vacation to recuperate from the extreme burden of caring for a critically ill family member.

### General Inpatient Care

Hospitals receive approximately $635 daily when an admission is for control of symptoms related to a hospice diagnosis. This is one reason it is important for the inpatient team and the hospice team to coordinate closely regarding the goals of care and appropriate effective treatments.

Admissions for aggressive life-prolonging care related to a hospice diagnosis require disenrollment from hospice, sometime with re-enrollment on discharge.

For hospital admissions not related to a hospice diagnosis, patients can remain enrolled in hospice, but billing bypasses the hospice agency and goes directly through Medicare. Routine treatments based on patients' goals of care should be pursued. For example, a patient with end-stage COPD who falls and breaks a hip could be admitted and treated surgically, without disenrolling from hospice, with billing for surgery and imaging going directly through Medicare.

## BENEFIT LIMITS

A small percentage of private insurers have limits on hospice coverage, but under Medicare patients can be certified for an indefinite number of 2-month periods as long as they meet criteria for terminal illness.[17] A few patients stay in hospice for several years, but the average length of stay was 69 days in 2008; median length of stay is lower (21 days), because most patients die within a few weeks in hospice.[5]

## PHYSICIAN BILLING

Hospice Conditions of Participation (COPs) designate 3 categories of physician—attending, consulting, or hospice employed—and 2 types of treatment—related or not related to hospice diagnosis—that determine billing (**Table 1**). Whether or not a treatment is related to a hospice diagnosis can sometimes be a complex judgment but usually there is a clear distinction.

At the time of enrollment, patients are asked who their primary physician is, defined in the COPs (COP 418.3) as:

*Attending physician means a physician who—*
*1. Is a doctor of medicine or osteopathy; and*

**Table 1**
**Physican billing for hospice patient's treatment related to the hospice diagnosis**

| | Type of Physician | | |
|---|---|---|---|
| | **Attending Physician** | **Consulting Physician (Needs Contract)** | **Hospice Medical Director (Volunteer or Paid)** |
| Type of Service | | | |
| Professional services | Bill Medicare Part B with modifier GV[a] | Bill hospice agency, (which bills Medicare Part A) | Bill hospice agency, (which bills Medicare Part A) |
| Administrative services | Bill Medicare Part B For CPO[b] | N/A | Not separately billable |
| Technical services e.g. Radiology, radiation, chemotherapy, laboratory | Bill hospice (paid out of per diem benefit) | Bill hospice | Covered by hospice out of per diem rate |

*Abbreviation:* N/A, not applicable.
[a] GV indicates the attending physician is not employed or paid under agreement by the patient's hospice provider.
[b] CPO, Care Plan Oversight includes substantive discussions with hospice nurses by phone, and must exceed 30 minutes per month for the patient. Billing is complex; more information is available from NHPCO or local hospice agencies.

2. Is identified by the individual, at the time he or she elects to receive hospice care, as having the most significant role in the determination and delivery of the individual's medical care.[11]

An attending physician does not have to be a primary care physician; often it is the specialist who has been managing the terminal diagnosis. Alternatively, some patients have received disjointed care and elect to designate the hospice's physician as their attending physician. Often, however, the attending physician is a patient's primary care physician.

Depending on if a doctor is the primary attending physician, consulting physician, or hospice medical director, the doctor bills the hospice or Medicare for any care related to the hospice diagnosis and bills Medicare Part B with a modifier for any care not related to the hospice diagnosis.[18,19] Consulting physicians need to arrange a contract with the hospice agency, allowing them to bill for hospice-related services. Physicians employed by hospice can bill for clinical care but not for general supervision or participation in interdisciplinary group meetings.[19]

## HOSPICE CORE SERVICES
### Nursing

Minimum frequency of nursing assessments is every 2 weeks; usually, visits are once weekly and can be more frequent if needed for symptom management or wound care (**Fig. 1**). The primary nurse is referred to in Centers for Medicare & Medicaid Services parlance as the coordinator of care and takes on the primary responsibility for assessment, education, supply of drugs and equipment, and coordinating care across all providers. Many hospice nurses have advanced training and extensive experience in the care of terminally ill patients and are in a position to provide treatment suggestions to patients, families, and supervising physicians.

### Physician

The COPs place responsibility for patient care on neither the attending physician nor the hospice physician only, but on both, and they specify that the care must be coordinated. As long as there is communication, the primary attending physician can choose any degree of involvement, from management of every detail, with the hospice physician involved only for documentations of certification, to a hands-off approach, reviewing reports of treatment provided by the hospice team. Often, the hospice medical director takes responsibility for symptom management and goals of care, whereas the primary attending physician continues to manage core medical issues. The degree of participation by a hospice doctor depends on local hospice structures and sizes, because many hospices do not employ full-time medical directors.

### Social Work

Medical social workers are required to assess and then provide services based on needs and preferences of patients and families. Hospice social workers can provide expertise in advance care planning, funeral arrangements, and plans for the future care of minor children in addition to supportive counseling.

### Bereavement Counseling

Hospices are required not simply to employ bereavement counselors but to have a bereavement program in place that is available to family members for at least a year after the death of a patient. This usually includes group sessions and memorial services as well as individual counseling at home or in the office.

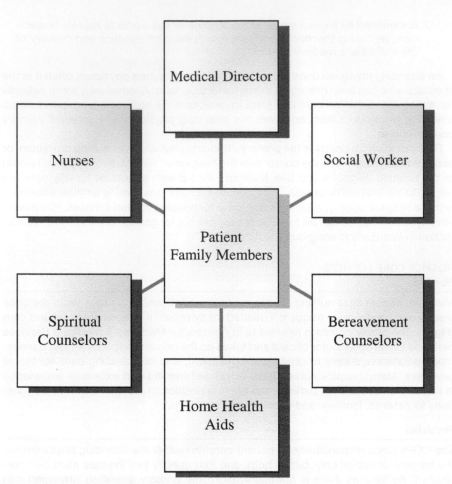

**Fig. 1.** Hospice interdisciplinary team and core services.

### *Dietary Counseling*

Dietary counseling must be available from an appropriately trained dietitian or nurse.

### *Spiritual Counseling*

Hospices are required at minimum to make a spiritual assessment and coordinate visits by local clergy or counselors if desired by a patient or family, but almost all hospices have dedicated employed or volunteer chaplains who participate in this spiritual assessment and counseling.

### *Noncore Services*

Services provided by many but not all hospices include physical therapy, occupational therapy, speech-language pathology, home aide services, and volunteer services. Typical volunteer services include massage, pet therapy, music therapy, and simple companionship visits.

## COVERED TREATMENTS

In the past decade, some hospice agencies have attempted to expand the scope of palliative treatments they can cover, and some larger hospices have been able to enroll patients regardless of the costs of their treatment, an approach known as open access. Currently, however, particular hospices are able or willing to provide varying levels of complex and costly treatments, and specific treatments, such as palliative radiation, should be discussed with the hospice medical director at the time of referral.

## SUMMARY

Hospice affirms the concept of palliative care as an intensive program that enhances comfort and promotes the quality of life for individuals and their families. When cure is no longer possible, hospice recognizes that a peaceful and comfortable death is an essential goal of health care. Hospice believes that death is an integral part of the life cycle and that intensive palliative care focuses on pain relief, comfort, and enhanced quality of life as appropriate goals for the terminally ill. Hospice also recognizes the potential for growth that often exists within the dying experience for individuals and their families and seeks to protect and nurture this potential.

Simple steps for incorporating hospice into primary care practice to enhance end-of-life care for terminally ill patients include:

1. Determination of prognosis. Pursuing conventional treatments rather than facing facts often deprives patients and families of the most effective palliative approaches.
2. Communication about goals of care. This can be emotionally difficult but consistently pays off; good communication skills can help avoid blame, guilt, and hopelessness for both physician and patient.
3. Referral to a hospice program. Even referrals that may be too early or too late lead to more familiarity with hospice criteria and services for physicians and the community.
4. Use hospice as a resource. Hospice staff can be trusted allies in the anxiety-provoking atmosphere of caring for a dying patient, enabling primary care doctors to extend their skill and compassion right up through death and bereavement.

## ACKNOWLEDGMENTS

The author would like to acknowledge the following people for their help with the preparation and editing of this article: Robert Morrow, MD; Darren Esposito, MD; Patricia Vigilante, BSN; Jessie Hutcheson; and Serife Eti, MD.

## REFERENCES

1. Saunders C. The care of the terminal stages of cancer. Ann R Coll Surg Engl 1967;41(Suppl):162–9.
2. Saunders C. Cicely saunders: selected writings 1958–2004. New York: Oxford University Press; 2006.
3. Kübler-Ross E. On death and dying. New York: Simon and Schuster; 1969.
4. Siebold C. The hospice movement: easing death's pains. New York: Twayne; 1992.
5. NHPCO facts and figures: hospice care in America. Alexandria (VA): National Hospice and Palliative Care Organization; 2009.

6. Beresford L. Does hospice have an image problem? Larry Beresford. 2009. Available at: http://growthhouse.typepad.com/larry_beresford/2009/04/does-hospice-have-an-image-problem.html. Accessed July 26, 2010.

7. Miller SC, Mor V, Teno J. Hospice enrollment and pain assessment and management in nursing homes. J Pain Symptom Manage 2003;26:791–9.

8. Greer DS, Mor V, Morris JN, et al. An alternative in terminal care: results of the National Hospice Study. J Chronic Dis 1986;39:9–26.

9. Seale C. A comparison of hospice and conventional care. Soc Sci Med 1991;32: 147–52.

10. Christakis NA, Iwashyna TJ. The health impact of health care on families: a matched cohort study of hospice use by decedents and mortality outcomes in surviving, widowed spouses. Soc Sci Med 2003;57:465–75.

11. The Medicare Conditions of Participation for Hospice Care. Prepared by NHPCO, August 2009. Available at: www.nhpco.org/files/public/COPS_RevisedSubpartBFG_0106.pdf. 2009. Accessed July 26, 2010.

12. Medicare Regulations 1983, 42 CFR §418.22.

13. Lynn J. Caring at the end of our lives. N Engl J Med 1996;335:201–2.

14. Fox E, Landrum-McNiff K, Zhong Z, et al. Evaluation of prognostic criteria for determining hospice eligibility in patients with advanced lung, heart, or liver disease. JAMA 1999;282(17):1638–45.

15. National Hospice and Palliative Care Organization. Hospice billing: local coverage determinators. NHPCO; 2009. Available at: http://www.nhpco.org/i4a/pages/index.cfm?pageid=5580. Accessed July 26, 2010.

16. Hospice Payment System. Fact Sheet. CMS. 2010. Available at: https://www.cms.gov/MLNproducts/downloads/hospice_pay_sys_fs.pdf. Accessed July 26, 2010.

17. Hospice Association of America. Facts and statistics. Washington, DC: Hospice Association of America; 2009.

18. Chamberlain B. Hospice medical director billing guide. Glenview (IL): American Academy of Hospice and Palliative Medicine; 2006.

19. Maxwell T, Martinez J, Knight C. UNIPAC 1: The hospice and palliative medicine approach to life-limiting illness. In: Porter Storey C Jr, editor. UNIPAC Hospice and palliative care training for physicians: a self-study program. 3rd edition. Glenview (IL): American Academy of Hospice and Palliative Medicine; 2006.

# Ethical Issues in Palliative Care

Danielle N. Ko, MBBS, LLB[a,b,c,1], Pedro Perez-Cruz, MD[a,b,d,1],
Craig D. Blinderman, MD, MA[e,*]

KEYWORDS

• Palliative care • Ethics • End of life • Autonomy
• Palliative sedation

*Not a week passes in the practice of the ordinary physician but he is consulted about one or more of the deepest problems in metaphysics and religion–not as a speculative enigma, but as part of human agony.*

Richard Cabot, MD[1]

Ethical problems in medicine are common, especially when caring for patients at the end of life. However, many of these issues are not adequately identified in the outpatient setting.[2,3] Primary care providers (PCPs) are in a unique and privileged position to identify ethical issues, prevent future conflicts, and help patients make medical decisions that are consistent with their individual values and preferences. This article describes some of the more common ethical issues faced by PCPs caring for patients with life-limiting illness.

## AUTONOMY, INFORMED CONSENT, AND DECISION-MAKING CAPACITY

Autonomy can be defined as the human capacity for self-determination. This concept supports the idea that each person has the right to select among the best alternatives according to a self-chosen plan.[4] Informed consent is the procedure through which patients' autonomy is respected, legally and ethically. The patient must be informed about the risks and benefits of a specific treatment or intervention to freely accept or refuse it. If the patient lacks capacity, then any form of consent is not valid, even

The authors have no financial interests or conflicts to disclose.
[1] Dr Ko and Dr Perez-Cruz are lead authors and have contributed equally to this work.
[a] Division of General Internal Medicine, Massachusetts General Hospital, 55 Fruit Street, Boston, MA 02114, USA
[b] Palliative Care Service, Massachusetts General Hospital, 55 Fruit Street, Boston, MA 02114, USA
[c] Division of Medical Ethics, Harvard Medical School, 641 Huntington Avenue, Boston, MA 02115, USA
[d] Department of Internal Medicine, School of Medicine, Catholic University, Lira 44, Santiago, Chile
[e] Adult Palliative Medicine, Department of Anesthesiology, Columbia University, 622 West 168th Street, PH5-530B, New York, NY 10032, USA
* Corresponding author.
*E-mail address:* cdb21@columbia.edu

Prim Care Clin Office Pract 38 (2011) 183–193
doi:10.1016/j.pop.2011.03.003      **primarycare.theclinics.com**

if the patient agrees with the physician's suggestions.[5] For these reasons, the assessment of a patient's ability to make decisions is a fundamental component of every physician–patient interaction.

Physicians often start with the assumption that all patients have capacity unless evidence suggests otherwise.[6] In general, physicians make a relatively cursory assessment of a patient's ability to make decisions, and only tend to explore the matter more deeply when conflict arises regarding medical management. Physicians are often biased toward believing a patient has capacity (when they do not),[7] and are frequently unaware of a patient's incapacity to make a decision,[5] or judge their capacity to be greater than it is in reality.[8] Another common problem is assuming that certain diagnoses (eg, depression, cerebral metastases) are associated with the inability to make decisions. Although this is not the case, these diagnoses may indicate who should be screened.[9]

Several strategies are available to assess decision-making capacity. In the medical setting, the most frequently used formal criteria include the assessment of a patient's ability to (1) communicate a choice, (2) understand the relevant information, (3) appreciate the situation and its consequences, and (4) manipulate relevant information in a rational way[5] (**Table 1**).

Some authors have suggested a sliding scale approach when evaluating capacity.[10] That is, the patient's ability to make a decision should be understood relative to the decision at hand, and whether the patient is refusing or accepting the advice of his physicians should be clear. More capacity is needed to consent to medical treatments with high risk and a low likelihood of success (eg, palliative chemotherapy) than to an intervention with low risk and a high likelihood of success (eg, penicillin for group A streptococcus infection). Refusing a low-risk, life-saving treatment should raise suspicion that perhaps the patient does not have capacity. Further evaluation and an opinion of a psychiatrist may be beneficial. Finally, the assessment of capacity should be restricted to a particular decision,[10] rather than evaluating a patient's capacity in general. For instance, one might ask whether the patient has capacity to refuse this specific life-prolonging therapy, rather than whether the patient has decision-making capacity.

PCPs are in a unique position for identifying patients' decision-making capacity: the outpatient setting is a relatively nonstressful environment for patient evaluation, with the absence of severe acute illness that affects patients' cognitive abilities[11]; the long-term patient–physician relationship can also be used to detect subtle cognitive impairment or changes of the patient's capacity over time; and the assessment can

**Table 1**
**Questions for assessing patient capacity to make decisions**

| Ability | Example Questions |
| --- | --- |
| Communicate a choice | Can you tell me what your decision is? |
| Understand the relevant information | Can you tell me in your own words what you understand about your health problem and the treatments being offered? |
| Appreciate the situation and its consequences | What do you believe will happen if you undergo the treatment? How might this impact your health? |
| Manipulate relevant information in a rational way | What makes treatment X better than Y? |

*Data from* Appelbaum PS. Clinical practice. Assessment of patients' competence to consent to treatment. N Engl J Med 2007;357(18):1834–40.

be complemented by family members' perspectives. For all of these reasons, and whenever possible, PCPs should perform a basic capacity assessment on every patient, especially for those near the end of life.

When a patient is deemed to lack decision-making capacity, then the physician should try to identify the causes of impairment and remedy them, if they are reversible. When the cause is fear or anxiety, introducing a confidant or an adviser to the consent process may permit the patient to make competent decisions.[5] If doubts exist when assessing the capacity of a patient or when a case is likely to be resolved in court, special assessment tools should be used[12] and consultation with psychiatry may be necessary. If the patient has no possibility to regain capacity, then a living will detailing patient preferences or assistance from a surrogate decision-maker becomes necessary to protect patient autonomy.[5] The surrogate decision-maker should ideally be designated by the patient prior to the loss of decision-making capacity, or in the absence of such an advance directive, the person with the strongest genetic and/or emotional ties to the patient.[6] This strategy has been supported by courts and legislation.[13]

## ADVANCE CARE PLANNING

Advance care planning (ACP) can be defined as the process of planning for future medical care. ACP was developed in an attempt to address the problem of decision-making in patients without capacity and to improve care at the end of life.[14] An advance directive directs the provision of life-sustaining treatment when the patient no longer has capacity to make decisions. Two types of advance directives are available: (1) a health care proxy document, in which a person is legally appointed as a health care decision-maker, and (2) a living will, in which a patient defines instructions regarding future medical care. A durable power of attorney is a legal instrument that allows a person to make decisions regarding financial or legal matters, and is not used for medical issues and therefore is not considered an advance directive.

The usefulness of advance directives has been debated.[15,16] Supporters of advance directives consider them valuable instruments for several reasons. First, they are believed to help guide health providers and family members in making decisions for incapacitated patients.[17] The underlying assumption is that the patient is the person who can best define the circumstances in which life should continue. Second, advance directives increase a patient's empowerment in medical decision-making and promote discussions about death planning and conversations between patients and their families.[16] For example, these instruments have helped increase the likelihood that patients will die in the place they prefer.[18] Third, talking about planning helps alleviate patients' anxiety regarding the future. Having open discussions about these issues and establishing a trustful patient–physician interaction reduces a patient's uncertainty and provides peace about who and how decisions will be made in the future.[19]

However, despite concerted efforts to extend the use of advance directives, the number of people who have completed one is still extremely variable. Studies have shown that anywhere from 5% and 67% of patients complete some form of advance directive.[15–17,20–25] This wide range can be partly explained by the heterogeneity of the populations studied, but in most studies the frequency of completed advance directives is less than 30%. Furthermore, these documents often are not easily available when physicians or the family need them.[26] When available, living wills may be too vague to interpret or are only occasionally followed.[27] Some physicians argue that ACP is time-consuming[28] and often requires more than one consult to discuss the different possibilities and their medical, social, legal, and ethical implications. Opponents of ACP also point out that once living wills are defined, the assumption is that the patient's preferences are stable over time, and that they accurately represent a patient's preference when facing serious medical situations.[29] However, what one may prefer in a premorbid, healthy state is likely to differ from what one would choose when actually faced with a life-threatening illness.[30] In addition, it is common for patients to change their minds about treatment preferences through the course of illness. Factors such as mood disorders, physical decline, and hospitalizations have been identified as influences that could partly explain this instability.[29] Therefore, patient predictions of preferences and reactions to hypothetical future events is both inaccurate and unstable over time.[31]

Regarding surrogate decision-makers, other problems arise. Studies have shown that surrogates often do not know how the patient would have decided in a certain situation,[32] and that decisions correlate more with the surrogate's own preferences rather than the preferences of incapable patients.[33] Researchers have also shown that family members of patients in the intensive care unit are often too impaired by depression and anxiety to make decisions regarding their loved ones.[34] Despite these facts, United States courts have supported the idea that surrogates and family members are in the best position to make medical decisions because of their deep investment in the patient's best interests.

It is the authors' view that PCPs are in a privileged position to initiate ACP with patients. Studies have shown that patients expect that their PCP to begin the discussion about advance directives.[35] PCPs can guide this process over several visits in a calm setting, focusing on patient values and beliefs. In our experience, this is an intensely rewarding endeavor. The goal of ACP is to respect patient autonomy when the patient is no longer able to make decisions. Through clarifying and documenting patient preferences, PCPs can provide important guidance regarding the future use of medical interventions at the end of life.

## WITHHOLDING AND WITHDRAWING TREATMENTS

Discussions about future treatment preferences are essential in ACP and should include discussions regarding withholding and withdrawing life-sustaining treatments. In many instances these decisions are morally troublesome for physicians, patients, and families. Therefore, it is essential for PCPs to be familiar with these topics, understand the ethical implications of these decisions, and recognize some of the moral concerns that might arise through the discussions with patients and families.[36]

Current technological advances in medicine allow patients to be kept alive who would have previously died, leading to a culture that seems to believe that every possible intervention should be attempted to extend a patient's life, despite the burdens that this decision would carry, and ultimately obscuring the ability to recognize when a patient is actually dying.[36] An additional factor affecting the decision to withhold or withdraw treatments is the fear of abandonment. Some families are uncomfortable withholding or withdrawing treatments from their loved ones because they are afraid of not doing "everything possible" or "giving up too soon," and that the subsequent death could be considered abandoning, or even worse, killing the patient. Some evidence also suggests that both African American and Hispanic families are less likely to discontinue life-supportive therapies, perhaps as a response to their distrust of the health care system resulting from the history of racism in medicine.[37] These facts make decisions regarding withholding and withdrawing treatment very complex, even for families that have extensively discussed these issues.

Attempting to clarify some of the ethical issues associated with withholding and withdrawing treatments may help mitigate some of the concern from families and clinicians. Firstly, a patient has the right to refuse any and all treatments, even if the removal of the treatment results in hastened death. Secondly, withdrawal of life support after which a patient subsequently dies should be distinguished from intentionally causing a patient's death. A general consensus exists that the former is morally permitted, whereas the latter is unacceptable. Thirdly, it is also widely accepted that withholding and withdrawing life-sustaining treatments are ethically and legally the same,[38,39] despite the fact that many physicians believe there is a difference between these two actions, particularly related to the proximity of withdrawing a treatment and the subsequent death.[40]

The decision to withhold or withdraw any life-sustaining therapy should be made together with the patient, whenever possible, or with the patient's family and/or surrogate decision-maker. Using guidance from ACP or other documented conversations with providers or family members in which patients have articulated their preferences is the best evidence to provide ethical justification for the withholding or withdrawing of life support. When the treatment is determined to be too burdensome or harmful in proportion to the likely outcome, clinicians should initiate discussions with patients and families regarding withholding and withdrawing life-sustaining treatments.

## PROVIDING ADEQUATE PAIN AND SYMPTOM RELIEF

Despite quality improvement efforts and educational initiatives to enhance the assessment and management of cancer pain, the problem of inadequate pain treatment persists.[41,42] Multiple barriers affect the clinician's ability to adequately address pain, including insufficient education and knowledge, patient and family factors, insurers' limitations placed on medication choices and amounts, regulatory scrutiny from government and legislative bodies, potential prescription drug abuse, and fear of litigation for overtreatment.[43]

Since the time of Hippocrates, relieving pain and suffering has been a primary goal and duty of physicians. Failure to adequately treat a patient's pain not only would violate the principle of nonmaleficence but also can diminish autonomy and the right-to-self determination, because unremitting pain can have significant effects on one's quality of life and ability to make reasonable decisions.[44,45] Pain relief is also important from the perspective of justice, because at the individual level it allows patients the opportunity to function normally within society.[46] Rawls[47] had considered "freedom from physical pain" as a possible candidate for an expansion of his list of primary goods (ie, those basic conditions that were necessary for a just society).

Federal and state legislative bodies have enacted statutes and regulations that impact on the treatment of pain. Some directly address how caregivers should treat pain, such as the Pain Relief Act of 1996,[48] whereas others regulate the distribution of controlled substances.[49] The latter, in conjunction with medical negligence cases and medical board disciplinary action for overtreatment of pain, have unfortunately deterred many medical practitioners from prescribing adequate pain relief.[50] More recently, the legal system has deliberated on cases asserting undertreatment of pain in terminally ill patients. In *Bergman v Chin*, a doctor's failure to adequately treat the pain of a terminally ill 85-year-old man who was discharged from a hospitalization with a pain score of 10 a few days before his death was found to constitute elder abuse.[51]

Some have argued that the treatment of pain is a fundamental human right and should be a priority for international public health programs.[52] The United Nations International Covenant on Economic Social and Cultural Rights articulates the right to "enjoyment of the highest attainable standard of physical and mental health." Although pain is not explicitly referred to, it has been argued that freedom from pain can be inferred in this right.[53] This view is gaining increasing acceptance as both developed and developing countries continue to struggle with the issue of undertreated pain.

Regardless of whether one views the treatment of pain as simply good clinical practice, an ethical obligation, or a legal or human right, the fact that pain is one of the most frequent reasons for consultation in the outpatient setting is sufficient justification for physicians to prioritize pain assessment and management in their practice.

## PALLIATIVE SEDATION

Despite high-quality palliative care, a small minority of patients experience intolerable suffering at the end of life. Although palliative sedation is largely in the domain of palliative care specialists, PCPs must be aware of palliative sedation to allow appropriate patients access to this therapy when indicated.

Palliative sedation, a useful but contentious treatment of last resort, is broadly defined as using sedative medications to relieve intolerable suffering caused by refractory symptoms via a reduction in patient consciousness.[54] Refractory symptoms have been defined as symptoms that cannot be adequately treated using standard palliative interventions within an acceptable time frame.[55] Suffering, intolerability, and adequate relief are of course subjective and can only be defined by the patient.

The issue of palliative sedation has been somewhat complicated by the fact that no agreed-on nomenclature exists to describe the process of sedation for refractory suffering at the end of life, and no widespread agreement exists as to what acts actually constitutes palliative sedation, its goals, and what medications are appropriate.[54,56] These factors, along with differing cultural and religious beliefs surrounding death and dying and the retrospective nature of relevant studies, have contributed to a wide discrepancy in reports of the prevalence of palliative sedation, with estimates varying from 3% to 51% of all palliative care deaths.[57,58]

Palliative sedation has traditionally been justified by the doctrine of double effect, which maintains that it is the intention of the moral actor that matters. The doctrine of double effect originally formulated by Thomas Aquinas applies to moral dilemmas in which it is impossible for a person to avoid all harmful actions. The doctrine of double effect requires that (1) the nature of the act must be good or at least morally neutral (prescribing sedatives is a morally neutral acts), (2) the harmful effect must be foreseen but not intended (hastened death), (3) the harmful effect must not be a way of producing the good effect (the good effect—less suffering—is a result of loss of consciousness with sedation), and (4) the good effect must outweigh the harmful effect, proportionately (in terminally ill patients with refractory suffering this is believed to be the case). Thus, the doctrine of double effect has been used to justify the administration of both high-dose opioids and sedatives for the purposes of pain and symptom relief, notwithstanding the unintended but foreseen risk of hastening the patient's death. Many critics have argued that the focus on intention is problematic; focusing on the requirements of informed consent and proportionality in seeking ethical justification for this practice may be more useful.[59] Informed consent for palliative sedation requires that the patient or surrogate be fully informed about the rationale for using palliative sedation and about the associated risks, and agree to the procedure.[60] Proportionality helps to balance the conflict between the duty to relieve the patient's suffering and the duty not to cause death. In other words, the risk of hastening death is justified if standard approaches have failed to relieve the severe symptoms. The authors give higher priority to relieving symptoms than to continuing a life filled with suffering.[61]

General consensus exists on the appropriateness of sedation for suffering caused by intractable physical symptoms such as pain, delirium, and dyspnea in terminally ill patients.[62] The argument for palliative sedation in these circumstances has been strengthened by studies indicating that palliative sedation does not appear to hasten death,[63] and by the 1997 US Supreme Court decision rejecting physician-assisted suicide as a constitutional right, based on the concept that palliative sedation is a valid alternative treatment option for suffering at the end of life.[64]

Palliative sedation for existential distress or severe psychosocial distress as an ethically acceptable treatment option is controversial, and is likely to remain so in light of the fact that there is still no widespread agreement regarding what constitutes existential distress or when it becomes refractory to standard approaches. The National Hospice and Palliative Care Organization (NHPCO) defines it as "suffering that arises from a sense of meaninglessness, hopelessness, fear and regret in patients who knowingly approach the end of life."[65] The arguments for and against palliative sedation for existential distress are complex and beyond the scope of this article.[66–68]

Various individuals and organizations have proposed or set out position statements and practical guidelines for palliative sedation, some of which endorse palliative sedation for existential suffering.[62,69] Guidelines, such as those of the European Association of Palliative Care, include (1) the indications in which sedation may be considered, (2) the necessary evaluation and consultation procedures, (3) consent requirements, (4) medications and dose titration, (5) patient monitoring, (6) guidance regarding hydration and nutrition during sedation, and (6) how to address the problem of using sedation for refractory existential distress.[70]

## PHYSICIAN-ASSISTED SUICIDE AND EUTHANASIA

Palliative sedation can be distinguished from physician-assisted suicide and euthanasia in that the specific intent of these practices are to end life with either the deliberate use of lethal doses of medication or therapeutically unjustified dose escalation.

Physician-assisted suicide is defined as a physician providing, at the patient's request, a lethal medication that the patient can take by his own hand to end otherwise intolerable suffering. In the United States, physician-assisted suicide is legal only in Oregon, Washington, and Montana. Each year, the Oregon Department of Human Services publishes an annual report on its use.[71] In 2009, 95 prescriptions for lethal medications were written, with 53 patients taking those medications. As in previous years, most participants were well educated, had cancer, and were insured. The most frequently mentioned end-of-life concerns were loss of autonomy (96.6%), loss of dignity (91.5%), and decreasing ability to participate in activities that made life enjoyable (86.4%).[72]

Euthanasia, defined from the Greek word *euthanatos* meaning "good death," refers to the active intentional ending of life by a physician. Euthanasia is the subject of intense ethical debate and is beyond the scope of this article. Although legal in the Netherlands, euthanasia is currently not an option in the United States.

## SUMMARY

Physicians encounter many ethical issues when caring for patients at the end of life. Their obligation to patient autonomy requires that they consider how and to what extent medical treatments should be used in the face of a life-threatening illness. These conversations ideally should happen while patients have the capacity to decide for themselves. Documentation of patient wishes in a living will and assignment of a surrogate decision-maker are proactive steps that can be taken to protect patients from undergoing treatments they may not want to endure in the future when they no longer have capacity. Ultimately, the patient's values should guide the use of medical interventions. Regardless of patient preferences, physicians should always strive to alleviate suffering, whether it is physical, psychological, or existential. With patient consent and the principle of proportionality, physicians are ethically justified in using medications and therapies to alleviate pain and suffering, even if these treatments carry a risk of hastening death. This approach should be differentiated from physician-assisted suicide and euthanasia. Consultation with palliative care specialists or clinical ethicists may help address the potential moral ambiguity and discomfort when addressing some of these issues.

## REFERENCES

1. Cabot RC. Training and rewards of the physician. Philadelphia: J.B. Lippincott Co; 1918. p. 15.
2. Yung VY, Walling AM, Min L, et al. Documentation of advance care planning for community-dwelling elders. J Palliat Med 2010;13(7):861–7.
3. Hawkins H, Cartwright C. Advance health care planning and the GP. Is it time to move forward? Aust Fam Physician 2000;29(7):704–7.
4. Beauchamp TL, Childress JF. Principles of biomedical ethics. Oxford (NY): Oxford University Press; 1989.
5. Appelbaum PS. Clinical practice. Assessment of patients' competence to consent to treatment. N Engl J Med 2007;357(18):1834–40.
6. Truog RD. End-of-life decision-making in the United States. Eur J Anaesthesiol Suppl 2008;42:43–50.
7. Etchells E, Darzins P, Silberfeld M, et al. Assessment of patient capacity to consent to treatment. J Gen Intern Med 1999;14(1):27–34.
8. Casarett DJ, Karlawish JH, Hirschman KB. Identifying ambulatory cancer patients at risk of impaired capacity to consent to research. J Pain Symptom Manage 2003;26(1):615–24.
9. Markson LJ, Kern DC, Annas GJ, et al. Physician assessment of patient competence. J Am Geriatr Soc 1994;42(10):1074–80.
10. Roth LH, Meisel A, Lidz CW. Tests of competency to consent to treatment. Am J Psychiatry 1977;134(3):279–84.
11. Messinger-Rapport BJ, Baum EE, Smith ML. Advance care planning: beyond the living will. Cleve Clin J Med 2009;76(5):276–85.
12. Dunn LB, Nowrangi MA, Palmer BW, et al. Assessing decisional capacity for clinical research or treatment: a review of instruments. Am J Psychiatry 2006;163(8):1323–34.
13. Volicer L, Cantor MD, Derse AR, et al. Advance care planning by proxy for residents of long-term care facilities who lack decision-making capacity. J Am Geriatr Soc 2002;50(4):761–7.
14. Patient Self-Determination Act, 42 USC §18 (1990).
15. Winter L, Parks SM, Diamond JJ. Ask a different question, get a different answer: why living wills are poor guides to care preferences at the end of life. J Palliat Med 2010;13(5):567–72.
16. Perkins HS. Controlling death: the false promise of advance directives. Ann Intern Med 2007;147(1):51–7.
17. Silveira MJ, Kim SY, Langa KM. Advance directives and outcomes of surrogate decision making before death. N Engl J Med 2010;362(13):1211–8.
18. Newton J, Clark R, Ahlquist P. Evaluation of the introduction of an advanced care plan into multiple palliative care settings. Int J Palliat Nurs 2009;15(11):554–61.

19. Singer PA, Martin DK, Lavery JV, et al. Reconceptualizing advance care planning from the patient's perspective. Arch Intern Med 1998;158(8):879–84.
20. Eiser AR, Weiss MD. The underachieving advance directive: recommendations for increasing advance directive completion. Am J Bioeth 2001;1(4):W10.
21. Teno J, Lynn J, Wenger N, et al. Advance directives for seriously ill hospitalized patients: effectiveness with the patient self-determination act and the SUPPORT intervention. SUPPORT Investigators. Study to Understand Prognoses and Preferences for Outcomes and Risks of Treatment. J Am Geriatr Soc 1997;45(4):500–7.
22. Resnick HE, Schuur JD, Heineman J, et al. Advance directives in nursing home residents aged >or=65 years: United States 2004. Am J Hosp Palliat Care 2008;25(6):476–82.
23. Dow LA, Matsuyama RK, Ramakrishnan V, et al. Paradoxes in advance care planning: the complex relationship of oncology patients, their physicians, and advance medical directives. J Clin Oncol 2010;28(2):299–304.
24. Kish SK, Martin CG, Price KJ. Advance directives in critically ill cancer patients. Crit Care Nurs Clin North Am 2000;12(3):373–83.
25. The Pew Research Centre for the People & The Press. More Americans discussing–and planning–end-of-life treatment. Washington, DC: The Pew Research Centre for the People & the Press; 2006.
26. Gillick MR. Reversing the code status of advance directives? N Engl J Med 2010;362(13):1239–40.
27. A controlled trial to improve care for seriously ill hospitalized patients. The study to understand prognoses and preferences for outcomes and risks of treatments (SUPPORT). The SUPPORT Principal Investigators. JAMA 1995;274(20):1591–8.
28. Roter DL, Larson S, Fischer GS, et al. Experts practice what they preach: a descriptive study of best and normative practices in end-of-life discussions. Arch Intern Med 2000;160(22):3477–85.
29. Ditto PH, Hawkins NA. Advance directives and cancer decision making near the end of life. Health Psychol 2005;24(Suppl 4):S63–70.
30. Redelmeier DA, Rozin P, Kahneman D. Understanding patients' decisions. Cognitive and emotional perspectives. JAMA 1993;270(1):72–6.
31. Loewenstein G. Hot-cold empathy gaps and medical decision making. Health Psychol 2005;24(Suppl 4):S49–56.
32. Uhlmann RF, Pearlman RA, Cain KC. Physicians' and spouses' predictions of elderly patients' resuscitation preferences. J Gerontol 1988;43(5):M115–21.
33. Fagerlin A, Ditto PH, Danks JH, et al. Projection in surrogate decisions about life-sustaining medical treatments. Health Psychol 2001;20(3):166–75.
34. Pochard F, Azoulay E, Chevret S, et al. Symptoms of anxiety and depression in family members of intensive care unit patients: ethical hypothesis regarding decision-making capacity. Crit Care Med 2001;29(10):1893–7.
35. Hickman SE, Hammes BJ, Moss AH, et al. Hope for the future: achieving the original intent of advance directives. Hastings Cent Rep 2005;(Spec No):S26–30.
36. Reynolds S, Cooper AB, McKneally M. Withdrawing life-sustaining treatment: ethical considerations. Surg Clin North Am 2007;87(4):919–36, viii.
37. Krakauer EL, Crenner C, Fox K. Barriers to optimum end-of-life care for minority patients. J Am Geriatr Soc 2002;50(1):182–90.
38. Gostin LO. Deciding life and death in the courtroom. From Quinlan to Cruzan, Glucksberg, and Vacco—a brief history and analysis of constitutional protection of the 'right to die'. JAMA 1997;278(18):1523–8.

39. Vincent JL. Cultural differences in end-of-life care. Crit Care Med 2001; 29(Suppl 2):N52–5.
40. Seymour JE. Negotiating natural death in intensive care. Soc Sci Med 2000;51(8): 1241–52.
41. Von Roenn JH, Cleeland CS, Gonin R, et al. Physician attitudes and practice in cancer pain management. A survey from the Eastern Cooperative Oncology Group. Ann Intern Med 1993;119(2):121–6.
42. Zenz M, Zenz T, Tryba M, et al. Severe undertreatment of cancer pain: a 3-year survey of the German situation. J Pain Symptom Manage 1995;10(3):187–91.
43. Altilio T. Pain and symptom management clinical, policy, and political perspectives. J Psychosoc Oncol 2006;24(1):65–79.
44. Katz N. The impact of pain management on quality of life. J Pain Symptom Manage 2002;24(Suppl 1):S38–47.
45. Cain JM, Hammes BJ. Ethics and pain management: respecting patient wishes. J Pain Symptom Manage 1994;9(3):160–5.
46. Gureje O, Von Korff M, Simon GE, et al. Persistent pain and well-being: a World Health Organization Study in Primary Care. JAMA 1998;280(2):147–51.
47. Rawls J. Political liberalism. New York: Columbia University Press; 1995.
48. Johnson SH. Disciplinary actions and pain relief: analysis of the Pain Relief Act. J Law Med Ethics 1996;24(4):319–27.
49. Controlled Substances Act 21 USC §802 (2007).
50. Joranson DE, Gilson AM. Controlled substances, medical practice and the law. In: Schwartz HI, editor. Psychiatric practice under fire: the influence of government, the media and special interests on somatic therapies. Washington, DC: American Psychiatric Press, Inc; 1994. p. 173–94.
51. Bergman v Chin, H205732–1 (Alameda County Superior Court, 2001).
52. Brennan F, Carr DB, Cousins M. Pain management: a fundamental human right. Anesth Analg 2007;105(1):205–21.
53. United Nations International Covenant on Economic Social and Cultural Rights. GA res. 2200A (XXI), 21 UN GAOR Supp. (No. 16) at 49, UN Doc. A/6316 (1966); 993 UNTS 3; 6 ILM 368 (1967) Article 12. Available at: http://www. hrweb.org/legal/escr.html. Accessed August 17, 2010.
54. de Graeff A, Dean M. Palliative sedation therapy in the last weeks of life: a literature review and recommendations for standards. J Palliat Med 2007; 10(1):67–85.
55. Cherny NI, Portenoy RK. Sedation in the management of refractory symptoms: guidelines for evaluation and treatment. J Palliat Care 1994;10(2):31–8.
56. Morita T, Tsuneto S, Shima Y. Proposed definitions for terminal sedation. Lancet 2001;358(9278):335–6.
57. Kohara H, Ueoka H, Takeyama H, et al. Sedation for terminally ill patients with cancer with uncontrollable physical distress. J Palliat Med 2005;8(1):20–5.
58. Rietjens J, van Delden J, Onwuteaka-Philipsen B, et al. Continuous deep sedation for patients nearing death in the Netherlands: descriptive study. BMJ 2008; 336(7648):810–3.
59. Quill TE, Lo B, Brock DW. Palliative options of last resort: a comparison of voluntarily stopping eating and drinking, terminal sedation, physician-assisted suicide, and voluntary active euthanasia. JAMA 1997;278(23):2099–104.
60. Rousseau P. The ethical validity and clinical experience of palliative sedation. Mayo Clin Proc 2000;75(10):1064–9.
61. Lo B, Rubenfeld G. Palliative sedation in dying patients: "we turn to it when everything else hasn't worked". JAMA 2005;294(14):1810–6.

62. National Ethics Committee VHA. The ethics of palliative sedation as a therapy of last resort. Am J Hosp Palliat Care 2006;23(6):483–91.
63. Sykes N, Thorns A. Sedative use in the last week of life and the implications for end-of-life decision making. Arch Intern Med 2003;163(3):341–4.
64. Vacco v Quill, 117 SCt 2293 (1997).
65. Kirk TW, Mahon MM. National Hospice and Palliative Care Organization (NHPCO) position statement and commentary on the use of palliative sedation in imminently dying terminally ill patients. J Pain Symptom Manage 2010;39(5):914–23.
66. Morita T. Palliative sedation to relieve psycho-existential suffering of terminally ill cancer patients. J Pain Symptom Manage 2004;28(5):445–50.
67. Morita T, Tei Y, Inoue S. Ethical validity of palliative sedation therapy. J Pain Symptom Manage 2003;25(2):103–5.
68. Cassell EJ, Rich BA. Intractable end-of-life suffering and the ethics of palliative sedation. Pain Med 2010;11(3):435–8.
69. Rousseau P. Palliative sedation in the management of refractory symptoms. J Support Oncol 2004;2(2):181–6.
70. Cherny NI, Radbruch L. European Association for Palliative Care (EAPC) recommended framework for the use of sedation in palliative care. Palliat Med 2009;23(7):581–93.
71. Available at: http://www.oregon.gov/DHS/ph/pas/. Accessed August 17, 2010.
72. Oregon Death with Dignity Act Annual report. Available at: http://www.oregon.gov/DHS/ph/pas/docs/year12.pdf. Accessed August 17, 2010.

# Assessment and Management of Pain in the Terminally Ill

Shalini Dalal, MD*, Eduardo Bruera, MD

**KEYWORDS**

• Palliative care • Opioids • Pain management • Terminal illness

In the United States, most deaths occur in a hospital or nursing home facility, and in the context of a chronic illness.[1,2] The period of chronic illness and time before death are frequently characterized by pain, other distressful symptoms, increasing functional impairments, and disability.[3] Hospitalized patients usually receive costly aggressive treatments, even immediately before death.[4,5] Unfortunately, the same aggressive care and use of resources does not seem to be directed toward palliation of symptom distress and suffering. Among hospitalized patients, 25% to 40% experience uncontrolled pain at the end of life, even 3 days before death.[4,6,7] Pain is experienced by most patients with advanced cancer, and is associated with unnecessary suffering and decreased quality of life (QoL).[8–10] The lack of pain assessment and failure to recognize the multidimensional nature of pain are some common causes of overall poor symptom control and decreased QoL in terminally ill patients.

Palliative care has the goal of reducing pain and suffering, and improving the QoL of patients diagnosed with terminal illness. The hospice model is the most developed and recognized but requires patients to "sign on" to services and often relinquish care by medical providers who have treated them for a long time. Approximately 40% of patients who die in the United States choose hospice care, but do so late in their illness trajectory (median hospice stay is approximately 3 weeks).[11] Over the years, United States hospital-based palliative care programs have dramatically increased; however, patient referrals to these programs are variable, mostly occurring in the last few weeks of life.[12,13] Thus, most terminally ill patients are cared for in a generalist rather than a specialist palliative care setting. Primary care physicians are uniquely positioned to provide palliative care to their patients, because they have an ongoing patient–physician relationship, which can be strengthened as

Eduardo Bruera is supported in part by National Institutes of Health grant numbers: RO1NR010162-01A1, RO1CA122292-01, and RO1CA124481-01.
Department of Palliative Care and Rehabilitation Medicine – Unit 1414, The University of Texas MD Anderson Cancer Center, 1515 Holcombe Boulevard, Houston, TX 77030, USA
* Corresponding author.
*E-mail address:* sdalal@mdanderson.org

patients navigate through their last moments of life. This delivery of palliative care, referred to as *primary* palliative care, requires basic skills and competencies in end of life care, including the management of pain. With adequate training, resources, and referral to specialist palliative care when needed, primary care physicians can improve the care of terminally ill patients.

This article addresses pain assessment and management in terminally ill patients. Pain in patients with cancer is often used as an example, but the principles of pain management are applicable to a multitude of conditions that patients experience at the end of life. The concept of individualizing therapy to the patient's evolving needs and circumstances is fundamental to successful pain management in the terminally ill, and requires a systematic and comprehensive approach (**Fig. 1**).

## MULTIDIMENSIONAL PAIN ASSESSMENT IN THE TERMINALLY ILL

Pain is subjective, and in patients who are terminally ill it is not simply a physical experience. Pain expression is impacted by the terminal nature of illness that also results in other sources of distress, functional decline, dependence, family disruption, and financial burdens that threaten QoL.[14] Dame Cecily Saunders,[15] founder of the modern hospice movement, was the first to use the term *total pain* to describe the physical, emotional, social, and spiritual components of distress and suffering in terminally ill patients (**Fig. 2**). These four dimensions, either individually or in combination, affect patients' perception of their total pain, and should be explored in all terminally ill patients. In addition, patients frequently experience other concurrent symptoms (eg, dyspnea, nausea, fatigue) that contribute to overall symptom burden and should be simultaneously explored and treated.

A formal systematic assessment of pain is beneficial, because it relays to patients/ families that their complaints are legitimate, are being quantified and documented, and will be used to evaluate treatments, thereby allowing them to become active participants in their care. However, impaired cognition, whether caused by delirium or dementia, is frequently present in advanced stages of illness, and can compromise assessments. Therefore, screening tests for cognitive impairments should be implemented early, preferably before detailed symptom assessments are performed.

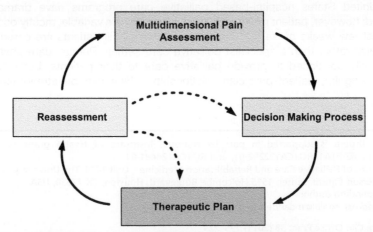

**Fig. 1.** Comprehensive approach to assessment and management of pain in terminally ill patients.

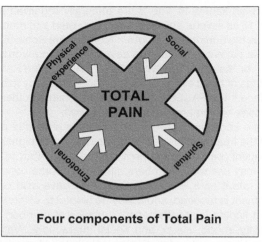

**Four components of Total Pain**

**Fig. 2.** Total pain is the sum of four components: the patient's physical experience, and psychological, social, and spiritual components to distress.

## Screening for Pain, "The Fifth Vital Sign"

In the United States, most health care organizations have followed the American Pain Society's lead to make pain assessment routine and "visible" as a vital sign, and the frequent assessment of pain is now considered standard of care. This assessment is particularly applicable in vulnerable terminally ill patients, who will benefit from timely therapeutic interventions. Patients and caregivers should be informed that pain management is a key component of care, and that its presence should be promptly reported to the medical team. Patients should be asked regularly if they have any pain or discomfort, hurt anywhere, or have any aching or soreness.

## Pain Characteristics and Severity

Patients should be asked about pain severity, quality, location, and temporal features, such as onset, duration, diurnal variation, or aggravating/relieving factors. Pain can be localized by asking patients to pinpoint its location on their body or a body diagram (part of some pain assessment tools, such as the Brief Pain Inventory [BPI]), including areas where the pain radiates. Some patients may only have episodic pain, precipitated by activity (incidental pain), or may experience spontaneous pain, such as cramping abdominal pain or neuropathic pain. The patient's descriptive words about the quality of pain may provide clues to its causes. Somatic nociceptive pain is usually described as sharp or dull, well-localized, aching, or a squeezing sensation. Visceral nociceptive pain is usually poorly localized, and described as a deep pressure-like sensation. Neuropathic pain is described as burning, tingling, electrical, stabbing, or "pins and needles." Pain may be caused by a complex mixture of nociceptive and neuropathic factors.

Validated scales for measuring pain severity include the numeric rating scale (NRS), verbal rating scale, visual analog scale, and the picture scale. For consistency, the same scale should be used for the patient throughout treatment. Each scales has advantages and limitations, depending on the patient's age, communication skills, and cognition.[6] The NRS, most commonly used, is a line with 0 (no pain) at one end and 10 (worst pain possible) at the opposite end. It is available in large type for visually impaired patients. Pain scores of 1 to 3 are generally regarded as mild, 4 to 6 as moderate, and 7 to 10 as severe. The NRS is incorporated into multisymptom assessment scales, such as the Edmonton Symptom Assessment Scale (ESAS).[16] The verbal rating scale requires patients to rate pain severity by using words such as "none," "mild," "moderate," or "severe." The Wong-Baker FACES Pain Rating Scale consists of a series of drawings of facial expressions ranging from happy to sad, with a number assigned to each face.[8] The FACES scale is ideal for children older than 3 years, and adults unable to speak or who are cognitively impaired.

Pain severity is the dominant factor determining the effects of pain on the patient and the urgency of the treatment process. Scores of 4 to 5 or higher have been shown to predict subsequent pain management complexity, and to impair QoL.[17-19] However, patients may use these numbers differently. Some patients may complain of severe pain but rate it as 5, whereas others may have mild pain and rate it the same. Clinical judgment is required, and it may be helpful to clarify the patient's sense of the pain (without finding fault with patient's choice of number) and its impact on QoL, physical activity, mood, sleep, and social interactions. Validated scales that rate pain severity and its impact on functioning include the Memorial Pain Assessment Card and the BPI.[20,21] If possible, determining the patient's personal goals for pain relief can be useful. A simple method may be to ask the patient to describe on a scale of 0 to 10 the level/intensity of pain that will allow the patient to achieve comfort in physical, functional, and psychosocial domains. Although this assessment has not been validated, support exists for pain management to be personalized, tailored to patients' individual needs for comfort and functioning.[22,23] Using terms such as "acceptable" or "tolerable" pain may have a negative connotation, suggesting that patients must accept or tolerate the pain. One way to ascertain personal pain goal may be to say, "We would like for you to have no pain, and we will strive for that. However, what is the level of pain, on a scale of 0 to 10, we can strive for that would provide you with good comfort and pain relief, and also allow you to function well and carry out your daily activities?"

### Pain Assessment in Patients With Cognitive Impairments

In patients with advanced cancer, delirium is present in 28% to 40% overall and, in most, hours to days before death.[24,25] Delirium is diagnosed based on cognitive impairment, particularly disordered attention, along with other features such as altered awareness, perceptual disturbances, acute onset, and fluctuant course.[26] Delirium may be missed when no objective cognitive testing is performed,[27] leading to incorrect assessments and therapies. The Mini Mental State Examination (MMSE) screens for cognitive impairment in patients with advanced illness, and provides useful information regarding the reliability of patient self-report scores.[28] The Memorial Delirium-Assessment Scale, a 10-item delirium rating scale, integrates objective cognitive testing and behavioral symptoms, and is validated to screen for and quantify delirium severity.[29]

Patients with mild to moderate cognitive impairments can usually respond to self-reported pain scales.[30,31] However, in severely impaired patients, it may be possible to only ask a few questions, observe behaviors (**Box 1**),[9] and gather information from family/caregivers. Caregivers should be educated to report behaviors that may indicate pain. Staff-administered behavioral pain assessment tools in older patients with dementia, such as the Face, Legs, Activity, Cry, and Consolability (FLACC) scale, are generally used in research settings.[32]

Although family and caregivers are often used as proxies, their reports may not always agree with a patient's. Among hospitalized seriously ill patients, surrogates

| Box 1 |
| Behavioral cues suggestive of pain in cognitively impaired patients |

*Verbal cues*
Crying
Moaning
Groaning
Grunting

*Facial expressions*
Grimacing
Biting lips
Blinking
Closing eyes tightly

*Body movements*
Clenching fists
Restlessness
Combativeness
Guarding

*Social interaction and activities*
Withdrawn
Silent
Wanting to spend time in bed
Irritability
Insomnia
Decreased appetite

accurately estimated presence of pain and its severity 74% and 53% of the time, respectively.[33] In patients with cancer, caregivers were accurate 71% of the time, with female caregivers having a higher percentage of agreement with patient reports. Among patients in hospice care, caregivers more likely overestimated pain.[34,35] Clinicians should use family/caregiver reports in combination with behavioral observations in severely impaired patients to determine the extent of pain. When doubt exists, a trial of analgesics is recommended to avoid the risk of undertreatment.

## Assessment of Concurrent Symptoms

Most terminally ill patients experience a multitude of symptoms.[36,37] Although some symptoms maybe volunteered, many (eg, fatigue, depression) are only detected through systematic questioning.[36–38] Using systematic assessment, the median number of symptoms was tenfold higher than what was volunteered among palliative care patients.[37] Frequently, management of one symptom may lead to improvements or aggravation of another. Opioids for pain relief may improve insomnia and anxiety but may exacerbate sedation, constipation, and nausea. Validated scales such as ESAS and the MD Anderson Brief Symptom Inventory simultaneously assess for the presence and severity of common physical and psychological symptoms.

## Functional Assessment

An objective assessment of physical functioning constitutes an important part of the multidimensional assessment of pain. Terminally ill patients may curtail their physical activity because of pain. Physical activity may also be restricted because of fatigue, cachexia, and drowsiness, common in end-stage illness, contributing to rapid deconditioning, with severe impairments in overall functional status. A systematic approach to identifying and treating the contributing factors to functional decline, such as pain, may help improve functional status. The BPI instrument assesses the effect of pain on patient functioning, including physical activity.[21]

### Medical Assessment

A physical examination helps identify focal neurologic signs, urinary retention, fecal impaction, and sources of infection, which can cause pain. Evaluation through blood tests or imaging studies must be guided by the patient's prior wishes, the clinical condition, and the benefits and risks of any subsequent therapeutic intervention. Physiologic changes play a small role in pain assessment, and patients with chronic pain often have normal vital signs.[39] Medications should be reviewed for potential drug interactions and side effects. Concurrent use of benzodiazepines and opioids may cause or worsen sedation and cognitive impairment. If patients used opioids previously, information should include duration of treatment, adverse effects, adherence, and outcomes.

### DECISION-MAKING PROCESS

Management of pain (and other symptoms) in terminally ill patients requires formulation of an individualized treatment plan, which involves understanding the patient's overall goals of medical care, determining patient and family resources and limitations, and identification of achievable objectives. This process is best achieved in a family meeting. The initial meeting can lay the groundwork for an end-of-life experience that is rewarding to all involved. Patients and family need guidance in their decision-making process and should be actively involved in the discussions. Clinicians should discuss the overall medical condition and potential contributors of symptoms, and describe potential treatments that may be appropriate, including the benefits and burdens of each option in the setting of the terminal illness. Together, reasonable priorities may be set. Patients and families should be reassured that in most instances, pain relief is obtainable, and part of the medical team's role is to provide that relief. Once adequately informed, patients and family will be in a better position to state their preferences and set their limits of care according to their personal values and goals. Patient preferences should weigh into final decision making. These discussions must be ongoing.

Family meetings may also provide an opportunity to discuss patient preference for the end-of-life care setting. For patients with life expectancy of less than 6 months, who are not receiving life-prolonging or disease-modifying treatments, referral to hospice care services should be considered. Hospice medical teams focus on treating symptoms, and provide much-needed bedside assistance and support to family caregivers.

### THERAPEUTIC PLAN FOR PAIN MANAGEMENT IN THE TERMINALLY ILL

Patients may have varying degrees of physical, psychological, spiritual, and social contributors to pain and suffering, which require simultaneous assessment and treatment. This multidimensional approach includes pharmacologic and nonpharmacologic options, individualized to the patient's evolving clinical circumstances.

## Pharmacologic Options for Pain Management

Medications used for treating pain include nonopioid and opioid analgesics, bisphosphonates for cancer-related bone pain, and a few select anticonvulsants and antidepressant agents as adjuvant analgesics. The World Health Organization's (WHO) method for treating pain involves a three-step ladder approach (**Fig. 3**), moving from nonopioids to weak opioids, and then to strong opioids, according to the severity of pain.[40,41] Numerous pain guidelines published since these are generally similar in principle, stress importance of prompt assessment, adopt the WHO approach when considering analgesics, and use multimodality approaches when appropriate.[42,43] However, two systematic reviews[44,45] raise questions about the usefulness of step 2 of the WHO ladder, because delayed introduction of strong opioids may result in periods of uncontrolled pain. Recent studies suggest that strong opioids may be safely initiated at low doses, and are more beneficial in cancer patients with mild to moderate pain.[46,47]

### Nonopioid analgesics

Acetaminophen and nonsteroidal anti-inflammatory drugs (NSAIDs) are recommended for use alone (step 1 WHO ladder), or in combination with opioids. Acetaminophen may be appropriate for patients with mild pain from osteoarthritis or nonspecific musculoskeletal pain. It is the most frequently used nonopioid in combination products with opioids (hydrocodone, codeine, tramadol, and oxycodone); however, the toxicity and ceiling dose of the acetaminophen component limits the total daily dose of opioid that can be administered. Acetaminophen should be avoided or reduced in patients with alcohol abuse or at risk for renal or liver insufficiency. Recently, the U.S. Food and Drug Administration (FDA) advisory committee expressed concern that hepatic function may be altered in some people at current maximum recommended doses of 3 to 4 g/d, and voted to eliminate combination products containing acetaminophen. However, the FDA has not yet implemented these recommendations. In terminally ill patients, if acetaminophen does not provide

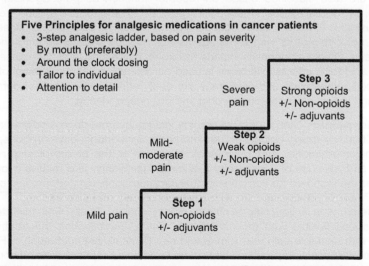

**Five Principles for analgesic medications in cancer patients**
- 3-step analgesic ladder, based on pain severity
- By mouth (preferably)
- Around the clock dosing
- Tailor to individual
- Attention to detail

**Step 3**
Severe pain
Strong opioids
+/- Non-opioids
+/- adjuvants

**Step 2**
Mild-moderate pain
Weak opioids
+/- Non-opioids
+/- adjuvants

**Step 1**
Mild pain
Non-opioids
+/- adjuvants

**Fig. 3.** World Health Organization principles for administering analgesic for cancer pain relief.

additional benefit, it should be discontinued to simplify the regimen and avoid potential toxicities.

NSAIDs mainly affect analgesia (and side effects) through inhibiting cyclooxygenase (COX) enzymes, thereby decreasing the prostaglandin production in the peripheral and central nervous systems. NSAIDs are considered more efficacious in inflammatory and bone pain,[48,49] Nonselective agents (eg, aspirin, ibuprofen, naproxen) inhibit both COX-1 and COX-2, whereas selective COX-2 inhibitors (celecoxib) spare COX-1 enzymes. NSAID adverse effects include gastrointestinal ulcerations and bleeding, renal dysfunction, and coagulation abnormalities, posing significant concerns in terminally ill patients, many of whom are elderly or may have coagulation/bleeding abnormalities or suboptimal organ functions. Selective COX-2 inhibitors offer some protection from gastrointestinal and platelet abnormalities, but several agents were withdrawn because of increased cardiovascular toxicity.[50,51] Celecoxib remains in use, but preliminary data have shown similar concerns.[52] Because long-term effects may not necessarily be a concern in terminally ill patients, celecoxib may be useful in selected patients with bone/inflammatory pain. If nonselective NSAIDs are used, the risk for gastrointestinal toxicity can be further reduced through coadministration of a proton pump inhibitor or misoprostol.[53] Patient and families nevertheless should be made aware of NSAID side effects.

### Opioids

Opioids are the mainstay of pain management in terminally ill patients because of their effectiveness in treating moderate to severe pain, lack of ceiling effect, and no direct effects on renal, hepatic, or coagulation functions. Opioids mediate analgesia through activating opioid receptors ($\mu$, $\kappa$, and $\delta$) present in the brain, spinal cord, and sensory neurons. $\mu$-Opioid receptor activation is considered most important for analgesia, and selective $\mu$-receptor agonists comprise the commonly used opioid analgesics.

Based on chemical structure, opioids are classified as phenanthrenes (morphine-like), phenylpiperidines (meperidine-like), and diphenylheptanes (methadone-like) (**Box 2**). Patients with a true opioid allergy may receive a structurally dissimilar opioid. Opioids are also classified based on receptor function as pure agonists, partial agonists, and partial agonist/antagonists (**Table 1**).[54] The latter two groups are generally not useful in terminal illness because of partial or ceiling effects for analgesia, and activation of $\kappa$-receptors with some agents that may be associated with undesired dysesthesia. Opioid antagonists include naloxone, naltrexone, and nalmefene, which have no analgesic effects. Naloxone is used parenterally for rapid reversal of opioid side effects. Naltrexone and nalmefene are orally effective, with longer duration of action, and are useful in treating alcohol and drug dependency.

$\mu$-**Receptor agonists** Step 2 or *weak* opioids include hydrocodone, codeine, and tramadol. Step 3 or *strong* opioids include morphine, oxycodone, oxymorphone, hydromorphone, methadone, and tapentadol. Morphine is the prototypical $\mu$-receptor agonist, and because of widespread availability, familiarity, and relatively low cost, is used as the standard for comparison.[55] Hydromorphone, oxycodone, and oxymorphone are semisynthetic agents, with similar analgesic and side effects.[56,57] Transdermal fentanyl is a lipophilic synthetic opioid and is usually well tolerated, but dosing is less flexible with the transdermal patch, complicating the treatment of patients with unstable pain in whom opioid requirements are fluctuating.[42] Fentanyl transmucosal/buccal preparations have more rapid onset of action than other nonparenterally administered opioids. Fentanyl is usually not recommended for initial therapy in opioid-naïve patients.

---

**Box 2**
**Classification of opioids based on chemical structure**

*Phenanthrenes, morphine-like*
Morphine
Codeine
Hydromorphone
Hydrocodone
Levorphanol
Oxycodone
Oxymorphone
Buprenorphine
Nalbuphine
Butorphanol

*Phenylpiperidines, meperidine-like*
Fentanyl
Alfentanil
Sufentanil
Meperidine

*Diphenylheptanes, methadone-like*
Propoxyphene
Methadone

---

In addition to μ-receptor agonism, some opioids exhibit additional analgesic mechanisms. Methadone is suggested to exhibit N-methyl-D-aspartate (NMDA) receptor antagonistic activity. NMDA, an excitatory amino acid, is implicated in neuropathic pain and opioid tolerance,[58] which may account for methadone's beneficial effects in neuropathic and cancer pain, and the lower need for opioid escalation.[59,60] Although, mainly used as a second-line strong opioid, increasing preliminary evidence supports its use as first-line agent for pain management.[61–63] Tramadol, a synthetic analog structurally related to codeine and morphine, inhibits norepinephrine and serotonin uptake.[64] Tapentadol also exhibits norepinephrine reuptake,[65] and is approved in the United States as a short-acting opioid for moderate to severe pain.

---

**Table 1**
**Classification of opioids based on actions at the opioid receptor**

| Group | Actions at Opioid Receptor | | Example of Opioids |
|---|---|---|---|
| | μ | Other | |
| Pure agonists | High Affinity High efficacy | — | Morphine, codeine, hydromorphone, hydrocodone, oxycodone, oxymorphone, fentanyl, and methadone |
| Partial agonists | High affinity Low efficacy | k-Antagonism | Buprenorphine |
| Partial agonist/ antagonists | High affinity Low efficacy | k-Agonist activity | Nalorphine, pentazocine, nalbuphine, and butorphanol |

**Opioid metabolism** Knowledge of opioid metabolism helps in initial opioid selection and making dose adjustments in terminally ill patients, many of whom are elderly and have increased likelihood of impaired organ functions. Most opioids undergo biotransformation in the liver and are primarily eliminated by kidneys as a mixture of the parent opioid and their metabolites.[42] Accumulation of active metabolites with analgesic or neurotoxic effects can result in significant opioid toxicity. For instance, 55% to 65% of morphine is metabolized to morphine-3-gluconate (M3G), which is neuroexcitatory, and 10% to 15% is converted to morphine-6-gluconate (M6G), which is significantly more potent than morphine. Hydromorphone-3-gluconate (H3G) is the main hydromorphone metabolite, and is also shown to have neurotoxic effects. Hydrocodone and codeine are metabolized by CYP2D6 to hydromorphone and morphine, respectively, which account for their analgesic benefits. Patients who are poor or ultrarapid metabolizers (10% each among Caucasians) may have minimal or amplified analgesic and toxic effects, respectively.

Meperidine is not recommended for chronic use because of its highly neurotoxic metabolite that has a prolonged half-life. Its accumulation may result in sedation, irritability, seizures, and myoclonus, which can be worse in patients with renal dysfunction. Fentanyl is mostly metabolized to norfentanyl and other minor metabolites, which are not active. However, cases of fentanyl-associated neurotoxicities have been reported.[66,67]

Methadone is highly lipophilic, with excellent oral bioavailability ($\sim$80%). Unlike other opioids, methadone does not have significant active metabolites, is mainly excreted via the gastrointestinal tract, and does not require dose adjustments in renal failure. However, its variable and unpredictable half-life can make it a difficult drug to manage by inexperienced clinicians. After oral administration it is rapidly absorbed and subject to extensive tissue distribution, from where it is slowly released. The half-life of the initial distribution phase is short ($\sim$2–3 hours), but the elimination phase β–half-life varies from 15 to 60 hours. This long half-life, however, does not match the observed analgesic duration ($\sim$6–12 hours) after steady state is reached, and therefore frequent doses (2–4 times per day) are usually required for pain management. Accumulation can result in prolonged sedation, or pain fluctuations may be difficult to manage with use of methadone alone. Methadone can also prolong the QT interval, and caution is required, especially when used concomitantly with other drugs known to cause the same.

**Physiologic and psychological responses to opioid use** Tolerance and physical dependence are expected physiologic responses to chronic opioid use. Tolerance is characterized by decreasing opioid analgesic effects, requiring increased opioid doses to achieve the same degree of pain relief. In terminally ill patients, knowing whether development of tolerance, disease progression, or both, is contributing to higher opioid requirement may not be possible. Tolerance also develops to several opioid side effects, including nausea and respiratory depression, but not to constipation. Physical dependence manifests as development of withdrawal symptoms on abrupt opioid cessation, such as increased pain, agitation, insomnia, diarrhea, sweating, and palpitations. Physical dependence is frequently and incorrectly considered addiction. Withdrawal symptoms can be prevented by gradually tapering opioids.

In contrast to the above physiologic responses, addiction and pseudoaddiction are psychological and behavioral responses toward opioids that patients may or may not develop. Addiction is compulsive use of drugs for nonmedical reasons, characterized by a craving for mood-altering drug effects, not pain relief. Suggestive aberrant behaviors include forgery of prescriptions, denial of drug use, stealing opioids from others, selling/buying opioids on the street, and using prescribed drugs to get "high." Addiction is uncommon in the chronic pain, postoperative, and cancer pain settings,[68–70] and opioids should not be withheld for fear that a patient will become addicted. When terminally ill patients request a strong analgesic, they probably have inadequate pain control. Pseudoaddiction is an "iatrogenic" phenomenon resulting from inadequate pain management by clinicians. Patient's behavior is geared toward obtaining pain relief, such as requesting stronger pain medications, asking several providers for opioids, and frequently visiting the emergency center for pain relief. The clinician response should always be to reassess the pain, reassure the patient, and treat pain adequately.

**Opioid side effects** All opioids have the potential for side effects, which may compel some patients to decrease or discontinue opioid use. Most common side effects include constipation, nausea, and sedation, whereas dose-limiting side effects typically involve the central nervous system. Greater compliance is likely if clinicians educate patients and family about anticipated side effects and how these may be managed. Side effects may be limited through using appropriate opioid doses, coadministration of adjuvant analgesics if indicated, and using medications to prevent or manage expected side effects (**Table 2**).

**Opioid-mediated gastrointestinal side effects** Constipation, the most common side effect, should be anticipated, monitored, and addressed throughout opioid therapy. Ideally, all patients treated with opioids should take laxatives unless contraindicated for the clinical setting, and these should be titrated to effect. Bowel stimulants such as senna, with or without a stool softener, are most commonly used. Other laxatives in combination and enemas may be indicated (see **Table 2**). Bulk-forming laxatives should be avoided in patients unable to maintain adequate fluid intake. Nausea and vomiting are prevalent in approximately 25% of patients treated with opioids.[71] In most, tolerance to nausea develops in a few days. Persistent nausea should trigger a search for coexisting contributors (eg, constipation, hypercalcemia). Dopamine antagonists such as metoclopromide and haloperidol are useful in management. Occasionally opioids may need to be switched. Transdermal fentanyl may have fewer constipating effects than other opioids.[72,73] Peripherally acting opioid antagonists such as methylnaltrexone may be considered for refractory constipation. **Table 3** provides a list of analgesics at doses, both oral and parenteral, that are approximately equal to each other in analgesic efficacy, and provides a conversion factor when switching opioids or the route of administration. **Box 3** provides a step-by-step guide for opioid rotation.

**Opioid-induced central nervous system side effects** Sedation is common after opioid initiation or significant increase in the opioid dose, and usually resolves after few days. Providing reassurance to the patient and family is usually sufficient. However, in the presence of comorbidities, such as dementia, metabolic encephalopathy, or brain metastases, or if the patient is taking other sedating medications, sedation is more likely to persist. Management should involve treatment of reversible causes of sedation and discontinuation of other sedating medications. If pain is well controlled, the opioid dose may be reduced. Opioid rotation and the addition of a psychostimulant may be appropriate if sedation is refractory.

Opioid-induced neurotoxicity (OIN) includes a constellation of neuropsychiatric symptoms, such as excessive sedation, cognitive impairment, delirium, hallucinations, myoclonus, and opioid-induced hyperalgesia (OIH).[58,74,75] OIH should be suspected when pain increases despite opioid escalation and in the presence of all-over pain

**Table 2**
**Prevention and management of common opioid side effects**

| Side Effect | Prevention | Management |
|---|---|---|
| Opioid-induced neurotoxicity | Consider stopping nonessential CNS-activating or -depressing drugs (eg, benzodiazepines)<br>Maintain adequate hydration | Consider reversible causes such as liver or renal dysfunction, dehydration, hypercalcemia, and organic brain disease; treat as appropriate for the clinical circumstance<br>Consider one or more of the following:<br>Opioid rotation (**Box 3**) or dose reduction<br>Stop other offending drugs (eg, benzodiazepines)<br>Hydration<br>Symptomatic treatment with haloperidol, 1–5 mg PO, IV/SC, or SC every 4 h PRN |
| Respiratory depression | Monitor sedation and respiratory status during the first 24 hours in opioid naive patients<br>Titrate opioids cautiously<br>Consider does reduction or opioid rotation if patient has excessive sedation | Stop the opioid, provide supplemental oxygen<br>If patient minimally responsive or unresponsive and respiratory rate ≤6, administer naloxone<br>Naloxone, 0.4 mg, diluted in 10 mL saline, 0.5 mL IV push, repeat 1–2 min until patient more awake and respiratory status improves<br>If no change with naloxone, rule out other causes for the respiratory depression<br>If patient is actively dying and receiving comfort care, it may not be appropriate to administer naloxone |
| Constipation | Unless contraindicated, start laxative regimen in all and titrate to effect<br>Stimulant laxatives (eg, Senna)<br>Fluids, dietary fiber, and exercise if feasible<br>Prune juice followed by warm beverage may be considered | Increase dose of laxative<br>May add one or more of following<br>Milk of magnesia, polyethylene glycol, lactulose<br>Consider digital rectal examination to rule out low impaction<br>If impacted, disimpact manually if stool is soft<br>May need to soften stool with mineral oil fleets enema before disimpaction<br>Follow-up with milk of molasses or fleets enemas<br>Consider use of rescue analgesics before disimpaction<br>Methylnatrexone SC injections |
| Nausea, vomiting | Make antiemetics available with opioid prescription (eg, metoclopramide)<br>For patients at high risk for nausea consider around-the-clock regimen for 5–7 d and then change PRN | Investigate for other causes of nausea (eg, constipation, bowel obstruction, chemotherapy or other medications) and treat per guideline<br>Initiate antiemetic regimen (eg, metoclopramide 5–10 mg PO, IV, or SC every 6 h)<br>Add or increase nonopioid or adjuvant medications for additional pain relief so that opioid dose can be reduced<br>If analgesia is satisfactory, reduce opioid dose by 25%<br>Consider opioid rotation if nausea remains refractory |

*Abbreviations:* CNS, central nervous system; IV, intravenous; PO, oral; PRN, as needed; SC, subcutaneous.

**Table 3**
**Initial equianalgesic conversion ratio**

| Opioid | Oral Dose | Parenteral (IV/SC) Dose | Conversion Factor for Changing Parenteral Opioid to Oral Opioid | Conversion factor for Changing Oral Opioid to Oral Morphine |
|---|---|---|---|---|
| Morphine | 15 mg | 6 mg | 2.5 | 1 |
| Oxycodone | 10 mg | Not applicable | Not applicable | 1.5 |
| Oxymorphone | 5 mg | 0.5 mg | 10 | 3 |
| Hydromorphone | 3 mg | 1.5 mg | 2 | 5 |

*Abbreviations:* IV, intravenous; SC, subcutaneous.

and increased sensitivity to touch. Mechanisms involved include increased excitatory nonanalgesic opioid metabolites and NMDA activation.[76,77] Terminally ill patients may already have high prevalence of cognitive decline because of their disease, use of psychoactive medication, dehydration, or renal and metabolic impairments, all of which are associated with a greater risk for opioid-induced delirium (**Fig. 4**).

OIN is frequently managed with opioid rotation, hydration, and symptomatic medications directed toward controlling patient distress (see **Table 2**). Haloperidol is considered first-line therapy for patients who have agitated delirium, because of its efficacy and low incidence of cardiovascular and anticholinergic side effects. Chlorpromazine can be used if sedation is required, although hypotension may be a concern. Benzodiazepines are best reserved for refractory situations, because in some patients it may paradoxically worsen delirium. Switching opioids and providing hydration allow the parent opioid and its toxic metabolites to be excreted.

**Respiratory depression** Although respiratory depression is potentially the most serious of opioid side effects, tolerance usually develops within days of opioid use.

**Box 3**
**Steps for opioid rotation**

Step 1: Calculate total 24-hour oral dose of current opioid (scheduled and breakthrough opioids). If patient is using parenteral opioids, convert from parenteral to oral opioid (see Table 3).

Step 2: Convert total 24-hour dose of current opioid (from step 1) to equianalgesic dose of oral morphine (morphine equivalent daily dose [MEDD]) using conversion factor for changing from oral opioid to oral morphine (see Table 3).

Step 3: Convert the calculated 24-hour oral MEDD (from step 2) to the 24-hour equianalgesic dose of the new opioid being considered.

Step 4: Adjust for lack of complete cross-tolerance between opioids. Usually decreasing the calculated dose of the new opioid (from step 3) by 25% to 50% is most appropriate.

Step 5: Divide the 24-hour dose of the final new opioid dose (from step 4) by the number of doses to be given over 24 hours and administer it as scheduled doses (usually every 12 or 8 hours around the clock). Calculate breakthrough opioid dose as 10% to 15% of the final calculated new opioid dose to administer as needed every 2 to 4 hours.

Step 6: Carefully titrate new opioid regimen until adequate analgesia is achieved.

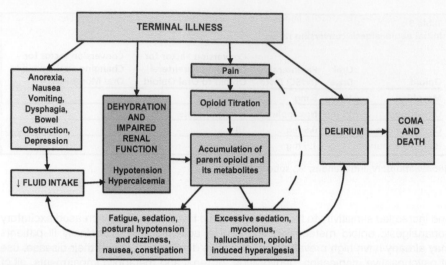

**Fig. 4.** Potential contributors to delirium and opioid-induced neurotoxicity in terminally ill patients.

This side effect is extremely rare in patients on chronic opioids. When respiratory compromise does occur, an alternative explanation is usually present, such as pneumonia or the use of benzodiazepines. Close monitoring in high-risk patients is advised. Because of the risk of opioid withdrawal, naloxone should only be used in impending or symptomatic respiratory depression (<8 breaths per minute), and in diluted doses (see **Table 2**).

**True versus pseudoallergy to opioids** Patients may report being "allergic" to opioids, and it is important to distinguish between "true" immune-mediated reactions (rare) and reactions that mimic an immune allergic response (nonallergic or pseudoallergy).

Pruritus, occurring in 2% to 10% of patients treated with opioids, is not an immune-mediated reaction. It is usually mild and self-limited, and can be treated with antihistaminics. The likely mechanism involves direct mast cell degranulation with histamine release, causing local itching and a typical weal and flare response. Although all opioids may cause direct histamine release, morphine, codeine, and meperidine are more potent offenders than others. If pruritis is severe, switching to an alternate opioid with lower potency of histamine release could be considered. Histamine release also may be associated with vasodilation, which is more common in volume-depleted patients. This reaction is not a contraindication to opioid use, and an alternative opioid may be well tolerated. Neuroaxially administered opioids, especially morphine, have higher pruritis risk, and do not seem to be mediated by histamine, but rather by µ-opioid receptors.[78] µ-Receptor antagonists therefore are more effective, whereas histamine antagonists do not usually help.

Unlike histamine-mediated nonallergic reactions, type 1 hypersensitivity reactions are IgE-mediated, resulting in the immediate systemic release of potent mediators and causing hypotension, bronchospasm, angiodemia, hives, and vascular collapse. These events are managed emergently with epinephrine, steroids, and histamine blockers, but fortunately are extremely rare. Patients who have had prior IgE-mediated allergic reactions should not be rechallenged with the offending opioid. For both of these immune-mediated reactions, an allergist may be consulted to identify appropriate alternatives. Opioids from an alternative chemical class may also be considered.

**Decision pathway for opioid therapy to manage pain in terminally ill patients** General treatment recommendations involve selecting the right opioid at the right dose, frequency, and route, and the prevention and treatment of opioid side effects. Careful opioid titrations with close monitoring of outcomes (eg, pain relief, side effects, physical and psychosocial functioning) is required to achieve an individualized analgesic response. The decision pathway algorithm for opioid therapy is illustrated in **Fig. 5**, and is discussed further later. The initial phase of opioid therapy depends on patient reports of pain, goals for pain relief, and whether the patient is currently on opioids or not.

In opioid naïve patients, treatment may begin with immediate-release opioids on an as needed (PRN) basis every 2 to 4 hours. Recommended initial opioid doses are shown in **Table 4**. If pain persists or requires frequent dosing, an extended-release opioid could be administered on a fixed schedule. Additional immediate-release opioids PRN should be allowed for breakthrough pain. Fentanyl patches are usually not recommended for opioid-naïve patients.

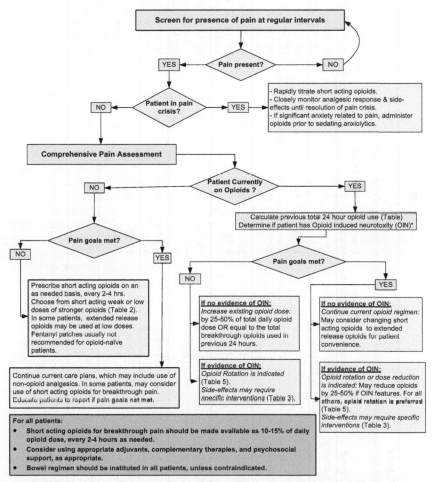

**Fig. 5.** Decision pathway for using opioids for pain management in terminally ill patients.

**Table 4**
Initial starting doses of commonly used opioids in opioid-naïve patients

| Opioid | Initial "Rescue" Dose in Opioid-Naïve Patients | Onset (min) | Peak Effect (h) | Duration (h) | Available Oral and Rectal[a] Formulations | Available Routes |
|---|---|---|---|---|---|---|
| Tramadol | PO: 25–50 mg<br>IV/SC: N/A | 30–60<br>— | 1.5 | 3–7 | IR: 50 mg (alone or with APAP)<br>ER: 100, 200, 300 mg | PO |
| Hydrocodone | PO: 5–10 mg<br>IV/SC: N/A | 10–20<br>— | 1–3 | 4–8 | IR: 5, 7.5, 10 mg; 2.5 mg/5 mL (all with APAP)<br>ER: N/A | PO |
| Codeine | PO: 30–60 mg<br>IV/SC: N/A | 30–60<br>— | 1–1.5 | 4–8 | IR: 15, 30, 60 mg (alone or with APAP)<br>ER: N/A | PO |
| Morphine | PO: 5–10 mg<br>IV/SC: 2–3 mg | 30<br>5–10 | 0.5–1 | 3–6 | IR: 15, 30 mg; 10 mg/5 mL, 20 mg/5 mL, 20 mg/mL<br>ER: 15, 30, 60, 100 mg<br>Rectal: 5, 10, 20 mg | PO<br>IV/SC<br>PR |
| Oxycodone | PO: 2.5–7.5 mg<br>IV/SC: N/A | 10–15<br>— | 0.5–1 | 3–6 | IR: 5, 15, 30 mg (5-mg dose with APAP);<br>5 mg/5 mL, 20 mg/mL<br>ER: 10, 20, 40, 80 mg | PO |
| Oxymorphone | PO: 5–10 mg<br>IV/SC: 0.5 mg | No data<br>5–10 | 0.5–1 | 3–6 | IR: 5, 10 mg tablet<br>ER: 5, 10, 20, 40 mg | PO, IV/SC |
| Hydromorphone | PO: 1–2 mg<br>IV/SC: 0.3–1 mg | 15–30<br>15–30 | 0.5–1 | 3–5<br>4–5 | IR: 2, 4, 8 mg tablet; 1 mg/mL liquid<br>ER: N/A<br>Rectal: 3 mg | PO, IV/SC<br>PR |
| Tapentadol | PO: 50–100 mg<br>IV/SC: N/A | <60<br>— | 1.25–1.5 | 4–6 | IR: 50, 75, 100 mg<br>ER: N/A | PO |

*Abbreviations:* APAP, acetaminophen; ER, extended-release; IR, immediate-release; IV, intravenous; N/A, not applicable; PO, oral; PR, per rectum; SC, subcutaneous.
[a] Rectal formulations, if available.

For patients already on opioids, whether any evidence of OIN exists is important to determine before increasing the dose. The 24-hour opioid dose should be calculated, including opioids used PRN for breakthrough pain.

If no evidence exists of OIN and pain is not adequately controlled, the dose of the scheduled opioid may be increased by 25% to 50%, or by an amount equal to the breakthrough opioids used in the previous 24 hours. The breakthrough opioid dose should be recalculated as 10% to 15% of the new scheduled dose, and prescribed every 2 to 4 hours as needed. For example, if a patient is taking 100 mg of extended-release morphine twice daily, and used six to seven 15-mg doses of immediate-release morphine for breakthrough pain in the past 24 hours, the scheduled morphine dose may be increased approximately by breakthrough opioid dose (90–105 mg). Therefore, extended-release morphine may be prescribed at 100 mg every 8 hours. The breakthrough opioid dose would be approximately 30 to 45 mg of immediate-release morphine PRN. Patients who are taking five to six acetaminophen/hydrocodone combination (or tramadol) tablets daily are not opioid-naive, and can be started on extended-release opioids equivalent to approximately 30 mg of morphine per day.

If pain is adequately controlled and the patient is not experiencing OIN, the medications need not be changed. Short-acting opioids may be converted to extended-release products for patient convenience. In addition, all patients should be prescribed short-acting opioids PRN for breakthrough pain episodes (usually 10%–15% of the 24-hour daily opioid dose).

If the patient has evidence of OIN, opioids should be changed (rotated) or reduced, and the OIN side effects should be treated. If the patient has good pain control and OIN features are mild (mild sedation or myoclonus), the dose of opioids may be reduced by 25% to 50%. In all other situations, opioid rotation is recommended (see **Box 3** and **Table 3**).

**Management of pain crisis** Although no standard definition of a pain crisis exists, it may be defined as severe uncontrolled pain, either of acute onset or exacerbation of chronic pain that is accompanied by significant distress for the patient or family.[79] A pain crisis requires an emergent response by the medical team. The treatment plan should begin with a thorough clinic assessment, as with any other medical emergency, with rapid titration of short-acting opioids and close monitoring of outcomes. Direct monitoring and supervision by the medical team is recommended until the crisis resolves. If the patient has significant anxiety, a trial of opioids is preferred before administration of any sedating medications, such as benzodiazepines. Short-acting opioids are preferably administered intravenously subcutaneously. Transmucosal fentanyl can be given in patients who are not opioid-naïve. Sublingual delivery of other opioids may be beneficial, but has not been formally tested.

**Opioid rotation and use of initial equianalgesic opioid conversion ratios** When switching opioids, or the route of administration, equianalgesic tables help in selecting the initial dose safely. **Table 3** shows comparative values for commonly used opioids. These values are approximate,[46] and the new opioid should be further titrated to patient response. Steps for opioid rotation are shown in **Box 3**. Because morphine is used as the standard for opioids, the initial step involves converting the current daily opioid dose to oral MEDD, and using equianalgesic tables to calculate the new opioid dose, which is then reduced by 25% to 50% for incomplete cross-tolerance between opioids.

**Morphine to methadone rotation** The morphine to methadone conversion ratio is based on the preswitch morphine dose range (**Table 5**). When the preswitch MEDD is higher than 100 mg, the switch to methadone should ideally be performed over several

**Table 5**
**Recommended initial morphine to methadone conversion ratios and methadone rotation schedule**

| Oral Morphine Equivalent Daily Dose (MEDD) | Conversion Ratio[a] |
|---|---|
| <100 mg | 3:1 |
| >100–300 mg | 5:1 |
| >300–600 mg | 10:1 |
| >600–800 mg | 12:1 |
| >800–1000 mg | 15:1 |
| >1000 mg | 20:1 |

[a] Dose of methadone is calculated by dividing the MEDD by the conversion ration. This dose should be decreased by 25% to 50% to accommodate for lack of incomplete tolerance.

days.[80] A 3-day phased rotation schedule is shown in **Box 4**. Longer schedules may also be used. Careful monitoring of side effects should continue for several days after successful rotation because of the possibility of late toxicity from methadone accumulation. Methadone to morphine rotation has received limited study, but is not bidirectional.

**Routes for opioid administration** Available routes for opioid administration, except for neuraxial administration, are described in the following sections.

**Oral route** The oral route is the least-invasive route and is generally preferred because of convenience, patient autonomy, and cost. For most short-acting opioids, time to onset and peak effects are 20 to 30 minutes and 60 minutes, respectively. Most oral opioids are also available as extended-release and liquid formulations (see **Table 4**).

**Enteral route** Liquid oral formulation of opioids can be administered through feeding tubes. For patients requiring a long-acting opioid, methadone or extended-release morphine in polymeric bead form (Kadian) may be used.

**Transdermal route** Fentanyl transdermal patch is an alternative noninvasive route for opioid delivery. The transdermal delivery system consists of a reservoir of fentanyl that provides continuous drug infusion for up to 72 hours. On initial application or dose change, a lag time occurs (12–16 hours) until steady-state drug levels are reached. The half-life of fentanyl after patch removal is approximately 14 to 24 hours. Therefore, fentanyl patches are not suitable for patients in pain crisis, requiring rapid titration of opioids, or who have fluctuating needs. The bioavailability of transdermal fentanyl

**Box 4**
**Recommended steps for a 3-day phased conversion from morphine to methadone**

Calculate methadone dose from **Table 5** and decrease by 25% to 50% for lack of incomplete tolerance. If the preswitch oral morphine dose is 700 mg, the calculated methadone dose will be approximately 30 mg/d (after a 50% reduction).

Day 1: Administer two-thirds of the preswitch morphine (~460 mg) and one-third of the planned methadone dose (10 or 5 mg twice daily).

Day 2: Administer one-third of the preswitch morphine dose (~230 mg) and two-thirds of the planned methadone dose (10 mg every 12 hours).

Day 3: Stop morphine. Administer all of the planned methadone dose (10 mg every 8 hours).

varies from 60% to 90%. Side effects of patches are usually mild and transient skin irritations, and rotation of skin sites is recommended.

**Parenteral routes** Intravenous or subcutaneous routes are options when rapid onset of analgesia is desired, or when less-invasive routes are not feasible. Intravenous and subcutaneous routes can be used to provide continuous opioid infusions, usually in conjunction with patient-controlled analgesia device. The major drawbacks of the intravenous route are the needs for continuous intravenous access, frequent maintenance, and nursing support, and limitations in patient mobility. The advantages of the subcutaneous route include its simplicity and lack of requirement for vascular access, with its associated risk for complications. A small 25- to 27-gauge butterfly needle is placed in an area on the chest, abdomen, or thigh, and is connected by tubing to the infusion pump. The injection site is changed weekly or as needed. Infusion rates of 2 to 4 mL/h have been found to be satisfactory without causing pain at the infusion site. To minimize the volume of fluid to be injected, concentrated opioid solutions should be used. Intramuscular injections should not be used in terminally ill patients because of the pain associated with injections, unreliable absorption, and relatively long interval to peak drug concentrations.

**Transmucosal/sublingual routes** Fentanyl is available as a solid sweetened lozenge and as a buccal tablet, which can provide rapid-onset analgesia. Bioavailability is variable, depending on the amounts absorbed through oral mucosa, or swallowed and absorbed through the gastrointestinal mucosa. In general, 15 minutes of lozenge use rapidly delivers one-fourth of the total dose into the systemic circulation through oral absorption, and the remaining undergoes first-pass metabolism after absorption from the gastrointestinal tract, with overall bioavailability of approximately 50%. The sublingual administration of other opioids, given in concentrated liquid formulations, is often used in patients who are too sick, unable to swallow, or lacking parenteral access. However, absorption and bioavailability are considered low, and dose should be individually titrated until adequate analgesia is achieved. In general, methadone (more lipophilic) is better absorbed than morphine (33% vs 22%, respectively).

**Rectal routes** The rectal route may be used if acceptable to the patient and family, if opioid doses are low to moderate, and patients do not have anal fissures or inflamed hemorrhoids. Rectal suppositories are available for some opioids (see **Table 4**), although most opioid extended- and immediate-release oral formulations are also readily absorbed rectally. The initial recommended rectal dose is the same as the oral route but should be individually titrated because absorption is highly variable.

**Adjuvant analgesics and common pain syndromes in terminally ill patients** Some pain syndromes may benefit from the use of adjuvant analgesics (**Table 6**). The decision to start any one or more of these agents should take into consideration the patient's pain syndrome, overall clinical condition, side effects of the adjuvant, drug interactions, availability, and costs. To reduce the risk of additive toxicity, it is best to initiate treatment with one drug at a time, with frequent monitoring of outcomes.

**Neuropathic pain** Neuropathic pain syndromes may include tumor-induced nerve or spinal cord compression, chronic back pain with radiculopathy, postherpetic neuralgia, or neuropathy secondary to diabetes or chemotherapy. Corticosteroids are indicated in patients with painful radiculopathies or spinal cord compression. Other additional therapies depend on the goals of care. For instance, spinal cord compression is a medical emergency in most instances, requiring emergent diagnostics and further treatment to reverse or prevent neurologic impairments. However,

**Table 6**
Adjuvant analgesics commonly used for neuropathic pain syndromes and chronic pain

| Drug Class and Uses | Medication | | Recommended Starting Dose | Usual Effective Dose | Comments |
|---|---|---|---|---|---|
| Anticonvulsants (various NP types) | Gabapentin | | 100–300 mg qd | 300–1200 mg in 2 or 3 divided doses | May cause drowsiness, dizziness, or peripheral edema Dose-adjust for renal impairment |
| | Pregabalin | | 25–75 mg bid | 75–200 mg in 3 divided doses | Carbamazepine has been associated with aplastic anemia, agranulocytosis, bone marrow suppression, severe dermatologic reactions, and hyponatremia Topiramate may cause acidosis, drowsiness, dizziness, or nausea Tiagabine may cause seizures |
| | Carbamazepine | | 100 mg bid | 300–800 mg bid | |
| | Oxcarbazepine | | 150–300 mg qd | 150–600 mg bid | |
| | Topiramate | | 25–50 mg bid | 50–200 mg bid | |
| | Tiagabine | | 4 mg at bedtime | 4–12 mg bid | |
| Antidepressants (NP, FM, chronic pain) | TCAs | Amitriptyline | 10–25 mg at bedtime | 50–150 mg at bedtime | Caution should be used in elderly and frail patients and those with glaucoma or arrhythmias |
| | | Nortriptyline | 10–25 mg at bedtime | 50–150 mg at bedtime | May cause sedation, arrhythmias, dry mouth orthostasis, or urinary retention |
| | | Desipramine | 10–25 mg at bedtime | 50–150 mg at bedtime | Caution should be used in patients with seizures; MAOIs and other SSRIs or SNRIs should be avoided because of potential for serotonin syndrome |
| | SSRIs | Citalopram | 20 mg qd | — | |
| | | Fluoxetine | 10–20 mg qd | — | |
| | | Paroxetine | 10–20 mg qd | — | |
| | SNRIs | Duloxetine | 20–30 mg qd | 60 mg qd | |
| | | Venlafaxine | 37.5 mg qd | 150–300 mg qd | |
| Muscle relaxants (muscle pain, spasm) | Baclofen | | 5 mg bid | 10–20 mg bid or tid | Caution should be used in patients with seizures, cardiovascular disease, glaucoma, myasthenia gravis, or renal or hepatic impairment; patients taking tricyclic antidepressants or MAOIs and elderly patients |
| | Cyclobenzaprine | | 5 mg tid | 10–20 mg tid | |
| | Metaxalone | | 400 mg tid | 800 mg tid or qid | |
| | Methocarbamol | | 500 mg qid | 500–750 mg qid | |
| | Tizanidine | | 2–4 mg at bedtime | 4–8 mg bid or tid | May cause anticholinergic effects and significant drowsiness |
| Corticosteroids (inflammation, nerve compression) | Dexamethasone | | 1–2 mg | Not defined | May cause impaired healing, infection, thrush, hyperglycemia, weight gain, myopathy, stomach upset, psychosis, or emotional instability |

*Abbreviations:* DN, diabetic neuropathy; FM, fibromyalgia; MAOI, monoamine oxidase inhibitors; NP, neuropathic pain; PHN, postherpetic neuralgia; SSRIs, selective serotonin reuptake inhibitors; SNRIs, serotonin-norepinephrine reuptake inhibitors; TCAs, tricyclic antidepressants; TGN, trigeminal neuralgia.

patients with life expectancy limited to less than several days to weeks, and when goals of care are comfort-oriented, steroids and opioids for pain may be considered exclusively. Specific anticonvulsants and antidepressants may be added PRN if pain remains uncontrolled.

For most other neuropathic pain syndromes, specific anticonvulsants or antidepressants may be considered. Gabapentin, the most commonly used anticonvulsant, has been well established in painful diabetic neuropathy and postherpetic neuralgia,[81,82] and is also widely used to treat cancer-related neuropathic pain.[83] In terminally ill patients, potential side effects and impact on renal function should be considered before starting this agent. The most common side effects of gabapentin are sedation, dizziness, unsteadiness, confusion, and nausea, especially when rapidly titrated. The usual starting dose is 100 to 300 mg at bedtime, which can be increased every 3 to 7 days, with close monitoring for side effects. Slower titrations may be prudent in terminally ill patients.

Pregabalin is a newer agent, and is reported to have greater potency and pharmacokinetic superiority but similar side effect profile to gabapentin. Pregabalin is also approved for the treatment of fibromyalgia. Other anticonvulsants (see **Table 6**) may be considered as alternatives to gabapentin. Parenteral administration of lidocaine and ketamine is not generally recommended in terminally ill patients, and should only be considered by experienced clinicians.

Select antidepressants, such as amitriptyline, desipramine (tricyclic drugs), or duloxetine (a serotonin-norepinephrine reuptake inhibitor), may be considered in patients with comorbid depression or whose past experience precludes the use of anticonvulsants.

NMDA receptors play a major role in chronic pain states through its participation in the induction and maintenance of central neuronal hyperexcitability.[84] Commercially available NMDA-receptor antagonists include ketamine, dextromethorphan, memantine, and amantadine. Although considered to have analgesic efficacy, these agents are associated with significant dose-limiting central side effects, such as auditory and visual hallucinations, feelings of unreality and detachment, dizziness, and sedation. A Cochrane systematic review[85] concluded that evidence was insufficient to make recommendations for the use of ketamine. Only two trials (N = 30) were eligible for this review.[85] Methadone has been proposed to have NMDA-receptor antagonistic activity, and may be useful for managing patients with neuropathic pain.

**Tumor-related bone pain** Patients with primary or metastatic bone tumors may benefit from addition of anti-inflammatory agents (NSAIDs or corticosteroids) and osteoclast inhibitors (bisphosphonates). The risk/benefit ratio of these agents should be individualized.

In patients with metastatic bone disease, bisphosphonates have shown to reduce the number of skeletal-related events.[86] Typically, opioids are simultaneously initiated because bisphosphonates have a delayed and variable efficacy in relieving pain.[87] Although generally well tolerated, bisphosphonates may be associated with a characteristic transient acute-phase response (fever, chills, bone pain, myalgias, and arthralgias), epigastric pain and esophagitis with oral agents,[88] and renal dysfunction with zoledronic acid and pamidronate,[80] which have not yet been observed with intravenous ibandronate. Osteonecrosis of the jaw has been increasingly described with the use of some bisphosphonates, with length of exposure, active dental disease, or recent dental procedures as significant risk factors.[90,91]

**Bowel obstruction** The management of bowel obstruction will depend on the cause, overall clinical setting, and goals of care. Symptoms of bowel obstruction secondary to malignancies can be managed with a combination approach, using agents that minimize bowel secretion and motility, such as anticholinergics (eg, scopolamine and hyoscyamine); octreotide; and opioids for pain. Corticosteroids may be used to decrease tumor-related inflammation and obstruction, especially if surgery is not appropriate.[92] Except in the very advanced setting, gastrointestinal drainage procedures, such as venting gastrostomies, may be considered.

**Role of cannabinoids in pain management** Cannabinoids refer to a group of more than 60 chemically active compounds present in the cannabis plant. The most prevalent and pharmacologically active compound is delta-9-tetrahydrocannabinol (THC), which has been suggested to have analgesic, orexigenic, and antiemetic properties. Dronabinol and nabilone are synthetic THC derivatives, and are approved in the United States for chemotherapy-associated nausea and appetite stimulation in HIV-related cachexia (dronabinol). Although cannabinoids have shown efficacy in several experimental models of inflammatory, neuropathic, and cancer pain,[93–95] their analgesic application in humans is uncertain. A systematic review of nine randomized controlled trials conducted before 1999 found cannabinoids to be no more effective than codeine, and were associated with significant central nervous system side effects.[96] Later trials of smoked cannabis,[97] dronabinol,[98] and nabilone[99] were also disappointing because of the predominance of side effects or unclear benefit in treating pain.

In Canada, a combination THC/cannabidiol oromucosal spray is approved as an adjunctive treatment for neuropathic pain in multiple sclerosis and moderate to severe pain in advanced cancer. Each spray contains 2.7 mg of THC and 2.5 mg of cannabidiol. Approval was primarily based on a randomized, double-blind, placebo-controlled trial in 66 patients with multiple sclerosis and central neuropathic pain.[100] However, compared with placebo, more patients in the cannabis-based group experienced dizziness, dry mouth, and somnolence.

## COMPLEMENTARY THERAPIES FOR PAIN MANAGEMENT

The combination of complementary modalities with mainstream conventional therapies is the practice of "integrative medicine." Integrative medicine programs have increased in United States cancer centers, and offer a range of services. Various nonpharmacologic therapies, including massage, transcutaneous electrical nerve stimulation, acupuncture, application of heat and cold, music therapy, cognitive interventions, and physical therapy, and rehabilitation, have been shown to be effective in alleviating pain for patients with advanced illness when used in conjunction with pharmacologic measures. The decision to try any of these approaches alone or in combination should consider a patient's overall physical condition and ability to work with a therapist, the source and severity of pain, safety, and availability and cost of the intervention.

In 2004, Tilden and colleagues,[101] through telephone interviews of 423 randomly selected caregivers of recently deceased patients, found that most (54%) patients had used complementary and alternative medicine therapies at the end of life. Massage was the most commonly used therapy (57%), followed by relaxation techniques (20%) and acupuncture (7%). A significant proportion of hospices offered a wide range of complementary therapies, with massage therapy also found to be most commonly used by patients at the end of life.[102,103]

## REASSESSMENT OF PAIN

Frequent reassessment of the patient's pain and related outcomes is crucial and considered the most important aspect of pain management. Depending on these assessments, opioids are titrated to maintain a favorable balance between efficacy and side effects. Examples of efficacy in pain management include decreases in pain intensity, achievement of pain relief goals, and improvements in physical and psychosocial functioning. These outcomes should not be at the expense of major opioid-induced side effects. A systematic approach that screens for common gastrointestinal and central nervous system side effects is recommended. If present, these should be treated appropriately based on the clinical circumstance. Asking patients if they are "satisfied" with their pain management is not useful, because studies show that patients sometimes have low expectations for pain control.[104] Assessment of patient compliance with changes in dosing and duration of opioid medications is essential. Noncompliance to opioids may be related to fears about addiction or avoidance of opioid side effects. Ongoing education may be necessary.

At some point, patients may have their pain satisfactorily controlled, so that their daily opioid doses remain relatively stable. Worsening pain after a period of stable opioid use may indicate disease progression, increased activity level, development of psychosocial stressors, tolerance, or development of hyperalgesia. Additional evaluation may be indicated to determine the cause. Furthermore, patients may experience unmanageable opioid-related side effects, warranting a decrease in opioid dosing (if pain is well controlled) or rotation to an alternative opioid. Consultation with pain and palliative care specialists should be sought for patients who have uncontrolled pain despite appropriate opioid-based therapies, in whom the cause of pain is likely multidimensional and, if unmanageable, lead to side effects.

### Palliative Sedation for Refractory Pain

In some patients, despite aggressive efforts with interventions directed toward relief, the pain may be intolerable. Palliative sedation is the use of sedating medications in terminally ill patients near the end of life to relieve pain and suffering that is refractory to treatments. This sedation is intended to decrease the patient's level of consciousness, but not hasten death.[105] The option of palliative sedation as a therapeutic option should be chosen as last resort after all other feasible interventions have been exhausted. Consultation with palliative care or pain specialists should be considered before palliative sedation is implemented. The US Supreme Court ruled in support of palliative sedation as a last resort for treating intractable suffering,[106,107] and is not considered euthanasia or physician-assisted suicide (PAS) by leading palliative care and hospice organizations.[108,109] The doctrine of double effect, with its roots in Roman Catholic theology, provides an ethical justification for palliative sedation.[110] The distinction between palliative sedation and euthanasia or PAS lies in the intent. The intent of the latter two is to end life, whereas the intent of palliative sedation is to relieve intractable distress, even though death may occur as an unintended effect of the intervention.

Commonly used sedating agents include neuroleptics, such as haloperidol, olanzapine, and chlorpromazine; benzodiazepines; barbiturates; and propofol. No controlled trials have compared the efficacy of one drug over the other, or the best method (continuous or intermittent use) for administrating sedation. The selection of the drug will depend on the clinical setting and available routes for administration. Initially, these agents may be prescribed on an intermittent basis, and then slowly titrated till the patient experiences comfort. For instance, haloperidol may be started at 1 to 2 mg (orally/intravenously/subcutaneously) every 4 to 6 hours around the clock, with additional doses as needed. Chlorpromazine is more sedating than haloperidol, but lowers blood pressure. Benzodiazepines may also be used intermittently. If intermittently administered agents do not provide satisfactory sedation or relief, continuous intravenous or subcutaneous sedation may be considered. Midazolam infusion can be started at 0.5 to 1 mg/h after a bolus dose of 1 to 5 mg, and then further titrated until the patient seems to be comfortable. During the administration of sedating agents, opioids should be continued to avoid opioid withdrawal and treat unobserved pain.

Several items must be addressed before implementing palliative sedation for refractory pain in patients with a terminal illness include. First, the patient and family must understand the options for treating pain with escalating doses of opioids, nonopioid analgesics, or adjuvants or why these are not applicable because of intolerable side effects. Second, the physician must discuss with the patient or designated medical power of attorney about the goal of sedating medication, and the risk of death associated with its use. Patients and family need to know that the use of sedation for refractory symptoms is ethical. Consent from the patient or designee and discussion regarding palliative sedation should be documented. Finally, patients must have a do-not-resuscitate order in place.

## REFERENCES

1. Xu J, Kochanek KD, Murphy SL, et al. Deaths: final data for 2007. Hyattsville (MD): National Center for Health Statistic; 2010.
2. Gruneir A, Mor V, Weitzen S, et al. Where people die: a multilevel approach to understanding influences on site of death in America. Med Care Res Rev 2007;64(4):351–78.
3. Teno JM, Weitzen S, Fennell ML, et al. Dying trajectory in the last year of life: does cancer trajectory fit other diseases? J Palliat Med 2001;4(4):457–64.
4. A controlled trial to improve care for seriously ill hospitalized patients. The study to understand prognoses and preferences for outcomes and risks of treatments (SUPPORT). The SUPPORT Principal Investigators. JAMA 1995;274(20):1591–8.
5. Hogan C, Lunney J, Gabel J, et al. Medicare beneficiaries' costs of care in the last year of life. Health Aff (Millwood) 2001;20(4):188–95.
6. Goodlin SJ, Winzelberg GS, Teno JM, et al. Death in the hospital. Arch Intern Med 1998;158(14):1570–2.
7. Teno JM, Clarridge BR, Casey V, et al. Family perspectives on end-of-life care at the last place of care. JAMA 2004;291(1):88–93.
8. Lesage P, Portenoy RK. Trends in cancer pain management. Cancer Control 1999;6(2):136–45.
9. Cleeland CS, Gonin R, Hatfield AK, et al. Pain and its treatment in outpatients with metastatic cancer. N Engl J Med 1994;330(9):592–6.
10. O'Mahony S, Goulet J, Kornblith A, et al. Desire for hastened death, cancer pain and depression: report of a longitudinal observational study. J Pain Symptom Manage 2005;29(5):446–57.
11. Inouye SK. The dilemma of delirium: clinical and research controversies regarding diagnosis and evaluation of delirium in hospitalized elderly medical patients. Am J Med 1994;97(3):278–88.
12. Brink-Huis A, van Achterberg T, Schoonhoven L. Pain management: a review of organisation models with integrated processes for the management of pain in adult cancer patients. J Clin Nurs 2008;17(15):1986–2000.
13. Morrison RS, Dietrich J, Meier DE. America's Care of serious illness: a state-by-state report card on access to palliative care in our nation's hospitals. New York: Center to Advance Palliative Care; 2008.
14. Turk DC, Monarch ES, Williams AD. Cancer patients in pain: considerations for assessing the whole person. Hematol Oncol Clin North Am 2002;16(3):511–25.

15. Saunders C. The management of terminal malignant disease. 1st edition. London: Edward Arnold; 1978.
16. Bruera E, Kuehn N, Miller MJ, et al. The Edmonton Symptom Assessment System (ESAS): a simple method for the assessment of palliative care patients. J Palliat Care 1991;7(2):6–9.
17. Fainsinger RL, Fairchild A, Nekolaichuk C, et al. Is pain intensity a predictor of the complexity of cancer pain management? J Clin Oncol 2009;27(4):585–90.
18. Wagner-Johnston ND, Carson KA, Grossman SA. High outpatient pain intensity scores predict impending hospital admissions in patients with cancer. J Pain Symptom Manage 2010;39(2):180–5.
19. Hsu H, Lacey DL, Dunstan CR, et al. Tumor necrosis factor receptor family member RANK mediates osteoclast differentiation and activation induced by osteoprotegerin ligand. Proc Natl Acad Sci U S A 1999;96(7):3540–5.
20. Fishman B, Pasternak S, Wallenstein SL, et al. The memorial pain assessment card. A valid instrument for the evaluation of cancer pain. Cancer 1987;60(5):1151–8.
21. Daut RL, Cleeland CS, Flanery RC. Development of the Wisconsin Brief Pain Questionnaire to assess pain in cancer and other diseases. Pain 1983;17(2):197–210.
22. Quality improvement guidelines for the treatment of acute pain and cancer pain. American Pain Society Quality of Care Committee. JAMA 1995;274(23):1874–80.
23. Gordon DB, Dahl JL, Miaskowski C. American pain society recommendations for improving the quality of acute and cancer pain management: American pain society quality of care task force. Arch Intern Med 2005;165(14):1574–80.
24. Lawlor PG, Gagnon B, Mancini IL, et al. Occurrence, causes, and outcome of delirium in patients with advanced cancer: a prospective study. Arch Intern Med 2000;160(6):786–94.
25. Minagawa H, Uchitomi Y, Yamawaki S, et al. Psychiatric morbidity in terminally ill cancer patients. A prospective study. Cancer 1996;78(5):1131–7.
26. Association AP. Delirium, dementia and amnestic and other cognitive disorders. Diagnostic and statistical manual of mental disorders. Washington, DC: American Psychiatric Assocation; 1994.
27. Armstrong SC, Cozza KL, Watanabe KS. The misdiagnosis of delirium. Psychosomatics 1997;38(5):433–9.
28. Pereira J, Hanson J, Bruera E. The frequency and clinical course of cognitive impairment in patients with terminal cancer. Cancer 1997;79(4):835–42.
29. Breitbart W, Rosenfeld B, Roth A, et al. The Memorial Delirium Assessment Scale. J Pain Symptom Manage 1997;13(3):128–37.
30. Ferrell BR. The impact of pain on quality of life. A decade of research. Nurs Clin North Am 1995;30(4):609–24.
31. Closs SJ, Barr B, Briggs M, et al. A comparison of five pain assessment scales for nursing home residents with varying degrees of cognitive impairment. J Pain Symptom Manage 2004;27(3):196–205.
32. Herr K, Bjoro K, Decker S. Tools for assessment of pain in nonverbal older adults with dementia: a state of the-science review. J Pain Symptom Manage 2006;31(2):170–92.
33. Desbiens NA, Mueller-Rizner N. How well do surrogates assess the pain of seriously ill patients? Crit Care Med 2000;28(5):1347–52.
34. Redinbaugh EM, Baum A, DeMoss C, et al. Factors associated with the accuracy of family caregiver estimates of patient pain. J Pain Symptom Manage 2002;23(1):31–8.

35. Allen RS, Haley WE, Small BJ, et al. Pain reports by older hospice cancer patients and family caregivers: the role of cognitive functioning. Gerontologist 2002;42(4):507–14.

36. Coyle N, Adelhardt J, Foley KM, et al. Character of terminal illness in the advanced cancer patient: pain and other symptoms during the last four weeks of life. J Pain Symptom Manage 1990;5(2):83–93.

37. Homsi J, Walsh D, Rivera N, et al. Symptom evaluation in palliative medicine: patient report vs systematic assessment. Support Care Cancer 2006;14(5): 444–53.

38. Stromgren AS, Groenvold M, Pedersen L, et al. Does the medical record cover the symptoms experienced by cancer patients receiving palliative care? A comparison of the record and patient self-rating. J Pain Symptom Manage 2001;21(3):189–96.

39. Glover J, Dibble SL, Dodd MJ, et al. Mood states of oncology outpatients: does pain make a difference? J Pain Symptom Manage 1995;10(2):120–8.

40. Ahles TA, Blanchard EB, Ruckdeschel JC. The multidimensional nature of cancer-related pain. Pain 1983;17(3):277–88.

41. World Health Organization. Cancer pain relief. 2nd edition. Geneva (Switzerland): World Health Organization; 1996.

42. Hanks GW, Conno F, Cherny N, et al. Morphine and alternative opioids in cancer pain: the EAPC recommendations. Br J Cancer 2001;84(5):587–93.

43. Jacox A, Carr DB, Payne R, et al. Management of cancer pain. Clinical practice guideline no. 9 AHCPR Pub. No. 94–0592. Rockville (MD): Agency for Health Care and Research, US Department of Health and Human Services, Public Health Service; 1994.

44. McNicol E, Strassels SA, Goudas L, et al. NSAIDS or paracetamol, alone or combined with opioids, for cancer pain. Cochrane Database Syst Rev 2005;1: CD005180.

45. Eisenberg E, Berkey CS, Carr DB, et al. Efficacy and safety of nonsteroidal anti-inflammatory drugs for cancer pain: a meta-analysis. J Clin Oncol 1994;12(12): 2756–65.

46. Mercadante S, Porzio G, Ferrera P, et al. Low morphine doses in opioid-naive cancer patients with pain. J Pain Symptom Manage 2006;31(3):242–7.

47. Marinangeli F, Ciccozzi A, Leonardis M, et al. Use of strong opioids in advanced cancer pain: a randomized trial. J Pain Symptom Manage 2004;27(5):409–16.

48. Woolf CJ. Pain: moving from symptom control toward mechanism-specific pharmacologic management. Ann Intern Med 2004;140(6):441–51.

49. Sabino MA, Ghilardi JR, Jongen JL, et al. Simultaneous reduction in cancer pain, bone destruction, and tumor growth by selective inhibition of cyclooxygenase-2. Cancer Res 2002;62(24):7343–9.

50. Davies NM, Jamali F. COX-2 selective inhibitors cardiac toxicity: getting to the heart of the matter. J Pharm Pharm Sci 2004;7(3):332–6.

51. Mukherjee D, Nissen SE, Topol EJ. Risk of cardiovascular events associated with selective COX-2 inhibitors. JAMA 2001;286(8):954–9.

52. NIH Office of Communications. Use of non-steroidal anti-inflammatory drugs suspended in large Alzheimer's disease prevention trial. 2004. Available at: http://www.nih.gov/news/pr/dec2004/od-20.htm. Accessed October 19, 2006.

53. Hawkey CJ, Karrasch JA, Szczepanski L, et al. Omeprazole compared with misoprostol for ulcers associated with nonsteroidal antiinflammatory drugs. Omeprazole versus Misoprostol for NSAID-induced Ulcer Management (OMNIUM) Study Group. N Engl J Med 1998;338(11):727–34.

54. Helm S, Trescot AM, Colson J, et al. Opioid antagonists, partial agonists, and agonists/antagonists: the role of office-based detoxification. Pain Physician 2008;11(2):225–35.
55. Kaltenback BL, Becker A. Use of opioids in adults with chronic cancer pain. Health Care 2002;1:1–7.
56. Houde R. Clinical analgesic studies of hydromorphone. In: Foley K, Inturrisi C, editors. Advances in pain research and therapy. New York: Raven Press; 1986. p. 129–35.
57. Gabrail NY, Dvergsten C, Ahdieh H. Establishing the dosage equivalency of oxymorphone extended release and oxycodone controlled release in patients with cancer pain: a randomized controlled study. Curr Med Res Opin 2004; 20(6):911–8.
58. Walsh D, Donnelly S, Rybicki L. The symptoms of advanced cancer: relationship to age, gender, and performance status in 1,000 patients. Support Care Cancer 2000;8(3):175–9.
59. Fainsinger RL, Nekolaichuk CL, Lawlor PG, et al. A multicenter study of the revised Edmonton Staging System for classifying cancer pain in advanced cancer patients. J Pain Symptom Manage 2005;29(3):224–37.
60. Mercadante S, Casuccio A, Agnello A, et al. Morphine versus methadone in the pain treatment of advanced-cancer patients followed up at home. J Clin Oncol 1998;16(11):3656–61.
61. Bruera E, Palmer JL, Bosnjak S, et al. Methadone versus morphine as a first-line strong opioid for cancer pain: a randomized, double-blind study. J Clin Oncol 2004;22(1):185–92.
62. Mercadante S, Porzio G, Ferrera P, et al. Sustained-release oral morphine versus transdermal fentanyl and oral methadone in cancer pain management. Eur J Pain 2008;12(8):1040–6.
63. Walker PW, Palla S, Pei BL, et al. Switching from methadone to a different opioid: what is the equianalgesic dose ratio? J Palliat Med 2008;11(8):1103–8.
64. Bamigbade TA, Davidson C, Langford RM, et al. Actions of tramadol, its enantiomers and principal metabolite, O-desmethyltramadol, on serotonin (5-HT) efflux and uptake in the rat dorsal raphe nucleus. British Journal of Anaesthesia 1997;79(3):352–6.
65. Chizh BA, Headley PM, Tzschentke TM. NMDA receptor antagonists as analgesics: focus on the NR2B subtype. Trends Pharmacol Sci 2001;22(12):636–42.
66. Bruera E, Pereira J. Acute neuropsychiatric findings in a patient receiving fentanyl for cancer pain. Pain 1997;69(1–2):199–201.
67. Adair JC, el-Nachef A, Cutler P. Fentanyl neurotoxicity. Ann Emerg Med 1996; 27(6):791–2.
68. Fishbain DA, Rosomoff HL, Rosomoff RS. Drug abuse, dependence, and addiction in chronic pain patients. Clin J Pain 1992;8(2):77–85.
69. Porter J, Jick H. Addiction rare in patients treated with narcotics. N Engl J Med 1980;302(2):123.
70. McQuay HJ. Opioid use in chronic pain. Acta Anaesthesiol Scand 1997;41(1 Pt 2): 175–83.
71. McNicol E, Horowicz-Mehler N, Fisk RA, et al. Management of opioid side effects in cancer-related and chronic noncancer pain: a systematic review. J Pain 2003;4(5):231–56.
72. Allan L, Hays H, Jensen NH, et al. Randomised crossover trial of transdermal fentanyl and sustained release oral morphine for treating chronic non-cancer pain. BMJ 2001;322(7295):1154–8.

73. Staats PS, Markowitz J, Schein J. Incidence of constipation associated with long-acting opioid therapy: a comparative study. South Med J 2004;97(2):129–34.

74. Bruera E, Neumann CM. Management of specific symptom complexes in patients receiving palliative care. CMAJ 1998;158(13):1717–26.

75. Mercadante S. Opioid rotation for cancer pain: rationale and clinical aspects. Cancer 1999;86(9):1856–66.

76. Bowsher D. Paradoxical pain. BMJ 1993;306(6876):473–4.

77. Mercadante S, Ferrera P, Villari P, et al. Hyperalgesia: an emerging iatrogenic syndrome. J Pain Symptom Manage 2003;26(2):769–75.

78. Szarvas S, Harmon D, Murphy D. Neuraxial opioid-induced pruritus: a review. J Clin Anesth 2003;15(3):234–9.

79. Moryl N, Coyle N, Foley KM. Managing an acute pain crisis in a patient with advanced cancer: "this is as much of a crisis as a code". JAMA 2008; 299(12):1457–67.

80. Bruera E, Rico M, Bertolino M, et al. A prospective, open study of oral methadone in the treatment of cancer pain. In: Devor M, Rowbotham M, Weisenfeld-Hallin Z, editions. Proceedings of the 9th World Congress on Pain. Seattle (WA): IASP Press; 2000. p. 957–63.

81. Backonja M, Beydoun A, Edwards KR, et al. Gabapentin for the symptomatic treatment of painful neuropathy in patients with diabetes mellitus: a randomized controlled trial. JAMA 1998;280(21):1831–6.

82. Rowbotham M, Harden N, Stacey B, et al. Gabapentin for the treatment of postherpetic neuralgia: a randomized controlled trial. JAMA 1998;280(21): 1837–42.

83. Caraceni A, Zecca E, Martini C, et al. Gabapentin as an adjuvant to opioid analgesia for neuropathic cancer pain. J Pain Symptom Manage 1999;17(6): 441–5.

84. Petrenko AB, Yamakura T, Baba H, et al. The role of N-methyl-D-aspartate (NMDA) receptors in pain: a review. Anesth Analg 2003;97(4):1108–16.

85. Bell R, Eccleston C, Kalso E. Ketamine as an adjuvant to opioids for cancer pain. Cochrane Database Syst Rev 2003;1:CD003351.

86. Ross JR, Saunders Y, Edmonds PM, et al. Systematic review of role of bisphosphonates on skeletal morbidity in metastatic cancer. BMJ 2003; 327(7413):469.

87. Wong R, Wiffen PJ. Bisphosphonates for the relief of pain secondary to bone metastases. Cochrane Database Syst Rev 2002;2:CD002068.

88. Body JJ. Dosing regimens and main adverse events of bisphosphonates. Semin Oncol 2001;28(4 Suppl 11):49–53.

89. Rosen LS, Gordon D, Kaminski M, et al. Long-term efficacy and safety of zoledronic acid compared with pamidronate disodium in the treatment of skeletal complications in patients with advanced multiple myeloma or breast carcinoma: a randomized, double-blind, multicenter, comparative trial. Cancer 2003;98(8):1735–44.

90. Bamias A, Kastritis E, Bamia C, et al. Osteonecrosis of the jaw in cancer after treatment with bisphosphonates: incidence and risk factors. J Clin Oncol 2005;23(34):8580–7.

91. Hoff AO, Toth BB, Altundag K, et al. Frequency and risk factors associated with osteonecrosis of the jaw in cancer patients treated with intravenous bisphosphonates. J Bone Miner Res 2008;23(6):826–36.

92. Feuer DJ, Broadley KE. Corticosteroids for the resolution of malignant bowel obstruction in advanced gynaecological and gastrointestinal cancer. Cochrane Database Syst Rev 2000;2:CD001219.

93. Martin WJ, Loo CM, Basbaum AI. Spinal cannabinoids are anti-allodynic in rats with persistent inflammation. Pain 1999;82(2):199–205.

94. Fox A, Kesingland A, Gentry C, et al. The role of central and peripheral Cannabinoid1 receptors in the antihyperalgesic activity of cannabinoids in a model of neuropathic pain. Pain 2001;92(1–2):91–100.

95. Kehl LJ, Hamamoto DT, Wacnik PW, et al. A cannabinoid agonist differentially attenuates deep tissue hyperalgesia in animal models of cancer and inflammatory muscle pain. Pain 2003;103(1–2):175–86.

96. Campbell FA, Tramer MR, Carroll D, et al. Are cannabinoids an effective and safe treatment option in the management of pain? A qualitative systematic review. BMJ 2001;323(7303):13–6.

97. Abrams DI, Jay CA, Shade SB, et al. Cannabis in painful HIV-associated sensory neuropathy: a randomized placebo-controlled trial. Neurology 2007; 68(7):515–21.

98. Svendsen KB, Jensen TS, Bach FW. Does the cannabinoid dronabinol reduce central pain in multiple sclerosis? Randomised double blind placebo controlled crossover trial. BMJ 2004;329(7460):253.

99. Beaulieu P. Effects of nabilone, a synthetic cannabinoid, on postoperative pain. Can J Anaesth 2006;53(8):769–75.

100. NSativex [product information]. Toronto, Canada: Bayer Inc; 2008.

101. Tilden VP, Drach LL, Tolle SW. Complementary and alternative therapy use at end-of-life in community settings. J Altern Complement Med 2004;10(5):811–7.

102. Demmer C. A survey of complementary therapy services provided by hospices. J Palliat Med 2004;7(4):510–6.

103. Kozak LE, Kayes L, McCarty R, et al. Use of complementary and alternative medicine (CAM) by Washington State hospices. Am J Hosp Palliat Care 2008; 25(6):463–8.

104. Hwang SS, Chang VT, Kasimis B. Dynamic cancer pain management outcomes: the relationship between pain severity, pain relief, functional interference, satisfaction and global quality of life over time. J Pain Symptom Manage 2002;23(3): 190–200.

105. Medicine AAoHaP. AAHPM position statement on sedation at the end of life. American Academy of Hospice and Palliative Medicine; 2006. Available at: http://www.aahpm.org/positions/default/sedation.html. Accessed March 2, 2011.

106. Vacco v Quill, 117 Wests Supreme Court Report. 2293, 2312 (1997).

107. Washington v Glucksberg, 117 Wests Supreme Court Report. 2258, 2293 (1997).

108. American Academy of Hospice and Palliative Medicine. AAHPM position statement: statement on palliative sedation. Available at: www.aahpm.org/positions/ sedation.html. Accessed September 17, 2010.

109. Hospice and Palliative Nurses Association. HPNA position statement: palliative sedation at end of life. Available at: www.hpna.org/DisplayPage.aspx?Title= Position%20Statements. Accessed September 17, 2010.

110. Sulmasy DP, Pellegrino ED. The rule of double effect: clearing up the double talk. Arch Intern Med 1999;159(6):545–50.

# Assessment and Management of Gastrointestinal Symptoms in Advanced Illness

Marlene E. McHugh, DNP, FNP-BC, RN[a,b],*,
Debbie Miller-Saultz, DNP, FNP-BC, RN[a,c]

## KEYWORDS

- Nausea • Vomiting • Constipation • Anorexia • Cachexia

In daily practice, the primary care clinician increasingly encounters patients with advanced illness, many suffering from symptoms other than pain. The management of these symptoms can be burdensome for the clinician, the patient, and the caregiver.

Key principles that guide palliative care are important to incorporate into a plan of care for each patient and family. Although medical management continues to be the mainstay of treatment, the generalist in palliative care needs to be familiar with the patient's preferences and goals of care to help guide treatment in advanced illness.

This article provides an overview of specific gastrointestinal (GI) symptoms that may be encountered by a generalist in palliative care: anorexia, cachexia, nausea, vomiting, and constipation. For the purposes of this article, advanced progressive illnesses are defined as conditions for which there is no cure and which have significant morbidity in the later stages of illness.[1]

## ANOREXIA

In advanced disease, a decline in nutritional status, a loss of muscle mass, and impaired function affect quality of life. These signs are commonly identified as risk factors for increased morbidity and mortality, and as indicators for poor prognosis.[2]

The authors have nothing to disclose.

[a] Columbia University, School of Nursing, 630 West 168th Street, New York, NY 10032, USA
[b] Palliative Care Service, Department of Family Medicine, Montefiore Medical Center, 3347 Steuben Avenue, Bronx, NY 10467, USA
[c] Department of Anesthesiology, Divison of Pain Medicine and Palliative Care, New York Presbyterian Medical Center, 622 West 168th Street, PH5, New York, NY 10032, USA
* Corresponding author. Columbia University School of Nursing, New York, NY.
E-mail address: mm234@columbia.edu

Prim Care Clin Office Pract 38 (2011) 225–246
doi:10.1016/j.pop.2011.03.005
0095-4543/11/$ – see front matter © 2011 Elsevier Inc. All rights reserved.

The significance of not eating has a deep impact on both patients and families, based on the premise that food is necessary for survival and a symbol of nurturing and caring.[3] However, anorexia is a symptom that is frequently ignored and untreated.[2]

### Definition

Anorexia is simply defined as a loss of appetite or desire to eat. Unintentional weight loss is defined as a loss greater than 10% of preillness body weight. In patients with cancer and advanced illness, unintentional weight loss is attributed to changes in metabolic rate and energy expenditure, causing an imbalance that is not corrected by increasing food intake.[4]

### Prevalence

Anorexia is prevalent in patients with multisystem organ failure (heart, kidney, liver, lung), chronic obstructive pulmonary disease (COPD), rheumatoid arthritis, acquired immune deficiency syndrome (AIDS), or cancer. The presence of anorexia is indicates disease progression, depression, fatigue, and anorexia-cachexia syndrome (discussed later) or occurs as a side effect of chemotherapy and/or radiation therapy. It has been reported in 50% of patients with advanced disease at the time of diagnosis, and in as many as 85% of patients with advanced cancer.[3,4]

Teunissen and colleagues[5] conducted a systematic review of symptom prevalence in patients who have terminal cancer and found that the 5 most prominent symptoms in the last 2 weeks of life were fatigue, pain, lack of energy, weakness, and appetite loss.

### Pathophysiology

Cancer anorexia is attributed to multifactorial physiologic responses to tumor growth: by-product secretion from both tumor and host, with an overproduction of interferons; tumor necrosis factor (TNF) synthesized by immune system cells; and inflammatory cytokines. Cytokines are hormonelike proteins that act as chemical messengers; they rarely act as a single substance, but are typically found with several substances, acting as antagonists or synergists (**Table 1**). The hypothalamus and brainstem integrate nutritional information from peripheral signals received via fat, liver, and gut hormones, which in turn are integrated and translated by means of peptidergic neurons (feedback loop). The result manifests as clinical symptoms of loss of appetite, early satiety, and unintentional weight loss.[6,7]

When cytokines are released, there is an increase in hypothalamic concentrations of neuropeptide Y (NPY) and hypothalamic serotonergic neurotransmitters, resulting in an inhibition of the feeding mechanism.[4] NPY is an amino acid found in the brain and hypothalamus. It also has an interconnected network to other orexigenic peptides, among them galanin, opioid peptides, melanin-concentrating hormone, orexin, and agouti-related peptide (**Table 2**). In animal studies, the level of NPY was found to be decreased in rats with tumors, but increased levels were found in rats that were starved and those that were calorie restricted, confirming the complex nature of anorexia-cachexia as opposed to starvation.[8]

Tumor-related changes in protein metabolism exacerbate anorexia, directly affecting food intake and nutritional status. Peripheral signals from adipose tissue that indicate food intake come from hormones such as insulin, leptin, and ghrelin. Leptin produces a negative influence on food intake, and ghrelin, synthesized by the stomach, stimulates growth hormone release from the pituitary, which has a strong

**Table 1**
**Cytokines associated with anorexia**

| Cytokine | Site of Origin/Response | Site of Action/Response |
|---|---|---|
| TNF-$\alpha$ | Blood monocytes<br>Tissue macrophages/tumor response | CNS (glucose-sensitive neurons in ventromedial nucleus and lateral hypothalamic area)/anorexia |
| IL-1 | Macrophages<br>Lymphocytes/acute and chronic disorders | CNS (linked to serotonergic action)/decreased food intake; early satiety |
| IL-6 | Astrocytes<br>Microglia<br>Neurons/tumor specific (lung, colon or lymphoma) | CNS/decreased food intake; inhibits tumor growth; increases cachexia |
| Interferon $\alpha$/$\gamma$ | — | CNS/<br>$\alpha$, antitumor activity; $\gamma$, decreased food intake<br>Progressive weight loss |

*Abbreviations:* CNS, central nervous system; IL, interleukin.

influence on the stimulation of food intake and the activity of feeding-regulating regions of the hypothalamus.

Weight loss stimulates appetite and food intake, but, in patients with cancer and advanced disease, this adaptive mechanism is lost. Anorexia found in patients who have cancer and those with advanced disease is not the result of simple starvation.[4,9]

### Signs of Anorexia

Commonly reported signs of anorexia are early satiety, taste and/or smell alterations, and nausea with or without vomiting. Patients also may experience uncontrolled pain or abdominal discomfort from ascites, breathlessness, or hiccups.[2]

Intractable hiccups interfere with eating, and thus are a major contributor to anorexia. Hiccups lasting for more than 48 hours are defined as persistent and intractable. They are the result of an involuntary spasm of the diaphragm and intercostal muscles, which is followed by a sudden closure of the glottis. Hiccups may be caused by a variety of factors, among them irritation of the vagus nerve, chemotherapy-induced release of 5-hydroxytryptamine (5-HT), trigeminal nerve irritation, and

**Table 2**
**Neuropeptides associated with anorexia**

| Anorexigenic Neuropeptides | Orexigenic Neuropeptides |
|---|---|
| Hypothalamic Neuropeptides<br>$\alpha$MCH<br>CRF | Hypothalamic Neuropeptides<br>NPY<br>MCH<br>AGRP |
| Hormones<br>Leptin | Hormones<br>Ghrelin<br>Galanin<br>Orexin |

*Abbreviations:* AGRP, agouti-related peptide; CRF, corticotropin-related factor; MCH, melanin-concentrating hormone; $\alpha$MCH, $\alpha$-melanocyte-concentrating hormone; NPY, neuropeptide Y.

innervation of the phrenic nerve. Hiccups frequently occur after endoscopy because of gastric distention, or from gastric outlet or small bowel obstruction.

Hiccups are associated with tumors of the esophagus or esophageal strictures, food impaction, or achalasia. Intractable hiccups cause an energy expenditure increase through contraction of the skeletal muscles. They interfere with food and fluid intake, which may result in poor caloric intake as well as aspiration, with the possible consequences of aspiration pneumonia, airway obstruction, or respiratory failure.[10]

## Assessment

Anorexia is assessed based on the patient's self-report of appetite and early satiety. Patients with advanced disease, including those with cancer, should be screened for weight changes, functional status, and treatment-related adverse impacts on nutritional status.

Assessment tools used to clarify symptom distress and severity in palliative care and to guide treatment include the Edmonton Symptom Assessment System (ESAS), a 9-item, patient-rated symptom visual analog scale (VAS), and the Memorial Symptom Assessment Scale (MSAS), a 32-item, patient-rated scale that is a multidimensional quality-of-life instrument.[2,11–13] Tools specific to anorexia-cachexia are the Functional Assessment of Anorexia/Cachexia Therapy (FAACT) questionnaire, a 28-item, general patient-rated measure of quality of life,[14] and the Patient-generated Subjective Global Assessment (PG-SGA), a nutritional screening tool for patients who have cancer self-report and health care provider assessment.[15]

## Treatment

Treatment of anorexia should be designed to eliminate the underlying disease. When that is not possible, treatment involves drug therapies that interfere with the downregulation of cytokine synthesis and release. In addition, treatment is designed to correct underlying physiologic mechanisms such as gastric dysmotility (decreased GI motility, decreased gastric emptying because of disease progression). Decreased gastric motility also may result from opioid therapy, a side effect of which may be constipation, leading to bloating and the feeling of fullness. All of these interfere with appetite and food intake. Esophageal reflux, mucositis, and oral candidiasis affect taste; poor dentition or ill-fitting dentures and intractable hiccups affect the ability to eat.[4]

Clinicians may use pharmacologic and nonpharmacologic therapies to prevent exaggeration of symptoms or to treat symptoms to minimize effect.

### Pharmacologic treatment

Megestrol acetate and medroxyprogesterone acetate (progestagens) are used as first-line therapy, particularly for cancer anorexia (**Table 3**). Maltoni and colleagues[16] conducted a systematic review of randomized controlled trials (RCTs) involving progestagens; they reported that use of high-dose progestagens improved food intake but had less of an impact on weight gain. Clinicians should be aware that progestagens are contraindicated in patients with hormone-dependent tumors and have side effects that include fluid retention, deep venous thrombosis, menstrual irregularities, and sexual dysfunction.

Other therapies that have been used include cannabinoids (in particular, dronabinol), which have been shown to affect cytokine expression (see **Table 3**). Corticosteroids are commonly used to suppress immune response and cytokine activity. The prokinetic agent metoclopramide is a 5-HT$_4$ receptor agonist that stimulates gastric and duodenal motility, predominantly via an action on efferent myenteric cholinergic neurons releasing acetylcholine, with some effect because of its property as

**Table 3**
**Agents for the treatment of anorexia-cachexia**

| Progesterones | |
| --- | --- |
| Megesterol acetate | 800 mg daily |
| Medroxyl-progesterone acetate | 1000 mg daily |
| Cannabinoids | |
| Dronabinol | 5–20 mg/d |
| Corticosteroids | |
| Dexamethasone | 0–75 mg 4 times daily |
| Prokinetic agent | |
| Metoclopramide | 10 mg every 6 hours |
| Hormones | |
| Ghrelin | 0.7–13 µg/kg daily |

a dopamine antagonist. Prokinetic agents affect lower esophageal sphincter pressure, increase frequency of transient lower esophageal sphincter relaxations and delayed gastric emptying, and mechanisms leading to esophageal motor dysfunction, such as disrupted peristaltic contractions.

Studies are being conducted on other promising therapies such as macrolides (which bind to motilin receptors located in the gastric antrum and proximal duodenum, increasing lower esophageal sphincter pressure, enhancing gastric emptying); cholecystokinin antagonists (which lower esophageal sphincter pressure); and mixed µ/K opioid agonists.[17,18]

### Nonpharmacologic treatment

**Food diaries, nutritional assessment, and support** Patients with anorexia should keep daily food diaries to assess caloric intake. The goal is to minimize the symptom burden of anorexia-cachexia, with the intent to preemptively treat symptoms and improve quality of life. Family members or caregivers should be involved, particularly with patients who suffer from cognitive impairment or depression, to obtain an accurate account of caloric intake. Assessment should include factors that point to desire to eat, early satiety, food aversion, and number of meals and amount consumed at each meal. The diary also should include the emotional components around meal preparation and the emotional connection to food, with particular attention to the family or caregiver at meal time.

**Behavioral therapy** Mood changes in patients with anorexia, particularly depression, interfere with quality-of-life activities. Behavioral therapy may help enhance appetite and prevent food aversion.

### CACHEXIA

Cachexia in patients who have cancer is found to have consequences beyond the physical and psychological; it is suggestive of poor prognosis and as a predictor of chemotherapy toxicity.[4] The cause of death in 20% of patients with cancer has been attributed to cachexia.[2]

### Definition

The term cachexia is derived from the Greek kakos (bad) and hexis (condition). Cachexia in general is characterized by the clinical presentation of anorexia, chronic nausea, early satiety, unintentional progressive weight loss, loss of muscle mass with muscle wasting, and poor functional status.[9]

Involuntary weight loss (despite adequate food intake) of more than 5% of premorbid weight in a 6-month period, particularly when combined with muscle wasting, a body mass index (BMI) of less than 20 in patients younger than 65 years and less than 22 in patients older than 65 years, albumin of less than 3.5 g/dL, decreasing total protein levels, anemia, and increasing triglyceride, glucose, and lactic acid levels, should raise strong suspicion for the presence of primary cachexia.[19,20]

Secondary cachexia results in unintentional weight loss but from different origins: inadequate oral intake with alteration in the GI tract (mechanical, intrinsic, or extrinsic). Factors that add to the malabsorption of nutrients are fistulae involving the GI tract and diarrhea, with increased loss of protein and decreased energy expenditures; changes in catabolic states because of infection (acute and/or chronic), chronic heart failure, chronic renal failure, COPD, cirrhosis, poorly controlled diabetes, or hyperthyroidism; deconditioning[19]; and muscle atrophy.[1]

Sarcopenia is defined as significant skeletal muscle wasting, and depletion of skeletal muscle can occur independent of adiposity. A muscle mass of more than 2 standard deviations less than that typical for healthy adults is one current definition of sarcopenia.[21] In cancer, tumor growth triggers metabolic changes through proteolysis-inducing factor (PIF), which induces degradation of skeletal muscle through upregulation of the ubiquitin/proteasome proteolytic pathway, and proinflammatory cytokines.[22]

## Prevalence

The prevalence of cachexia is variable, ranging from 15% to 40% of patients with cancer; because of the insidious nature of the aforementioned symptoms, patients do not usually seek treatment of cachexia itself, but for other symptoms, such as pain, dyspnea, and fatigue.[20] Cachexia is present in more than 80% of patients with advanced illnesses other than cancer, is more commonly found in the elderly and in children with cancer, and becomes more pronounced in end-stage disease and as cancer progresses.[2]

Recent studies have suggested that there are different phenotypes of cancer cachexia, resulting from distinct mechanisms, such as pronounced muscle wasting (brain-liver axis phenotype, predominantly secondary to proinflammatory cytokine activity), early satiety and anorexia (gut-brain axis phenotype, apparently caused by altered enterohormonal production), and anorexia without marked cachexia (brain-muscle axis phenotype, likely secondary to low serum anabolic steroids).[23]

## Assessment

A patient's weight is the most common factor used to determine nutritional status. Body composition is an important determinant in identifying lean body mass. Skinfold thickness and midarm circumference are used to estimate body fat and muscle mass in healthy individuals; these should not be used in the initial assessment of patients with cancer or those with advanced illness, but can be used in longitudinal follow-up. The most accurate assessment tool is dual energy x-ray absorptiometry (DEXA) with an estimation of extracellular water volume. DEXA works on the principle that 2 different energy level photons are linearly related to the percentage of fat and soft tissue mass.[20]

## Anorexia-Cachexia Syndrome

An involuntary weight loss of more than 10% of a patient's predisease weight meets the criterion for anorexia-cachexia syndrome.[24] The hallmark signs and symptoms of anorexia-cachexia syndrome are severe loss of weight, including loss of muscle with or without loss of fat mass; loss of appetite; nausea; early satiety; anemia; weakness and fatigue; food aversions; depression or anxiety; and breathlessness.

Esper and Heidrich[25] explored the phenomenon of symptom clusters; that is, 3 or more symptoms that are related to each other. These symptoms typically do not occur as 1 entity but as a grouping or clustered together, such as pain, constipation, and confusion; anxiety, agitation, and delirium; cough, dyspnea, and fatigue; and anorexia, cachexia, and dehydration. The clustering of anorexia, cachexia and dehydration is often found in patients with advanced disease. Physiologic connections between symptoms seem to be the result of autonomic failure. Autonomic failure presents as gastroparesis, early satiety, anorexia, and nausea. Hyperglycemia increases anorexia, polyuria, and hypercalcemia, commonly found in patients with cancer, which then promote nausea and anorexia, inhibiting oral intake with worsening dehydration.[25,26]

## Treatment

Treatment is designed to correct any underlying disease and reversible causes of anorexia-cachexia syndrome. Symptoms and conditions that can be treated to lessen symptom burden include pain; gastrointestinal dysfunction including constipation and gastroesophageal reflux disease; xerostomia; infection; depression; or iatrogenic causes.

Anorexia-cachexia syndrome could be reversed with the complete elimination of tumor burden. When oncologic treatment does not resolve the condition, then treatment is designed to provide early nutritional support, adequate hydration, and pharmacologic interventions to stimulate appetite.[27]

### Pharmacologic treatment

Treatment is targeted to adjust metabolic, neuroendocrine, and anabolic imbalances to decrease symptom burden and improve quality of life. Presently, quality of life and survival have not improved with the addition of enteral or parental nutrition.

The drug therapies used are the same as previously described in the treatment of anorexia: hormones, corticosteroids, prokinetic agents, cannabinoids, and antidepressants (see **Table 3**).[28]

Newer therapies include an orexigenic peptide, ghrelin, which is synthesized in the upper third of the stomach. Ghrelin acts as a potent appetite enhancer and increases food intake and body weight.[29–31] Ghrelin has endocrine growth hormone–releasing activity, as well as autocrine/paracrine factors that regulate cell proliferation apoptosis, inflammation, gastric functions (gastric acid secretion, gastric motility, turnover of gastric and intestinal mucosa), cardiovascular functions (improve cardiac structure and function, cardiac output, blood pressure, particularly in patients with congestive heart failure), and play a role in sleep, memory retention, anxiety, embryo development, reproduction, and lactation. In the treatment of cachexia, ghrelin regulates metabolic functions associated with appetite, energy expenditure, adiposity, and blood glucose/insulin release. As a consequences of these relationships, metabolic functions between ghrelin production and disease states, such as obesity, diabetes, inflammatory conditions, cardiovascular disease, and cancer, have caused a heightened interest in this peptide.[32,33]

Eicosapentaenoic acid (EPA) is an anti-inflammatory agent that stabilizes the acute protein phase response, as measured by C-reactive protein (CRP); interleukin-6 (IL-6) is involved in inducing the acute protein phase response. In a study by Read and colleagues,[34] use of an EPA supplement before the start of chemotherapy resulted in a significant correlation between IL-6 and survival, and IL-6 and CRP in the mediation of the acute phase response.

Treatment with β2-adrenoceptor agonists may affect protein metabolism in skeletal muscle, allowing for protein deposits and preservation of skeletal muscle. Thalidomide inhibits TNF-α, improving mood, restlessness, and insomnia, as well as having an impact on weight gain. Melatonin decreases the level of circulating TNF-α and was found to reduce myelosuppression, cachexia, and neuropathy in specific cancer populations.

### Nonpharmacologic therapy

**Nutritional and psychological support** Food preparation and consumption allows patients and families to interact despite illness or surroundings. The goals of care in anorexia and cachexia management are to:

1. Educate patients and families to identify early signs and symptoms of anorexia and cachexia: early satiety, loss of appetite, food aversion and lack of interest in eating, or taste alteration
2. Keep track of calories, food intake, and output excess from vomiting and diarrhea
3. Assess mood for depression and anxiety
4. Provide nutritional counseling to patients and families from diagnosis through treatment and beyond.

## NAUSEA AND VOMITING
### Definition

Nausea is the objectionable sensation of the need to vomit. Nausea occurs in advanced illness both in relation to, and independent of, therapeutic treatments.[25] Chronic nausea is defined as the presence of nausea lasting more than 1 week in the population with advanced illness, in the absence of any self-limiting causes such as chemotherapy or radiation.[35] Vomiting is the forceful expulsion of the contents of the stomach through the oral or nasal cavities.[36]

Clinicians working with patients in palliative care also should be aware of the term retching and be able to differentiate between nausea, vomiting, and retching. Retching is described in the literature as the attempt to vomit without expulsion of contents.[36] Emesis is the word used to represent all 3 components of the symptom complex.[37]

### Prevalence

Chronic nausea and vomiting commonly complicate the lives of people with advanced illness. A recent systematic review in patients with incurable cancer found that nausea occurred in 17% (6 studies, 2219 patients) and vomiting in 13% (3 studies, 799 patients) of patients in the last 1 to 2 weeks of life.[5] Another study reported that nausea and vomiting occur in up to 70% of patients with cancer toward the end of life.[38] A review by Solano and colleagues[39] in 2006 compared symptom prevalence in different advanced illnesses, and reported that nausea was present in 6% to 68% of patients with cancer (19 studies, 9140 patients), 17% to 48% of patients with heart disease (3 studies, 146 patients), 30% to 43% of patients with renal disease (3 studies, 362 patients), and 43% to 49% of patients with AIDS (2 studies, 689 patients).

### Pathophysiology

Understanding what neurotransmitter receptors may have been activated by metabolites or chemotherapeutic agents is vital to pharmacologic management. The common causes of nausea and vomiting in patients with advanced illness and the various pathways of emesis are shown in **Box 1**.

Vomiting can be triggered by afferent impulses to the vomiting center (located in the medulla) from the chemoreceptor trigger zone, GI tract, and cerebral cortex. Vomiting occurs when efferent impulses are sent from the vomiting center to the salivation center, abdominal muscles, respiratory center, and cranial nerves.

There are many neurotransmitter receptors in the chemoreceptor trigger zone, vomiting center, and GI tract. The principle neuroreceptors involved in the emetic response are the serotonin and dopamine receptors (**Fig. 1**).[31] Other neuroreceptors involved include acetylcholine, corticosteroid, histamine, cannabinoid, opioid, and neurokinin-1.[40] Antiemetic drugs are predominantly blocking agents, effective at different receptor sites. Administering the most potent antagonist to the implicated receptor has been shown to be effective in up to 80% to 90% of patients near the end of life.[41]

## Assessment

Nausea and vomiting can be debilitating symptoms, creating a substantial source of physical and psychological distress for patients and families. A thorough assessment of these symptoms assists the clinician in understanding the severity and cause. Nausea is subjective and, therefore, the clinician must rely on patient report. Vomiting may be measured objectively, but the degree of distress is subjective and can only be reported by the individual.

As mentioned previously, multiple tools have been developed to identify symptom distress in patients in palliative care. The Cambridge Palliative Assessment Schedule (CAMPAS-R) is a validated, patient-rated tool that uses a set of VASs to rate symptoms and problems in terms of intensity and impact on daily life.[42] The MSAS and the ESAS are other tools used to assess common symptoms in the patient in palliative care. The tool identified should be initially used to assess severity and then, at regular intervals, to assess response to treatment. The International Association of Hospice and Palliative Care provides access to symptom assessment and research tools for use by clinicians in palliative care settings (http://www.hospicecare.com/resources/pain-research.htm). (See Appendix for other online palliative care information.)

The underlying physiologic mechanisms, metabolic causes, and medications that may be causing or contributing to the symptoms of nausea and vomiting should be identified by the clinician.[38] Given that these symptoms may resolve by the time a cause is identified, it is important that the clinician review all the mechanisms as soon as the symptoms appear. Examples of this would be opioid use, constipation, or electrolyte imbalance.

Assessment also needs to include a review of laboratory and radiologic testing results. In the palliative care setting, further testing should be based on the symptom burden, goals of care, and distress that testing may cause the patient and family. The National Comprehensive Cancer Network (NCCN) Clinical Practice Guidelines suggest that the evaluation of underlying abnormalities should be dictated by the patient's life expectancy.[40]

## Treatment

### Pharmacologic treatment

Development of the 5-HT$_3$ receptor antagonists has improved the management of nausea and vomiting. Evidence supports the use of these agents for chemotherapy-induced nausea and vomiting (CINV)[41] and radiation-induced nausea.[38] There are limited studies of the 5-HT$_3$ antagonists in nausea and vomiting outside the oncology literature; however, a 2002 study in chronic renal failure patients with uremia showed

---

**Box 1**
**Common causes of nausea and vomiting in advanced illness**

Drugs

- Chemotherapy
- Opioids
- Nonsteroidal anti-inflammatory drugs
- Medications with anticholinergic side effects
- Polypharmacy

Radiation induced

- Whole body
- Upper abdominal

Biochemical causes

- Renal or liver impairment or failure
- Hypercalcemia
- Hyponatremia
- Infection
- Tumor toxins

Gastrointestinal causes

- Impaired GI motility
- Gastrointestinal myopathies
- Gastrointestinal neuropathies
- Intestinal obstruction
- Constipation
- Hyperacidity
- Gastroesophageal reflux disease

Psychological causes

- Anxiety
- Depression
- Anticipatory (before treatment)

Neurologic causes

- Increased intracranial pressure
- Meningeal irritation
- Metastasis
- Stimulation of vestibular nerve

Myocardial dysfunction

- Ischemia
- Congestive heart failure

---

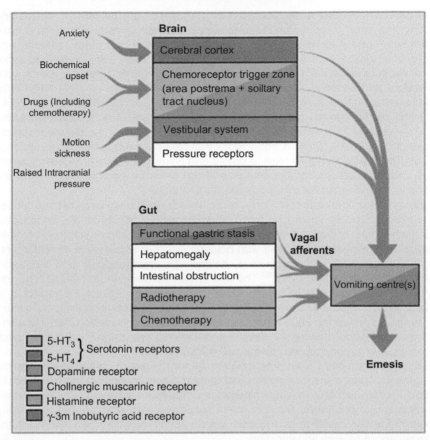

**Fig. 1.** The emetic process: pathways of emesis and the neurotransmitters involved. (*From* Baines MJ. Nausea, vomiting and intestinal obstruction. BMJ 1997;315:1148; with permission.)

improved symptom control with use of ondansetron. The data showed that ondansetron was more effective in controlling nausea and vomiting than metoclopramide, both objectively ($2.80 \pm 0.422$ vs $1.40 \pm 0.699$, $P<.005$) and subjectively ($4.10 \pm 0.738$ vs $2.10 \pm 0.994$, $P<.005$).[43]

Steroids also are commonly used for nausea and vomiting, primarily in patients with CINV. The mechanism of action of steroids for preventing nausea and vomiting is still not completely understood. It mainly involves reduction in the release of serotonin or activation of corticosteroid receptors in the central nervous system (CNS).[44] Dexamethasone is used primarily in the prevention of acute CINV when a highly emetogenic chemotherapeutic regimen is used. Steroid doses used for nausea and vomiting should be reviewed with a palliative care specialist. The side effects of steroids depend on the dose and duration of therapy; these side effects include insomnia and agitation.[45] For clinicians interested in obtaining further information on CINV, the NCCN Guidelines provide up-to-date, evidenced-based recommendations for acute nausea and vomiting associated with chemotherapy.

Metoclopramide is the most widely prescribed antiemetic for uncontrolled chronic nausea of advanced cancer.[46] It is a D2 receptor antagonist that reverses the dopaminergic brake in the upper gut only, leading to increased gastric emptying.[47] However, there are limited data available regarding its effectiveness in the advanced cancer population.[46]

Haloperidol is another antiemetic used by palliative care providers for nausea and vomiting; however, there are no RCTs to support its use. A review of multiple case reports has found it to be beneficial for patients.[48] In a recent study, patients with a score of at least 1 on a 4-point nausea and vomiting scale were prescribed either oral or subcutaneous haloperidol. On day 2, 33 of 42 (79%) treated patients were assessable for response. Eight (24%; 95% confidence interval [CI], 10%–39%) patients had complete control of nausea and vomiting, and 12 (36%; 95% CI, 20%–53%) had partial control, giving an overall response rate of 61% (95% CI, 44%–77%). On day 5, 23 patients were assessable for response. The overall response rate was 17 of 23 (74%; 95% CI, 56%–92%). If all patients are included in the response analysis, the overall response rates at days 2 and 5 were 47% and 40%, respectively. These data showed a favorable response in the palliative care population and the study may provide pilot data for future research studies.[49]

Although prescribed less commonly, cannabinoids have been used to treat nausea and vomiting (usually in an oral form). A systematic analysis of 30 randomized, comparative trials of cannabinoids (oral nabilone, 16 trials; oral dronabinol, 11 trials; intramuscular levonatrodol, 1 trial) with placebo or other antiemetics (prochlorperazine, metoclopramide, chlorpromazine, haloperidol, domperidone, and alizapride) confirmed their efficacy in CINV.[50] The use of cannabinoids in an inhaled form has been reported by patients to control nausea and vomiting. Clinician prescribing of cannabinoids for medical use varies from state to state. Providers seeking more information should review the 2003 Institute of Medicine consensus report, *Marijuana and Medicine: Assessing the Science Base,*[51] and the Web site: http://medicalmarijuana. procon.org,/view.resource.php?resourceID=000140.

Recent research has shown promising results for the use of olanzapine for nausea and vomiting. Olanzapine is currently used to treat mania and schizophrenia. It blocks multiple neurotransmitter (ie, dopaminergic, serotonergic, adrenergic, histaminergic, and muscarinic) receptors. Most of these receptors also are involved in causing emesis.[52] Further research is required before recommending olanzapine for the management of nausea and vomiting.

If symptoms are refractory despite adequate dosing and around-the-clock prophylactic administration, an empirical trial combining several therapies to block multiple emetic pathways should be attempted. Often, oral administration of medication is not feasible and alternative routes of administration, such as rectal suppositories, subcutaneous infusions, and orally dissolvable tablets, should be considered.[38] When complex symptom management issues arise, the primary care clinician should obtain further guidance through consultation with a palliative care specialist.

Clinicians should be aware that patients in palliative care may present with mechanical obstruction resulting in symptoms of nausea and vomiting, and that these symptoms may worsen with prokinetic agents.[35] Bowel obstruction produces refractory nausea with continuous abdominal pain, punctuated by colicky episodes that are relieved temporarily by vomiting. Opioid management is commonly used, but may lead to more nausea and vomiting. Opioid-sparing therapy with ketorolac or corticosteroids may prevent a partial obstruction from becoming complete with the influence of opioids.[35] Once a patient has a complete obstruction and is not a candidate for surgery, nasogastric pharmacologic management without either nasogastric tube or gastric tube suctioning should be attempted.[35] The success of this approach depends on the level of obstruction. A gastrostomy tube for decompression is another option for obstruction. The clinician may need to add an opioid regimen for abdominal pain.

**Table 4** details receptor sites, medications used, dosages, adverse effects, and costs of commonly used antiemetics.

**Table 4**
**Antiemetics**

| Antiemetic | Trade Name | Presumed Primary Receptor Site of Action | Dosage/Route | Major Adverse Effects | Cost ($)[a] |
|---|---|---|---|---|---|
| Metoclopramide | Reglan | $D_2$ (primarily in GI tract) or 5-$HT_3$ (only at high doses) | 5–20 mg orally or subcutaneously or IV before every meal and before bed | Dystonia, akathisia, esophageal spasm, and colic in GI tract obstruction | 1.21 per 10-mg pill |
| Haloperidol | Haldol | $D_2$ (primarily in CTZ) | 0.5–4 mg orally or subcutaneously or IV every 6 h | Dystonia and akathisia | 0.10 per 1-mg pill |
| Prochlorperazine | Compazine | $D_2$ (primarily in CTZ) | 5–10 mg orally or IV every 6 h or 25 mg rectally every 6 h | Dystonia, akathisia, and sedation | 0.43 per 10-mg pill |
| Chlorpromazine | Thorazine | $D_2$ (primarily in CTZ) | 10–25 mg Orally every 4 h, 25–50 mg IM or IV every 4 h, or 50–100 mg rectally every 6 h | Dystonia, akathisia, sedation, and postural hypotension | 0.30 per 25-mg pill |
| Promethazine | Phenergan | $H_1$, muscarinic acetylcholine receptor, or $D_2$ (primarily in CTZ) | 12.5–25 mg orally or IV every 6 h or 25 mg rectally every 6 h | Dystonia, akathisia, and sedation | 0.39 per 25-mg pill |
| Diphenhydramine | Benadryl | $H_1$ | 25–50 mg orally or IV or subcutaneously every 6 h | Sedation, dry mouth, and urinary retention | 0.13 per 25-mg pill |
| Scopolamine | Transderm scop | Muscarinic acetylcholine receptor | 1.5 mg transdermal patch every 3 d | Dry mouth, blurred vision, ileus, urinary retention, and confusion | 7.80 per patch |
| Hyoscyamine | Levsin | Muscarinic acetylcholine receptor | 0.125–0.25 mg sublingually or orally every 4 h or 0.25–0.5 mg subcutaneously or IV every 4 h | Dry mouth, blurred vision, ileus, urinary retention, and confusion | 0.82 per 0.125-mg tablet |
| Ondansetron[b] | Zofran | 5-$HT_3$ | 4–8 mg orally by pill or dissolvable tablet or IV every 4–8 h | Headache, fatigue, and constipation | 38.93 per 8-mg tablet |
| Mirtazapine | Remeron | 5-$HT_3$ | 15–45 mg Orally every night | Somnolence at low dose, dry mouth, and increased appetite | 3.20 per 15-mg tablet |

*Abbreviations:* CTZ, chemoreceptor trigger zone; $D_2$, dopamine type 2 receptor; GI, gastrointestinal; $H_1$, histamine type 1 receptor; IM, intramuscular; IV, intravenous; 5-$HT_3$, 5-hydroxytryptamine type 3 receptor.

[a] Cost per pill was calculated from prices listed on epocrates.com.

[b] Ondansetron is included as an example of 5-$HT_3$ antagonists because it was the first agent of this class and has been adopted in many hospital formularies. Its inclusion is not meant to indicate superiority compared with other members of the class, such as dolasetron, granisetron, and palonosetron.

*Data from* Wood G, Shega JW, Lynch B, et al. Management of intractable nausea and vomiting in patients at the end of life. JAMA 2007;288(10):1202.

*Nonpharmacologic treatment*

**Acupressure** In a systematic review, one relevant study evaluated acupressure to relieve nausea and vomiting in 6 hospice patients (mean age 68 years; range 36–84 years), using an N-of-1 design. Each patient underwent 3 treatments in alternating sequence: acupressure wrist band (at the commonly accepted P6 acupoint), placebo wrist band, and no band. Each treatment condition lasted 4 or 8 hours. No significant differences were found among the treatments, although the sample size was small and 2 patients had no nausea during the treatment period.

No large-scale trials of acupressure have been done in terminally ill patients with nausea and vomiting that have not been associated with chemotherapy.[53]

# CONSTIPATION
## *Definition*

Constipation is defined as a decrease in the passage of formed stool, and is characterized by stools that are hard and difficult to pass. Constipation may be accompanied by abdominal pain, nausea, vomiting, abdominal distention, loss of appetite, and headache.[54] It is a common problem in patients with advanced illness that can generate a considerable level of suffering for patients from both unpleasant physical symptoms and psychological preoccupations that may arise.[55]

## *Prevalence*

Constipation is common in patients receiving palliative care, and occurs in approximately half of all patients with advanced cancer, 63% of the elderly in hospitals, 22% of the elderly in the home, and nearly 95% of patients receiving opioids.[56]

## *Pathophysiology*

The causes of constipation may be categorized as[55]:

1. Lifestyle-related or primary constipation: associated with a low-fiber diet, decreased fluid intake, and inactivity, which result in a reduction in abdominal muscle activity and stimulation, producing a sluggish bowel (also referred to as slow-transit constipation). A slowing of physical activity also is a cause of primary constipation. In addition, environmental factors or a lack of privacy, or both, may inhibit bowel function and predispose debilitated patients to constipation.
2. Disease-related or secondary constipation: arises from a pathologic condition and includes a variety of disease processes, such as abdominal tumor, anal fissure, anterior mucosal prolapse, colitis, diabetes, diverticular disease, hypercalcemia, hemorrhoids, hernia, hypokalemia, hypothyroidism, and rectocele (**Box 2**).[57]
3. Drug-induced constipation: can result from a wide range of drugs, including opioids, anticholinergics, tricyclic antidepressants, antipsychotics, anticonvulsants, iron or calcium supplements, and antacids (calcium and aluminum compounds).

## *Assessment*

An assessment of patients with constipation includes taking a thorough history of the patient's current and premorbid bowel pattern, diet changes, and medications. The physical examination should include the presence or absence of bowel sounds, flatus, or abdominal distention. In patients with colostomies, the clinician should assess for increase or decrease in passage of stool. A digital rectal examination may be necessary to rule out fecal impaction, tumor, anal fissure, or hemorrhoids, or for those patients with new rectal discharge. The clinician should be aware that, in patients with neutropenia or thrombocytopenia, a rectal examination should only be done if

---

**Box 2**
**Causes of secondary constipation**

Endocrine and metabolic diseases

    Diabetes mellitus

    Hypercalcemia

    Hyperparathyroidism

    Hypothyroidism

    Uremia

Myopathic conditions

    Amyloidosis

    Myotonic dystrophy

    Scleroderma

Neurologic diseases

    Autonomic neuropathy

    Cerebrovascular disease

    Hirschsprung disease

    Multiple sclerosis

    Parkinson disease

    Spinal cord injury, tumors

Psychological conditions

    Anxiety

    Depression

    Somatization

Structural abnormalities

    Anal fissures, strictures, hemorrhoids

    Colonic strictures

    Inflammatory bowel disease

    Obstructive colonic mass lesions

    Rectal prolapse or rectocele

Other

    Irritable bowel syndrome

    Pregnancy

*Data from* Hsieh C. Treatment of constipation in older adults. Am Fam Physician 2005;72(11): 2277–84.

---

warranted.[3] A review of imaging studies and blood work may be appropriate based on the clinical condition of the patient and may be useful to rule out bowel obstruction, the amount of stool in the bowel, or electrolyte abnormalities. A consensus guideline from the American Gastroenterological Association also recommends that most patients with constipation have tests for a complete blood count and serum glucose, thyroid stimulating hormone, calcium, and creatinine levels.[58] The clinician working with patients with advanced cancer should recognize that sudden changes in bowel habits and motor weakness may indicate spinal cord compression; this is considered an oncologic emergency.[3] Clinicians should review the NCCN Practice Guidelines, which suggest that the evaluation of underlying abnormalities should be dictated by the patient's life expectancy.[40]

Although a diagnosis of constipation may be established with diagnostic tests, such as abdominal radiographs, assessing subjective symptoms by talking to the patient is the most efficient and cost-effective way to determine the presence of this common problem.[59,60]

## Treatment

Prevention and management of primary constipation usually includes increasing fluid and fiber intake; encouragement of physical activities; planning for regular bowel hygiene; and measures to remove factors that may inhibit defecation, such as lack of privacy and poor positioning. For further information on prevention, the clinician should review the National Cancer Institute PDQ on gastrointestinal complications (http://www.cancer.gov/cancertopics/pdq/supportivecare/gastrointestinalcomplications/HealthProfessional/page3).

### Pharmacologic treatment

**Laxatives** Although effective palliative care includes aggressive symptom management with the goal of comfort, a preventive approach to symptom management also is needed. In the case of constipation, such a preventive regimen involves the dose of laxatives being titrated against the clinical effect.

Two recent Cochrane reviews have been published, one addressing the effectiveness of laxatives for the management of constipation in patients in palliative care,[55] and one more specific to those with neurogenic bowel conditions.[61] The first review included 4 randomized trials involving 280 patients in palliative care with constipation. Outcomes included patient-reported data measuring changes in stool frequency and ease in passing stools. All of the laxatives used in the trials were ineffective for a significant number of patients and some patients required multiple rescue laxatives, indicating the severity of the problem. The report concluded that there is a lack of evidence to support the use of one laxative, or combinations of laxatives, rather than another.[55]

The second review examined the effectiveness of management strategies for fecal incontinence and constipation in people with neurologic diseases affecting the CNS. This review is relevant to patients with chronic and advanced illness. The 10 randomized trials that were identified all had small sample sizes and were mostly of poor quality. Four trials studied the effect of oral medications for constipation. Results indicated that cisapride did not seem to be clinically useful in people with spinal cord injuries (3 trials); psyllium was linked with increased stool frequency in people with Parkinson disease but not with changed colonic transit time (1 trial); and prucalopride did not prove beneficial in this patient group (1 study). One study of rectal preparations used to initiate defecation showed that some produced faster results than others, and 1 trial showed that different time schedules for administration of rectal medication produced different bowel responses. Another trial noted that mechanical evacuation (eg, digital stimulation, manual evacuation, abdominal massage, rectal irrigation) may be more effective than oral or rectal medication.[61]

**Methylnaltrexone** In one study,[62] subcutaneous (SC) methylnaltrexone induced laxation in 133 patients with advanced illness and opioid-induced constipation lasting more than 3 days. In this study, patients were randomly assigned to receive SC methylnaltrexone (at a dose of 0.15 mg per kilogram of body weight) or placebo every other day for 2 weeks. Forty-eight percent of patients in the methylnaltrexone group had laxation within 4 hours after the first study dose, compared with 15% in the placebo group; and 52% had laxation without the use of a rescue laxative within 4 hours after 2 or more of the first 4 doses, compared with 8% in the placebo group. The primary clinician should be aware that this management strategy should be considered only after consultation with a palliative care specialist.

**Table 5**[57] lists common medications used for the treatment of constipation.

### Nonpharmacologic treatment

**Abdominal massage** In 1999, Ernst[63] published a systematic review of the evidence to support abdominal massage for chronic constipation. In this study, 4 trials, with a total of 54 patients with chronic constipation, were reviewed. The control groups received an active treatment phase of abdominal massage compared with a control phase of no massage or treatment with laxatives. The outcomes included total GI/colonic transit time, stool frequency, number of days with bowel movements, episodes of fecal incontinence, number of enemas given, stool consistency, and patient well-being. The 4 trials included 1 randomized study of 32 patients: no significant differences were shown in outcomes (GI transit time, stool frequency and consistency, number of enemas given, patient well-being) between the different treatment phases (3-week run-in, regular massage for 7 weeks, 1 week wash-out, laxatives for 7 weeks). Two additional trials of 21 patients found no significant difference between massage and control phases for total colonic transit time and stool frequency, although 1 reported massage therapy to cause significant improvement in the number of days with bowel movements, episodes of fecal incontinence, and number of enemas given. The primary care clinician should be aware that there is no sound scientific evidence to determine whether massage is effective in patients with chronic constipation.

**Caregiver education** Caregiver education has been recognized as a means to aid patients with advanced illness manage the symptom of constipation. In one large RCT performed by McMillan and Small,[60] caregivers of patients with advanced-stage cancer in hospice (n = 329) were taught symptom assessment and management, including that of constipation. Caregiver involvement in symptom management significantly alleviated patients' symptom burden, although constipation intensity remained unchanged.

Suggestions for the patient's treatment plan may include the following[64]:

- Keep a record of all bowel movements
- Increase fluid intake by drinking eight 240-mL glasses of fluid each day (patients who have kidney or heart disease may need to limit fluid intake)
- Exercise regularly, including abdominal exercises in bed or moving from the bed to chair if the patient cannot walk
- Increase the amount of dietary fiber by eating more fruits (raisins, prunes, peaches, and apples), vegetables (squash, broccoli, carrots, and celery), and whole-grain cereals, whole-grain breads, and bran. Patients must drink more fluids when increasing dietary fiber or they may become constipated
- Patients who have had a bowel obstruction or have undergone bowel surgery (eg, a colostomy) should not eat a high-fiber diet.

- Drink a warm or hot drink about half an hour before the patient's usual time for a bowel movement
- Provide privacy and quiet time when the patient needs to have a bowel movement
- Help the patient to the toilet or provide a bedside commode instead of a bedpan
- Take only medications prescribed by the doctor
- Do not use suppositories or enemas unless ordered by the doctor. In some patients with cancer, these treatments may lead to bleeding, infection, or other harmful side effects.

**Table 5**
**Common medications for treatment of chronic constipation**

| Agent | Formula/Strength | Adult Dosage |
|---|---|---|
| **Bulk laxatives** | | |
| Methylcellulose (Citrucel) | Powder: 2 g (mix with 240 mL liquid) Tablets: 500 mg (take with 240 mL liquid) | 1–3 times daily 2 tablets up to 6 times daily |
| Polycarbophil (Fibercon) | Tablets: 625 mg | 2 tablets 1–4 times daily |
| Psyllium (Metamucil) | Powder: 3.4 g (mix with 240 mL liquid) | 1–4 times daily |
| **Stool softeners** | | |
| Docusate calcium (Surfak) | Capsules: 240 mg | Once daily |
| Docusate sodium (Colace) | Capsules: 50 or 100 mg Liquid: 150 mg per 15 mL Syrup: 60 mg per 15 mL | 50–300 mg[a] |
| **Osmotic Laxatives** | | |
| Lactulose | Liquid: 10 g per 15 mL | 15–60 mL daily[a] |
| Magnesium citrate | Liquid: 296 mL per bottle | 0.5–1 bottle per day |
| Magnesium hydroxide (Milk of Magnesia) | Liquid: 400 mg per 5 mL | 30–60 mL once daily[a] |
| Polyethylene glycol 3350 (Miralax) | Powder: 17 g (mix with 240 mL liquid) | Once daily |
| Sodium biphosphate (Phospho-Soda) | Liquid: 45 mL, 90 mL (mix with 120 mL water, then follow with 240 mL water) | 20–45 mL daily |
| Sorbitol | Liquid: 480 mL | 30–150 mL daily |
| **Stimulant Laxatives** | | |
| Bisacodyl (Dulcolax) | Tablets: 5 mg | 5–15 mg daily |
| Cascara sagrada | Liquid: 120 mL | 5 mL once daily |
| — | Tablets: 325 mg | 1 tablet daily |
| Castor oil | Liquid: 60 mL | 15–60 mL once daily[a] |
| Senna (Senokot) | Tablets: 8.6 mg | 2 or 4 tablets once or twice daily |
| **Prokinetic Agents** | | |
| Tegaserod (Zelnorm) | Tablets: 2 mg, 6 mg | Two times daily[b] |

[a] May be taken in divided doses.
[b] Used for constipation related to irritable bowel syndrome in women.
   *Data from* Hsieh C. Treatment of constipation in older adults. Am Fam Physician 2005;72(11): 2277–84.

## SUMMARY

The burden of gastrointestinal symptoms contributes to patient suffering throughout the course of advanced illness or cancer. It is important to address symptom control throughout the disease trajectory, and especially at the end of life. The primary care clinician must recognize these symptoms early, provide ongoing assessment, and keep abreast of evidenced-based management strategies, including valid clinical protocols. Open communication with patients and families can minimize the effects of disease progression and help to aggressively treat symptoms that affect quality of life. Primary care clinicians also should be aware of the palliative care specialists in their community and collaborate with these specialists on cases that are complex.

## APPENDIX: WEB RESOURCES FOR END-OF-LIFE CARE

End-of-Life/Palliative Education Resource Center (EPERC)
http://www.eperc.mcw.edu/EPERC/FastFactsIndex
Online resource that includes educational resources for end-of-life care.

The Center to Advance Palliative Care (CAPC)
http://www.capc.org
Online site that provides health care professionals with the tools, training, and technical assistance necessary to start and sustain successful palliative care programs in hospitals and other health care settings.

National Cancer Institute (NCI) Supportive Care
http://www.cancer.gov/cancertopics/pdq/supportivecare
Online site with educational resources for patients and health professionals. Various topics related to palliative care can be accessed through this site, including nausea and vomiting.

Department of Pain Medicine and Palliative Care, Beth Israel Medical Center, New York City
http://www.stoppain.org/main_site/content/about.asp
Online site that provides information for patients, families, caregivers, and health professionals on common topics in palliative care. The site also provides information on referrals for caregivers in need of assistance.

International Association of Hospice and Palliative Care
http://www.hospicecare.com/resources/
Online site that provides information on patient assessment tools, symptom management guidelines, and various other resources for patients, families, and health professionals.

## REFERENCES

1. Payne C, Martin S, Wiffen PJ. Interventions for fatigue and weight loss in adults with advanced progressive illness (Protocol). Cochrane Database Syst Rev 2010;3:CD008427. Accessed July 4, 2010.
2. Muscaritoli M, Anker SD. Consensus definition of sarcopenia, cachexia and pre-cachexia: joint document elaborated by Special Interest Group (SIG) "Cachexia-Anorexia in Chronic Wasting Diseases" and "Nutrition in Geriatrics." Clin Nutr 2010;29:154–9.
3. Reville B, Axelrod D, Maury R. Palliative care for the cancer patient. Prim Care 2009;36(4):781–810.
4. Laviano A, Meguid MM, Rossi-Fanelli F. Cancer anorexia: clinical implications, pathogenesis, and therapeutic strategies. Lancet Oncol 2003;4:686–94.

5. Teunissen SC, Wesker W, Kruitwagen C, et al. Symptom prevalence in patients with incurable cancer: a systematic review. J Pain Symptom Manage 2007; 34(1):94–104.
6. Ramos EJB, Suzuki S, Marks D, et al. Cancer anorexia-cachexia syndrome: cytokines and neuropeptides. Curr Opin Clin Nutr Metab Care 2004;7:427–34.
7. Dalal S, Del Fabbro E, Bruera E. Symptom control in palliative care–Part I: oncology as a paradigmatic example. J Palliat Med 2006;9(2):391–408.
8. Chance WT, Balasubramaniam A, Thompson H. Hypothalamic concentration and release of neuropeptide Y into microdialysates is reduced in anorectic tumor-bearing rats. Life Sci 1994;54:1869–74.
9. Inui A. Cancer anorexia-cachexia syndrome: current issues in research and management. CA Cancer J Clin 2002;52(2):72–91.
10. Marinella MA. Diagnosis and management of hiccups in the patient with advanced cancer. J Support Oncol 2009;7:122–7, 130.
11. Bruera E, Kuehn N, Miller MJ, et al. The Edmonton Symptom Assessment System (ESAS): a simple method for the assessment of palliative care patients. J Palliat Care 1991;7:6–9.
12. Portenoy RK, Thaler HT, Kornblith AB, et al. The Memorial Symptom Assessment Scale: an instrument for the evaluation of symptom prevalence, characteristics, and distress. Eur J Cancer Am 1994;30(9):1326–36.
13. Tisdale MJ. Biology of cachexia. J Natl Cancer Inst 1997;89:1763–73.
14. Chang VT, Xia Q, Kasimis B. The Functional Assessment of Anorexia/Cachexia Therapy (FAACT) appetite scale in veteran cancer patients. J Support Oncol 2005;3(5):377–82.
15. Brown JK. A systematic review of the evidence on symptom management of cancer-related anorexia and cachexia. Oncol Nurs Forum 2002;29(3):517–32.
16. Maltoni M, Nanni O, Pirovano M. Successful validation of the Palliative Prognostic Score in terminally ill cancer patients. J Pain Symptom Manage 1999; 17:240–7.
17. Akkermans LM, Smout AJPM. What are the actions of prokinetic agents? 1994. Available at: http://www.hon.ch/OESO/books/Vol_3_Eso_Mucosa/Articles/ART094.HTML. Accessed August 8, 2010.
18. Fraser RJ, Bryant L. Current and future therapeutic prokinetic therapy to improve enteral feed intolerance in the ICU. Nutr Clin Pract 2010;25:26–31.
19. Policzer J, Sobel J. Anorexia-cachexia in management of selected nonpain symptoms of life limiting illness. Glenview (IL): American Academy of Hospice and Palliative Medicine; 2008.
20. Bruera E, Strasser F. Update on anorexia and cachexia. Hematol Oncol Clin North Am 2002;16:589–617.
21. Antoun S, Birdsell L, Sawyer MB, et al. Association of skeletal muscle wasting with treatment with sorafenib in patients with advanced renal cell carcinoma: results from a placebo-controlled study. J Clin Oncol 2010;28:1054–60.
22. Boddert MS, Gerritsen WR, Pinedo HM. On our way to targeted therapy for cachexia in cancer? Curr Opin Oncol 2006;18:335–40.
23. Strasser F. The silent symptom early satiety: a forerunner of distinct phenotypes of anorexia/cachexia syndromes. Support Care Cancer 2006;14(7):689–92.
24. Prado CM, Lieffers JR, McCargar LJ, et al. Prevalence and clinical implications of sarcopenic obesity in patients with solid tumours of the respiratory and gastrointestinal tracts: a population-based study. Lancet Oncol 2008;9:629–35.
25. Esper P, Heidrich D. Symptom clusters in advanced illness. Semin Oncol Nurs 2005;21(1):20–8.

26. Tsai JS, Wu CH, Chiu TY, et al. Significance of symptom clustering in palliative care of advanced cancer patients. J Pain Symptom Manage 2010;39(4):655–62.
27. Berenstein G, Ortiz Z. Megestrol acetate for treatment of anorexia-cachexia syndrome. Cochrane Database Syst Rev 2005;2:CD004310.
28. Riechelmann RP, Burman D, Tannock IF, et al. Phase II trial of mirtazapine for cancer-related cachexia and anorexia. Am J Hosp Palliat Care 2010;27:106–10.
29. Lundholm K, Gunnebo L, Korner U, et al. Effects by daily long term provision of ghrelin to unselected weight-losing cancer patients. Cancer 2010;116:2044–52.
30. Garcia JM, Cata JP, Dougherty PM, et al. Ghrelin prevents cisplatin-induced mechanical hyperalgesia and cachexia. Endocrinology 2008;149(2):455–60.
31. Baines MJ. Nausea, vomiting and intestinal obstruction. BMJ 1997;315:1148–50.
32. Seim I, Amorim L, Walpole C, et al. Ghrelin gene-related peptides: multifunctional endocrine/autocrine modulators in health and disease. Clin Exp Pharmacol Physiol 2010;37:125–31.
33. Clark AL, Anker SD. Body mass, chronic heart failure, surgery and survival. J Heart Lung Transplant 2010;29:261–4.
34. Read JA, Beale PJ, Volker DH, et al. Nutrition intervention using an eicosapentaenoic acid (EPA)-containing supplement in patients with advanced colorectal cancer: effects on nutritional and inflammatory status: a phase II trial. Support Care Cancer 2007;15:301–7.
35. Davis M, Walsh D. Treatment of nausea and vomiting in advanced cancer. Support Care Cancer 2000;8:444–52.
36. Rhodes VA, Watson PM, Johnson MH, et al. Patterns of nausea, vomiting and distress in patients receiving antineoplastic drug protocols. Oncol Nurs Forum 1987;14:35–44.
37. Saxby C, Ackroyd R, Callin S, et al. How should we measure emesis in palliative care? Palliat Med 2007;21:369–83.
38. Wood GJ, Shega JW, Lynch B, et al. Management of intractable nausea and vomiting in patients at the end of life: "I was feeling nauseous all of the time nothing was working". JAMA 2007;298(10):1196–207.
39. Solano JP, Gomes B, Higginson IJ. A comparison of symptom prevalence in far advanced cancer, AIDS, heart failure, chronic obstructive pulmonary disease, and renal disease. J Pain Symptom Manage 2006;31:58–69.
40. National Comprehensive Cancer Network. Clinical practice guidelines in oncology. Antiemesis. Available at: http://www.nccn.org/professionals/physician_gls/PDF/antiemesis.pdf. Accessed July 14, 2010.
41. Kris MG, Hesketh PJ, Sommerfield MR, et al. American Society of Clinical Oncology guideline for antiemetics in oncology: update 2006. J Clin Oncol 2006;24(18):2932–47.
42. Ewing G, Todd C, Rogers M, et al. Validation of a symptom measure suitable for use among palliative care patients in the community: CAMPAS-R. J Pain Symptom Manage 2004;27:287–99.
43. Ljutić D, Perković D, Rumboldt Z, et al. Comparison of ondansetron with metoclopramide in the symptomatic relief of uremia-induced nausea and vomiting. Kidney Blood Press Res 2002;25(1):61–4.
44. Lohr L. Chemotherapy-induced nausea and vomiting. Cancer J 2008;14(2):85–93.
45. Jordan K, Schmoll HJ, Aapro MS. Comparative activity of antiemetic drugs. Crit Rev Oncol Hematol 2007;61(2):162–75.
46. Clark K, Agar MR, Currow D. Metoclopramide for chronic nausea in adult palliative care patients with advanced cancer. Cochrane Database Syst Rev 2010;2:CD008387.

47. Tonini M, Cipollina L, Poluzzi E, et al. Review article: clinical implications of enteric and central D2 receptor blockade by antidopaminergic gastrointestinal prokinetics. Aliment Pharmacol Ther 2004;19:373–90.

48. Perkins P, Dorman S. Haloperidol for the treatment of nausea and vomiting in palliative care patients. Cochrane Database Syst Rev 2009;2:CD006271. Available at: http://onlinelibrary.wiley.com.ezproxy.cul.columbia.edu/o/cochrane/clsysrev/articles/CD006271/frame.html. Accessed June 30, 2010.

49. Hardy JR, O'Shea A, White C, et al. The efficacy of haloperidol in the management of nausea and vomiting in patients with cancer. J Pain Symptom Manage 2010;40(1):111–6.

50. Tramer MR, Carroll D, Campbell FA, et al. Cannabinoids for control of chemotherapy-induced nausea and vomiting: quantitative systematic review. BMJ 2001;323:16–21.

51. Institute of Medicine. In: Joy JE, Watson SJ Jr, Benson JA Jr, editors. Marijuana and medicine: assessing the science base. Washington, DC: National Academies Press; 2003.

52. Licup N, Baumrucker S. Olanzapine for nausea and vomiting. Am J Hosp Palliat Care 2010;27(6):432–4.

53. Pan CX, Morrison RS, Ness J, et al. Complementary and alternative medicine in the management of pain, dyspnea, and nausea and vomiting near the end of life. A systematic review. J Pain Symptom Manage 2000;20(5):374–87.

54. Oncology Nursing Society. Definition of constipation. Available at: http://www.ons.org/Research/NursingSensitive/Summaries/media/ons/docs/research/summaries/constipation/definitions.pdf. Accessed March 3, 2010.

55. Miles C, Fellowes D, Goodman ML, et al. Laxatives for the management of constipation in palliative care patients. Cochrane Database Syst Rev 2006;4:CD003448.

56. Hartford Institute for Geriatric Nursing. Constipation in palliative care. Available at: http://consultgerirn.org/topics/palliative_care/want_to_know_more#item_8. Accessed October 28, 2009.

57. Hsieh C. Treatment of constipation in older adults. Am Fam Physician 2005;72(11):2277–84.

58. Locke GR III, Pemberton JH, Phillips SF. American Gastroenterological Association Medical Position Statement: guidelines on constipation. Gastroenterology 2000;119:1761–6.

59. Chambers K, McMillan SC. Measuring bowel elimination. In: Frank-Stromberg M, Olsen S, editors. Instruments for clinical healthcare research. 3rd edition. Sudbury (MA): Jones and Bartlett; 2004. p. 487–97.

60. McMillan SC, Small BJ. Using the COPE intervention for family caregivers to improve symptoms of hospice homecare patients: a clinical trial. Oncol Nurs Forum 2007;34(2):313–21.

61. Coggrave M, Wiesel P, Norton CC. Management of faecal incontinence and constipation in adults with central neurological diseases. Cochrane Database Syst Rev 2006;2:CD002115.

62. Thomas J, Karver S, Cooney GA, et al. Methylnaltrexone for opioid-induced constipation in advanced illness. N Engl J Med 2008;358(22):2332–43.

63. Ernst E. Abdominal massage for chronic constipation: a systematic review of controlled clinical trials. Forsch Komplementarmed 1999;6:149–51.

64. National Cancer Institute. Gastrointestinal complications PDQ® (patient version). Available at: http://www.cancer.gov/cancertopics/pdq/supportivecare/gastrointestinalcomplications/Patient/page3. Accessed September 28, 2010.

# Management of End-Stage Dementia

David Lussier, MD[a,b,c,d],*, Marie-Andrée Bruneau, MD[a,e],
Juan Manuel Villalpando, MD[a,b]

**KEYWORDS**

• Dementia • Palliative care • Tube feeding • Alzheimer

The aging of the population is a worldwide phenomenon. In the United States, for example, the proportion of the population older than 65 years is expected to increase from 12.6% in 2010 to 19.3% in 2030, whereas the proportion older than 80 years is expected to increase from 3.7% to 5.1% in the same period.[1] This increased proportion of older persons in the population will largely be caused by a significant increase in life expectancy, which has increased from 65 years in 1942 to 77.7 years in 2005 (75.1 years for men and 80.2 years for women),[2] and is expected to increase to 79.5 years by 2020.[2]

However, increased life expectancy does not always correlate with increased healthy life expectancy. The prevalence of chronic diseases, often associated with disability, will also increase significantly. For example, in Great Britain in 2006, men and women could expect to live 14.6 and 17.7 years, respectively, with a limiting illness or disability (compared with 12.8 and 16 years in 1981).[3]

The aging of the population has a significant impact on palliative care, for various reasons. First, because the incidence of cancer is increasing with age, the incidence and prevalence of cancer has increased, and continues to increase steadily. The average age of patients at cancer diagnosis is also increasing. Given the presence of several comorbidities and higher frailty in older patients, the treatment of cancer in these patients is often more complex than in younger ones.[4] Thanks to better cancer treatments, the survival of older patients has also increased, which means that a higher

The authors have nothing to disclose.
[a] Institut universitaire de gériatrie de Montréal, 4565 Queen-Mary, Montreal, QC, Canada H3W 1W5
[b] Department of Medicine, University of Montreal, C.P. 6128, Succursale Centre-Ville, Montreal, QC, Canada H3C 3J7
[c] Division of Geriatric Medicine, McGill University, 1650 Cedar Avenue, Montreal, QC, Canada H3G 1A4
[d] Alan-Edwards Centre for Research on Pain, McGill University, Suite 3100, Genome Building, 740 Doctor Penfield Avenue, Montreal, QC, Canada H3A 1A4
[e] Department of Psychiatry, University of Montreal, C.P. 6128, Succursale Centre-Ville, Montreal, QC, Canada H3C 3J7
* Corresponding author.
*E-mail address:* david.lussier@mcgill.ca

Prim Care Clin Office Pract 38 (2011) 247–264
doi:10.1016/j.pop.2011.03.006
0095-4543/11/$ – see front matter © 2011 Elsevier Inc. All rights reserved.

number of older persons are living with cancer or cancer complications. Patients who do not respond to treatment and die from cancer often do so at an older age than previously, which can also make the treatment of their symptoms more difficult because of their comorbidities, functional disability, and polypharmacy. Second, an increasing number of older patients die from nonmalignant terminal diseases, an area in which research and knowledge are less developed than for malignant diseases.

## PREVALENCE AND CLINICAL PRESENTATION OF DEMENTIA

Dementia is an acquired syndrome characterized by a significant deterioration in an individual's usual cognitive abilities, which provokes a functional decline severe enough to interfere with his everyday life.[5] Although dementia is not exclusive to the geriatric population, its prevalence increases exponentially with age, going from only 1% at 60 years old to more than 20% at 85 years and older.[6] With the aging of the population, the number of patients with dementia is expected to keep rising.

There are many medical and neurologic conditions that can manifest as a dementia syndrome. The most frequent causes in the geriatric population are Alzheimer disease, accounting for about 60% of all cases, followed by vascular dementia and dementia with Lewy bodies. Mixed dementia, usually defined as the coexistence of Alzheimer disease and vascular dementia, is also recognized as a major cause of cognitive impairment in older patients.[7]

Table 1 presents the main characteristics of the different types of dementia. Alzheimer disease is a neurodegenerative disease manifested by an insidious onset and slow progression for many years.[8] Vascular dementia is the second most frequent cause of dementia in the elderly, causing 25% to 30% of all cognitive problems in this age group. It is not a disease by itself, but rather a heterogeneous group of entities caused by different vascular mechanisms (occlusion, hypoperfusion, or hemorrhage). In the elderly, two-thirds of all vascular dementias can be attributed to subcortical ischemic vascular dementia (SIVD).[9] This is a small-vessel, white matter disease caused by lacunar infarcts and/or leukoaraiosis caused by diffuse chronic ischemia of the white matter. SIVD tends to have an insidious onset seemingly unrelated to a stroke, and it tends to have a slowly progressive course. Dementia following multiple cortical infarcts or a single strategic lesion is not as prevalent as SIVD, and usually occurs in patients with multiple vascular risk factors. Dementia with Lewy bodies (DLB) Is a slowly progressive neurodegenerative disease. Less than 50% of patients with DLB present a severe neuroleptic sensitivity, presenting as a sudden exacerbation of parkinsonism, impaired consciousness, or a neuroleptic malignant syndrome. This reaction is seen both with typical or atypical antipsychotics, and it can be immediate or seen within the first weeks of either first exposure or dose increase. Careful consideration before prescribing this type of medication is therefore warranted.

Pharmacologic treatments of Alzheimer and Lewy body dementia mostly consist of cholinesterase inhibitors (donepezil, rivastigmine, galantamine), which can slow the deterioration of the cognition in patients with mild to moderate dementia, delaying progression for approximately 6 months when effective.[10] Memantine, an antagonist of the $N$-methyl-D-aspartate (NMDA) receptor, sometimes reduces symptoms in patients with more advanced disease.[10] Although cholinesterase inhibitors and memantine have also been reported to delay the progression of vascular dementia,[11] the mainstay of therapy is prevention of vascular disease by reducing risk factors.

Although the type of dementia is important to predict its clinical course and select the appropriate pharmacologic treatment, the final stages, which are mostly of interest

**Table 1**
Characteristics of different types of dementia

| Type of dementia | Alzheimer Disease | Subcortical Ischemic Vascular Dementia | Vascular Dementia Secondary to Multiple Cortical Infarcts or Single Strategic Lesion | Dementia with Lewy Bodies |
|---|---|---|---|---|
| | Cortical | Subcortical | Cortical | Cortical |
| Memory impairment | Early impairment of episodic memory, later impairment of semantic memory | Caused by difficulties in retrieving stored information | Variable, depending on localization of lesion | Episodic memory impairment less present in early stages, becomes evident as disease progresses |
| Main features | Language impairment, progressing to mutism<br>Disorientation<br>Visuospatial and object manipulation difficulties<br>Impaired object recognition<br>Executive dysfunction | Psychomotor slowing<br>Inattention<br>Dysexecutive syndrome | Heterogeneous, varying depending on number, localization and/or extension of lesions<br>Abrupt onset, within 3 mo of cerebrovascular event<br>Stepwise progression | One-year rule: less than 1 year between onset of parkinsonism and dementia (vs dementia related to Parkinson disease, which occurs in late stages)<br>Might progress more rapidly than Alzheimer disease<br>Early executive and visuoperceptual impairment<br>Fluctuations in attention, cognition, or alertness |
| Neuropsychiatric symptoms | Present in moderate to advanced disease | Frequent: depression, apathy, emotional lability | | Detailed and recurrent visual hallucinations<br>REM sleep behavior disorder (50%) |
| Neurologic signs | May be present in later stages: opposition rigidity, paratonias, parkinsonism, myoclonus, tonicoclonic seizures | Soft or subtle: magnetic gait, loss of postural reflexes, urinary incontinence | Evident focal neurologic signs, varying depending on localization of lesions | Spontaneous parkinsonism (75% of cases)<br>Autonomic dysfunction early in disease, with postural hypotension that can cause syncope and falls<br>Severe neuroleptic sensitivity (<50%) |

for palliative care, are similar for all types of dementia. Because pharmacologic treatment is not curative but simply delays the progression, dementia is now recognized as a progressive terminal illness.[12,13] The clinical course depends on the type of dementia. Most epidemiologic studies have reported a median length of survival of approximately 6 years after diagnosis for patients with Alzheimer disease,[14] possibly slightly less and more variable for Lewy body disease,[15] and of 41 to 60 months for vascular dementia.[16]

## ADVANCED DEMENTIA

Advanced, severe, or late-stage dementia is characterized by severe cognitive impairment, inability to ambulate, swallowing difficulties, anorexia, decreased oral intake, weight loss, bowel and bladder incontinence, and consequent loss of functional autonomy, progressing to the patient being totally bedridden, with severe sensory deprivation and complete dependence for care.[17] Severe dementia corresponds to a stage 6 or 7 on the Global Deterioration Scale[18] and to Mini Mental State Examination (MMSE) scores of less than 9; very severe, or end-stage, dementia is seen in patients with an MMSE score of less than 3.[19]

Cognitive evaluations in these late stages are cumbersome and difficult to interpret because these patients perform at extremely low levels on traditional instruments. The Severe Impairment Battery[20] or the shorter Test for Severe Impairment[21] may be more useful in these cases.

Although dementia predisposes to several illnesses, it is a contributory factor to death rather than the actual cause. For this reason, it is difficult to determine the incidence of dementia-related deaths. Pneumonia and other infectious diseases, as well as eating problems, are the most common causes of death for patients with advanced dementia and are negative prognostic factors for survival.[22] On average, patients with moderate to severe dementia (MMSE<18) survive less than 4 years.[23]

The most common and distressing symptoms, increasingly frequent as death approaches, are dyspnea, pain, pressure ulcers, aspiration, and agitation.[22,24] These symptoms are similar to those experienced by patients with cancer and other terminal illnesses.[24] For this reason, there has been increasing awareness that a palliative care approach is appropriate for patients with advanced dementia, and can benefit both the patients and their families.[12,25]

## APPROPRIATE LEVEL OF CARE AND INTERVENTIONS

As with all progressive and noncurable illnesses, advanced care planning should be encouraged for all patients with dementia, and should start when the diagnosis is made, to facilitate decision making at the end of life. Because most patients with advanced dementia are no longer able to express wishes and preferences for level of care, the presence of a living will should be sought. If such a document is not available, decisions on the level of care and appropriateness of various interventions should be made with substitute decision makers or family members. Whenever possible, these decisions should be made in advance, to avoid having to make the decision during a crisis, and to avoid unnecessary suffering caused by inappropriate interventions. When discussing level of care, one should always keep in mind that, in the presence of advanced dementia, the advisable goal of treatment is comfort care, avoiding life-prolonging therapies and those associated with the patient's discomfort. The goal should always be to relieve suffering, and optimize quality of life and quality of dying.[26]

In a recent prospective study, 40.7% of nursing home residents with advanced dementia underwent at least 1 burdensome intervention (hospitalization, emergency room visit, parenteral therapy, tube feeding) in their last 3 months of life.[22] Patients whose proxies had a better understanding of the poor prognosis of advanced dementia were less likely to undergo such an intervention.[22]

## Cardiopulmonary Resuscitation

The likelihood of a successful cardiopulmonary resuscitation in an older patient is extremely low (0.8%), except for specific cases such as a witnessed in-hospital arrest caused by ventricular fibrillation.[27] In a patient with advanced dementia, the chances of being discharged alive from the hospital following a cardiopulmonary arrest are almost nil. In the rare cases that it might happen, the experience would surely be traumatic for the patient and family, associated with unnecessary pain and suffering, and leaving the patient with additional disabilities. However, as many as 45% of patients with dementia residing in a nursing home are administered cardiopulmonary resuscitation at the time of their death, compared with only 15% of patients with cancer.[28] This difference is probably related to a lack of knowledge and recognition of dementia as a terminal illness by both health care professionals and family members. It is therefore important that the decision makers be appropriately informed before making a decision regarding cardiopulmonary resuscitation. In most cases, they should be advised against it, to avoid unnecessary suffering to the patient.[29]

## Feeding

Feeding always becomes a difficult problem in patients with severe dementia, for several reasons. They often develop dysphagia, leading to poor oral intake, malnutrition, and weight loss, as well as pneumonia caused by aspiration. Patients also sometimes refuse to open their mouth and to eat. Although reduced oral intake might be partly related to a lower basal metabolic rate and decreased caloric needs,[30] many family members and health care professionals have difficulties leaving a patient without nutrition, which often triggers the placement of a percutaneous endoscopic gastrostomy (PEG) feeding tube. Such artificial nutrition has been reported in up to 34% of severely demented patients residing in a nursing home.[31]

The decision to place or withhold a PEG feeding tube is difficult, both for the family and the health care team, especially if there are no advance directives on that issue.[31] Family members are often unable to forgo tube feeding, afraid that patients will suffer from hunger, or that withholding feeding represents a form of abandonment. Several studies, including a Cochrane review, have shown that tube feeding does not prevent malnutrition or pressure sores, and does not improve survival or functional status.[32–34] PEG tube placement can also be associated with postoperative complications (in 32%–70% of cases) and discomfort, either from the procedure, the presence of the tube, or the need for restraints to prevent patients from pulling the tube out.[32,34] For these reasons, withholding feeding tubes is often recommended.[32,35,36] Comfort feeding is often more appropriate, using careful hand feeding when the patient agrees to open his/her mouth and shows no signs of distress, aiming to maximize comfort rather than maximize oral intake.[37] A tube feeding decision aid has been developed to help families make the decision regarding tube feeding (**Box 1**).[38]

## Hydration

The decision to use or withhold parenteral hydration in patients who are unable to maintain adequate oral hydration is as challenging as the decision on feeding tubes. When making this decision, one should be aware of the difference between dehydration and

---

**Box 1**
**Tube feeding decision aid**

Information to be provided to the resident and family should include:

- Common causes of eating and swallowing problems in older persons
- Technical considerations regarding the placement and use of PEG tubes
- Principles of substitute/proxy decision making
- Risks and benefits of tube feeding
- Option of supportive/comfort care
- Some considerations regarding future discontinuation of PEG tube (eg, when and how often will the need for the PEG tube be reviewed; who can request a review/discontinuation, and whether there is a process for this)

Steps to decision making include:

- Guiding residents and their families through what they have learned about PEG tubes
- How to apply this knowledge to the resident's preferences, personal values, and clinical situation
- What is the resident's situation?
- What would the resident want?
- How is the decision affecting the family?
- What questions need answering before the resident or family can make a fully informed decision?
- Who should decide about PEG placement?
- When should the PEG be disbanded?
- What is the resident's or the family's overall thoughts about the decision?

*Data from* Mitchell SL, Tetroe J, O'Connor AM. A decision aid for long-term tube feeding in cognitively impaired older persons. J Am Geriatr Soc 2001;49:313–6.

---

thirst. Dehydration refers to the loss of normal body water and manifests itself by dry skin and mucous membranes, thickened secretions, decreased urine output, postural hypotension, irritability, headaches, drowsiness, constipation, weight loss, and disorientation. Thirst is a symptom that usually does not respond to medical treatments, and is best treated by small amounts of fluid or ice chips, and keeping the resident's mouth and lips moist. There is currently no evidence that parenteral hydration can improve comfort or reduce symptoms associated with dehydration, such as pressure sores or constipation, in patients with end-stage cancer.[39,40] To our knowledge, there has been no study of parenteral hydration in patients with advanced dementia. Parenteral hydration, whether it is intravenous or subcutaneous, is associated with a risk of complications such as cellulitis at the site of catheter insertion, discomfort from catheter placement and presence, fluid overload, and need for restraints to maintain the catheter in place. Because of the lack of evidence for benefits of parenteral hydration, the decision on its use should be individualized and based on the patient's or family's wishes, as well as unique circumstances. For example, temporary hydration might be appropriate in the event of an acute illness such as diarrhea, vomiting, or infection. When decreased hydration is caused by patient's decreased oral intake, oral hydration can often be increased by using simple interventions and frequently encouraging the patient to drink small amounts of fluids when possible.[41,42]

## Acute Care Hospitalization

Admission to an acute care hospital or an emergency room can be detrimental to older patients, and even more so if demented. Complications of such an admission include delirium, falls, decreased oral intake, nosocomial infections, and iatrogenic complications (eg, urinary tract infection triggered by urinary catheterization). There is even scientific evidence that, rather than improving survival, transfer from a nursing home to an acute care hospital for the treatment of a pneumonia might increase the risk of mortality and functional deterioration in patients with advanced dementia,[43] as well as expose them to adverse consequences such as delirium and pressure ulcers.[28] Demented patients who die in an acute care hospital are also likely not to receive appropriate palliative care interventions.[44] For these reasons, risks and benefits should always be weighed when considering admitting a patient with advanced dementia to an acute care hospital, either from the community or a nursing home. The decision should be made in collaboration with a well-informed surrogate decision maker.

## Treatment of Acute Illnesses and Infections

The treatment of acute illnesses, such as cardiac events, pulmonary embolism, or infections, should always be done following an evaluation of the expected benefits, risks, and discomfort, and respecting the goals of care determined for the patient. An illness associated with discomfort should be treated to avoid suffering. A similar strategy should apply to cancer, with the decision to treat or not treat based on the likely consequences and discomfort of both options.

Pneumonia represents a particular challenge because it is common in patients with dementia because of a high prevalence of dysphagia, and might be responsible for up to 40% of deaths.[28] There is no consensus on the appropriateness of treating pneumonia in a patient with advanced dementia. Although some studies suggest that antibiotics do not improve survival or comfort,[45–48] others have shown better short-term survival in patients with more aggressive antibiotic therapy.[49] When successfully treated, a pneumonia has a high likelihood of recurrence given that the dysphagia will persist. Antibiotic therapy, even if effective, can be associated with adverse effects such as Clostridium difficile colitis, which causes added discomfort. Parenteral antibiotic therapy can also be uncomfortable for the patient, especially if requiring admission to an acute care hospital. There is a clear lack of scientific evidence in this area. The decision to treat or not to treat a pneumonia in a patient with advanced dementia should therefore be based on clinical judgment, which has been shown to be adequate in a high proportion of cases,[50] as well as on the patient's and surrogate decision-maker's wishes.

## Treatment of Chronic Diseases

The treatment of some chronic diseases might not be appropriate in patients with advanced dementia, because of limited life expectancy and consequent low long-term benefits of some therapy, such as treatment of dyslipidemia or osteoporosis. However, the decision to withhold a medication is often difficult to make, because of the lack of scientific evidence supporting one option or the other. A summary of the appropriateness of various medications, based on a recent literature review[51] and recommendations from a modified Delphi consensus panel,[52] is provided in **Box 2**.

## Specific Treatment of Dementia

As previously indicated, cholinesterase inhibitors have been shown to slow the deterioration of cognition in Alzheimer disease, Lewy body disease, and some cases of

**Box 2**
**Appropriateness of medication use in advanced dementia**

Always appropriate:

  Analgesics

  Antidiarrheals

  Antiemetics

  Laxatives

  Inhaled bronchodilators

  Anxiolytics

  Antiepileptics

  Expectorants

  Lubricating eye drops

  Pressure ulcer treatment

Sometimes appropriate:

  Proton pump inhibitors

  Histamine-2 receptor blockers

  Antihypertensives

  Anti-ischemic

  Diuretics

  Inhaled corticosteroids

  Antipsychotics

  Antidepressants

  Hypoglycemics

  Thyroid hormones

  Antithyroid

  Corticosteroids

  Colchicine and allopurinol

  Digoxin

Rarely appropriate:

  Antiandrogens

  Bisphosphonates

  Mineral and vitamin supplements

  Heparin

  Warfarin

  Appetite stimulants

  Bladder relaxants

Never appropriate:

  Lipid-lowering medications

  Antiplatelets excluding aspirin

  Antiestrogens

Sex hormones

Cytotoxic chemotherapy

Hormone antagonists

*Data from* Parsons C, Hughes CM, Passmore AP, et al. Withholding, discontinuing and withdrawing medications in dementia patients at the end of life: a neglected problem in the disadvantaged dying? Drugs Aging 2010;27:435–49, and Holmes HM, Sachs GA, Shega JW, et al. Integrating palliative medicine into the care of persons with advanced dementia: identifying appropriate medication use. J Am Geriatr Soc 2008;56:1306–11.

vascular dementia.[53] Memantine is effective and indicated in mild to moderate dementia.[53] There is much less evidence on the use of these disease-altering medications in advanced dementia. It is usually recommended that treatment should be continued as long as clinical benefit persists,[19,54] and should be stopped in the severe stage or when the cognitive status no longer corresponds to the approved indication (MMSE<10 for cholinesterase inhibitors, <3 for memantine). In a recently published survey, 80% of hospice medical directors surveyed recommend discontinuing cholinesterase inhibitors and memantine at the time of hospice enrolment.[55] However, approximately 30% have observed accelerated cognitive and functional decline or emergence of challenging behaviors with medication discontinuation. Family members are also frequently reluctant to discontinue these medications.[55]

## SYMPTOM MANAGEMENT

Symptom assessment is often difficult in patients with advanced dementia, because of severe cognitive impairment. Although self-reporting should be used as often as possible, behavioral observation and reports from staff or family members often have to be relied on. For this review, we only focus on issues that are more specific to patients with dementia compared with other types of terminal illnesses, including pain, depression, and agitation and other behavioral disturbances. Other symptoms common in those patients are shortness of breath and death rattle, constipation, and pressure sores. These symptoms should be managed using the same approach as for other patients in palliative care.

### Pain

Although pain complaints are less common in demented patients,[56] there is no evidence of decreased pain perception associated with dementia.[57] The problem is therefore underreporting of pain because of communication difficulties. When the presence of nonverbal pain behaviors or other indicators of pain (eg, osteoarthritis or another disease usually associated with pain) are used as suggestive of pain, the prevalence is estimated to be as high as 80% in nursing home patients with advanced dementia.[58] In those approaching death, pain is probably even more frequent. However, pain is also undertreated in patients with dementia, especially those at advanced stages who are prescribed fewer analgesics, even if expressing nonverbal pain behaviors.[59]

The first obstacle to better pain management is the difficulty in evaluating the presence of pain in these patients who cannot communicate. Pain assessment then has to rely on the observation of nonverbal pain behaviors, summarized in **Box 3**.[60] Several scales have been developed and evaluated for pain assessment in older patients with cognitive impairment. Of those, the Pain Assessment Checklist for Seniors with

**Box 3**
**Common pain behaviors in cognitively impaired older persons**

Facial expressions

Slight frown; sad, frightened face

Grimacing; wrinkling forehead, closed or tightened eyes

Any distorted expression

Rapid blinking

Verbalizations, vocalizations

Sighing, moaning, groaning

Grunting, chanting, calling out

Noisy breathing

Asking for help

Verbally abusive

Body movements

Rigid, tense body posture, guarding

Fidgeting

Increased pacing, rocking

Restricted movement

Gait or mobility changes

Changes in interpersonal interactions

Aggressive, combative, resisting care

Decreased social interactions

Socially inappropriate, disruptive

Withdrawn

Changes in patterns or routines

Refusing food, appetite change

Increase in rest periods

Sleep, rest pattern changes

Sudden cessation of common routines

Increased wandering

Mental status changes

Crying or tears

Increased confusion

Irritability or distress

*Data from* American Geriatrics Society panel on persistent pain in older persons. The management of persistent pain in older persons. J Am Geriatr Soc 2002;50:S205–24.

Limited Ability to Communicate (PACSLAC)[61] is often recommended,[62] because its validity and reliability has been shown.[63] Once the probable presence of pain has been identified, the cause should be sought with physical examination and appropriate investigation. Common causes of pain in patients with advanced dementia include musculoskeletal degenerative disease (osteoarthritis, degenerative disc disease, spinal stenosis), pressure sores, and contractures. If the change in the patient's status is sudden rather than progressive, an acute medical illness associated with acute pain should be ruled out (eg, pneumonia, angina, acute inflammatory arthritis, cholecystitis). Constipation, which is common in bedridden patients, might also present as pain.

If no acute reversible cause has been identified, the pain should be treated using a multidisciplinary and multimodality analgesic approach, including nonpharmacologic and pharmacologic treatments. Adequate positioning, prevention of contractures, and gentle approach for mobilization are especially important for this population. Analgesic therapy should be prescribed based on pain severity and using an appropriate combination of nonopioid, opioid, and adjuvant analgesics. To favor tolerability and decrease the risk of adverse effects, it is important to pay special attention to age-related changes in pharmacokinetic and pharmacodynamic properties, take into consideration the patient's comorbidities, start with low doses and titrate up according to clinical response and adverse effects, and identify potential drug-drug interactions.[64,65] Except from frequently requiring lower doses to achieve analgesia or produce adverse effects, pharmacologic pain management in end-stage dementia does not differ from other terminal illnesses. Because patients with advanced dementia often have swallowing difficulties, nonoral routes of administration frequently have to be used, including transdermal, transmucosal, subcutaneous, or via a feeding tube.

As in all palliative care, the optimal balance between pain control and adverse effects should be sought, taking into consideration the overall goals of treatment.

## Agitation and Behavioral Disturbances

Neuropsychiatric symptoms (NPSs) are present in every stage of dementia, and most NPSs increase in prevalence and severity with the progression of the disease.[66,67] Almost all patients with Alzheimer disease (80%–97%) present with NPSs at some point of their disease.[68] NPSs are associated with a more rapid cognitive decline, more functional incapacities, and increased mortality. They diminish the quality of life of both patients and their families and increase the care burden.[69] There have been few studies of NPSs in the latest stage of dementia. They have been reported to be present in 85% of hospice-eligible nursing home residents with advanced dementia,[70] the most common being aggression/agitation, depression, anxiety, aberrant motor behaviors, and apathy/withdrawal/lethargy.[70,71] Agitation, manifested by repetitive mannerisms and vocalizations or physical aggressiveness, seems to be associated mostly with resistiveness to care. This behavior happens during interaction between the severely demented person and a family member or caregiver, and is caused by a lack of understanding.[72] Because they do not understand the need to do an activity or care, they resist it. If the caregiver insists, the resistiveness might escalate to aggression and combative behavior. This behavior should first be managed with nonpharmacologic and environmental approaches, using a gentle approach and adapting to the patient's routine or pattern. Involvement of a significant person can often make patients feel more at ease, which will favor their cooperation with care. Resistiveness to care might also be related to depression or delusional ideation, and might improve after treatment of these diseases.[72]

In cases of end-stage behavioral disturbances or agitation that are not related to resistiveness to care, an underlying physical or medical cause should always be investigated. These causes include symptoms of thirst, hunger, sleep difficulties, constipation, sensory deprivation or overstimulation, social withdrawal, discomfort caused by bad position, or an intercurrent illness or infection (eg, pneumonia). Physicians must also exclude the adverse effects of delirium or medications.

Environmental and nonpharmacologic interventions should always be the first-step treatment of NPSs associated with advanced dementia.[19,54] Education of staff and caregivers on the appropriate approach to these patients is crucial, and should be used both to prevent and attenuate these behavioral disturbances.[19,54] The best evidence for efficacy provided by the literature concerns sensory-focused strategies, including aroma, preferred or live music, and multisensory intervention.[73] Snoezelen, an approach using controlled multisensory stimulation (lighting effects, color, sounds, music, scents) has been shown to reduce agitated and withdrawn behavior in patients with Alzheimer disease[74] during treatment sessions, but without evidence of longer-term benefits.[54] Emotion-oriented approaches, such as simulated presence, may also be effective but mainly for individuals with preserved verbal interactive capacity.[73]

Consensus expert guidelines recommend that pharmacologic interventions should be initiated concurrently with nonpharmacologic approaches in the presence of severe depression, psychosis, or aggression that puts the patient or others at risk of harm.[19] Pharmacologic interventions should be initiated at the lowest doses, titrated slowly, and monitored for effectiveness and safety. First-step agents for severe agitation, aggression, and psychosis are risperidone and olanzapine.[75] Aripiprazole can also be a good alternative.[76] The potential benefit of all antipsychotics must be weighed against the potential risks,[19,54] such as extrapyramidal symptoms, cerebrovascular adverse events, and mortality. Alternatives to antipsychotic medications are memantine,[77] citalopram,[78] sertraline,[79] trazodone,[80] and carbamazepine,[81] which have shown some benefits in the treatment of psychosis, agitation, and aggression associated with dementia. New therapeutic avenues include cannabinoid receptors agonists[82] and melatonine[83] for the sundowning syndrome.

Agitation and other neuropsychiatric symptoms might also be related to pain and the inability to express it. In the presence of agitation without any identifiable cause, it can be reasonable to empirically prescribe an analgesic regimen, including acetaminophen and opioid analgesics.[84] Low doses of long-acting opioids have been shown to decrease aggression in demented patients who did not respond to neuroleptics.[85] Benzodiazepines should usually be used only for short periods because of risks of physical dependency, cognitive blunting, and falls.[54]

Physical restraints should be avoided, unless there is an immediate danger for the patient or somebody else's well-being, and the agitation or aggressive behavior cannot be managed by other interventions.[19]

When approaching NPSs, one should keep in mind that final-stage dementia is a terminal illness and that NPSs are associated with great suffering for patients and their families. As with all patients in palliative care, treatment goals shift away from prolonging life and toward maximizing quality of life, dignity, and comfort. The priority should therefore be to treat these symptoms as well as possible, because the risks associated with the medication could be accepted by those concerned. Having an open and informed discussion with family members about treatment options and risks is mandatory. However, medication should never be an alternative to an insufficient ratio of personnel, staff education about NPS approaches, and a stimulating and adapted environment.

## Depression

Depression is frequent in Alzheimer disease and other types of dementia, even at late stages, in which it has been reported to affect between 6% and 27% of patients.[86] The diagnosis of depression is often difficult in demented patients, especially in late stages, for a variety of reasons. Severe cognitive impairment can impair the patient's ability to recall and report depressive symptoms. Many symptoms of depression, such as decreased sleep and appetite, weight loss, psychomotor retardation, and apathy, are also found in demented patients who are not depressed. To diagnose depression, dysphoric symptoms such as sadness, hopelessness, and guilt should be present.[87] Depression might also present as behavioral disturbances, including agitation, disturbed vocalization, physical aggression, and food refusal. When these symptoms appear de novo in a patient with advanced dementia, an empiric treatment of depression might be warranted.

Appropriate management of depression is important, even in advanced dementia, because it can increase cognitive and functional impairments, as well as behavioral disturbances. Furthermore, depression is associated with increased medical comorbidities, acute care admission, and an increased level of pain. A comprehensive treatment strategy should be implemented, including nonpharmacologic and pharmacologic interventions. Nonpharmacologic interventions that have been shown effective in treating depression in severely demented patients include snoezelen therapy, simulated presence, bright-light therapy, massage, and aromatherapy.[86] Scientific data on the use of antidepressants in severely demented patients with major depression are scarce. Selective serotonin reuptake inhibitors have been reported to improve depressive symptoms.[88] First-choice antidepressants are usually selective serotonin reuptake inhibitors (citalopram, sertraline), venlafaxine, bupropion, and mirtazapine, based on past effectiveness, medical comorbidities, potential side effects, and pharmacologic interactions. Although the optimal duration of treatment is uncertain, long-term maintenance might be reasonable in several cases, especially in the event of relapse after discontinuation.

## SUMMARY

There is a consensus among experts and in the literature that dementia is a progressive and noncurable illness, and that its management in late stages should follow a palliative care approach. However, this has not yet translated into clinical practice, with many patients with advanced dementia sustaining aggressive interventions that do not improve their survival and might hinder their comfort and quality of life.[59] This is likely explained by a lack of research on this population; a lack of knowledge from health care providers, patients, and family members; and lack of communication between those involved in the care of these patients. There is therefore an urgent need for research and education on this topic, as well as development of palliative care services devoted to this population.

## REFERENCES

1. US Census Bureau. International data base. Available at: www.census.gov/ipc/www/idb/groups.php. Accessed July 22, 2010.
2. US Census Bureau. Expectations of life at birth, 1970 to 2006, and projections, 2010 to 2020. Available at: www.census.gov/compendia/statab/2010/tables/10s0102.pdf. Accessed July 22, 2010.

3. National Statistics. Government actuary's department for expectation of life data. ONS for healthy life expectancy data. Published on 26 February 2010. Available at: www.statistics.gov.uk/cci/nugget.asp?id=934. Accessed August 18, 2010.

4. Rao AV, Cohen HJ. Oncology and aging: general principles. In: Halter JB, Ouslander JG, Tinetti ME, et al, editors. Hazzard's geriatric medicine and gerontology. 6th edition. New York: McGraw-Hill; 2009. p. 1123–35.

5. American Psychiatric Association Committee on Nomenclature and Statistics. Diagnostic and statistical manual on mental disorders, fourth edition (DSM IV). Diagnostic criteria. Washington, DC: American Psychiatric Association; 1994.

6. O'Connor DW. Epidemiology. In: Burns A, O'Brien J, Ames D, editors. Dementia. 3rd edition. London: Edward Arnold; 2005. p. 16–23.

7. Langa KM, Foster NL, Larson EB. Mixed dementia: emerging concepts and therapeutic implications. J Am Med Assoc 2004;292:2901–8.

8. McKahnn G, Drachman D, Flostein M, et al. Clinical diagnosis of Alzheimer's disease: report of the NINCDS-ADRDA work group under the auspices of the Department of Health and Human Services task force. Neurology 1984;47: 1113–24.

9. Roman GC, Erkinjuntti T, Wallin A, et al. Subcortical ischaemic vascular dementia. Lancet Neurol 2002;1:426–36.

10. Burns A, O'Brien J, Auriacombe S, et al. Clinical practice with anti-dementia drugs: a consensus statement from British association for psychopharmacology. J Psychopharmacol 2006;20:732–55.

11. Roman G. Therapeutic strategies for vascular dementia. In: Burns A, O'Brien J, Ames D, editors. Dementia. 3rd edition. London: Edward Arnold; 2005. p. 574–600.

12. Birch D, Draper J. A critical literature review exploring the challenges of delivering effective palliative care to older people with dementia. J Clin Nurs 2008; 17:1144–63.

13. Shuster JL Jr. Palliative care for advanced dementia. Clin Geriatr Med 2000;16: 373–86.

14. Corey-Bloom J, Fleisher AS. The natural history of Alzheimer's disease. In: Burns A, O'Brien J, Ames D, editors. Dementia. 3rd edition. London: Edward Arnold; 2005. p. 376–86.

15. McKeith IG, Ince P, Jaros EB, et al. What are the relations between Lewy body disease and AD? J Neural Transm Suppl 1998;54:107–16.

16. Rockwood K, Wentzel C, Hachinski V, et al. Prevalence and outcomes of vascular cognitive impairment. Vascular cognitive impairment investigators of the Canadian study of health and aging. Neurology 2000;54:447–51.

17. Newhouse P, Lasek J. Assessment and diagnosis of severe dementia. In: Burns A, Winblad B, editors. Severe dementia. Chichester (UK): John Wiley; 2006. p. 3–20.

18. Reisberg B, Ferris SH, de Leon MJ, et al. The global deterioration scale for assessment of primary degenerative dementia. Am J Psychiatry 1982;139: 1136–9.

19. Vellas B, Gauthier S, Allain H, et al. Consensus statement on dementia of Alzheimer type in the severe stage. J Nutr Health Aging 2005;9:330–8.

20. Saxton J, Swihart AA. Neuropsychological assessment of the severely impaired elderly patient. Clin Geriatr Med 1989;5:531–43.

21. Albert M, Cohen C. The test for severe impairment: an instrument for the assessment of patients with severe cognitive dysfunction. J Am Geriatr Soc 1992;40: 449–53.

22. Mitchell SL, Teno JM, Kiely DK, et al. The clinical course of advanced dementia. N Engl J Med 2009;361:1529–38.
23. Larson EB, Shadlen MF, Wang L, et al. Survival after initial diagnosis of Alzheimer disease. Ann Intern Med 2004;140:501–9.
24. McCarthy M, Addington-Hall J, Altmann D. The experience of dying with dementia: a retrospective study. Int J Geriatr Psychiatry 1997;12:404–9.
25. Casarett D, Takesaka J, Karlawish J, et al. How should clinicians discuss hospice for patients with dementia? Anticipating caregivers' preconceptions and meeting their information needs. Alzheimer Dis Assoc Disord 2002;16:116–22.
26. Koopmans RT, Roeline H, Pasman W, et al. Palliative care in patients with severe dementia. In: Burns A, Winblad B, editors. Severe dementia. Chichester (UK): John Wiley; 2006. p. 205–13.
27. Herlitz J, Eek M, Engdahl J, et al. Factors at resuscitation and outcome among patients suffering from out of hospital cardiac arrest in relation to age. Resuscitation 2003;58:309–17.
28. Mitchell SL, Kiely DK, Hamel MB. Dying with advanced dementia in the nursing home. Arch Intern Med 2004;164:321–6.
29. Volandes AE, Abbo ED. Flipping the default: a novel approach to cardiopulmonary resuscitation in end-stage dementia. J Clin Ethics 2007;18:122–39.
30. Hoffer LJ. Tube feeding in advanced dementia: the metabolic perspective. BMJ 2006;333:1214–5.
31. Mitchell SL, Teno JM, Roy J, et al. Clinical and organizational factors associated with feeding tube use among nursing home residents with advanced cognitive impairment. J Am Med Assoc 2003;290:73–80.
32. Gillick MR. Rethinking the role of tube feeding in patients with advanced dementia. N Engl J Med 2000;342:206–10.
33. Sampson EL, Candy B, Jones L. Enteral tube feeding for older people with advanced dementia. Cochrane Database Syst Rev 2009;2:CD007209.
34. Finucane TE, Christmas C, Travis K. Tube feeding in patients with advanced dementia: a review of the evidence. J Am Med Assoc 1999;282:1365–70.
35. Volicer L. Palliative medicine in dementia. In: Hanks G, Cherny NI, Christakis NA, et al, editors. Oxford textbook of palliative medicine. 4th edition. Oxford (UK): Oxford University Press; 2010. p. 1376–85.
36. Australia national palliative care program. Guidelines for a palliative approach in residential aged care, enhanced version. Available at: www.health.gov.au/palliativecare. Accessed July 22, 2010.
37. Palecek EJ, Teno JM, Casarett DJ, et al. Comfort feeding only: a proposal to bring clarity to decision-making regarding difficulty with eating for persons with advanced dementia. J Am Geriatr Soc 2010;58:580–4.
38. Mitchell SL, Tetroe J, O'Connor AM. A decision aid for long-term tube feeding in cognitively impaired older persons. J Am Geriatr Soc 2001;49:313–6.
39. Jenkins CA, Schulz M, Hanson J, et al. Demographic, symptom, and medication profiles of cancer patients seen by a palliative care consult team in a tertiary referral hospital. J Pain Symptom Manage 2000;19:174–84.
40. Viola RA, Wells GA, Peterson J. The effects of fluid status and fluid therapy on the dying: a systematic review. J Palliat Care 1997;13:41–52.
41. Simmons SF, Alessi C, Schnelle JF. An intervention to increase fluid intake in nursing home residents: prompting and preference compliance. J Am Geriatr Soc 2001;49:926–33.
42. Robinson SB, Rosher RB. Can a beverage cart help improve hydration? Geriatr Nurs 2002;23:208–11.

43. Thompson RS, Hall NK, Szpiech M, et al. Treatments and outcomes of nursing-home-acquired pneumonia. J Am Board Fam Pract 1997;10:82–7.
44. Afzal N, Buhagiar K, Flood J, et al. Quality of end-of-life care for dementia patients during acute hospital admission: a retrospective study in Ireland. Gen Hosp Psychiatry 2010;32:141–6.
45. Congedo M, Causarano RI, Alberti F, et al. Ethical issues in end of life treatments for patients with dementia. Eur J Neurol 2010;17:774–9.
46. Volicer L, Rheaume Y, Brown J, et al. Hospice approach to the treatment of patients with advanced dementia of the Alzheimer type. J Am Med Assoc 1986;256:2210–3.
47. van der Steen JT, Kruse RL, Ooms ME, et al. Treatment of nursing home residents with dementia and lower respiratory tract infection in the United States and The Netherlands: an ocean apart. J Am Geriatr Soc 2004;52:691–9.
48. van der Steen JT, Mehr DR, Kruse RL, et al. Treatment strategy and risk of functional decline and mortality after nursing-home acquired lower respiratory tract infection: two prospective studies in residents with dementia. Int J Geriatr Psychiatry 2007;22:1013–9.
49. Kruse RL, Mehr DR, van der Steen JT, et al. Antibiotic treatment and survival of nursing home patients with lower respiratory tract infection: a cross-national analysis. Ann Fam Med 2005;3:422–9.
50. van der Steen JT, Meuleman-Peperkamp I, Ribbe MW. Trends in treatment of pneumonia among Dutch nursing home patients with dementia. J Palliat Med 2009;12:789–95.
51. Parsons C, Hughes CM, Passmore AP, et al. Withholding, discontinuing and withdrawing medications in dementia patients at the end of life: a neglected problem in the disadvantaged dying? Drugs Aging 2010;27:435–49.
52. Holmes HM, Sachs GA, Shega JW, et al. Integrating palliative medicine into the care of persons with advanced dementia: identifying appropriate medication use. J Am Geriatr Soc 2008;56:1306–11.
53. Waldemar G, Dubois B, Emre M, et al. Recommendations for the diagnosis and management of Alzheimer's disease and other disorders associated with dementia: EFNS guideline. Eur J Neurol 2007;14:e1–26.
54. Herrmann N, Gauthier S. Diagnosis and treatment of dementia: 6. Management of severe Alzheimer disease. CMAJ 2008;179:1279–87.
55. Shega JW, Ellner L, Lau DT, et al. Cholinesterase inhibitor and N-methyl-D-aspartic acid receptor antagonist use in older adults with end-stage dementia: a survey of hospice medical directors. J Palliat Med 2009;12:779–83.
56. Sengstaken EA, King SA. The problems of pain and its detection among geriatric nursing home residents. J Am Geriatr Soc 1993;41:541–4.
57. Scherder E, Herr K, Pickering G, et al. Pain in dementia. Pain 2009;145:276–8.
58. Ferrell BA, Ferrell BR, Osterweil D. Pain in the nursing home. J Am Geriatr Soc 1990;38:409–14.
59. Morrison RS, Siu AL. A comparison of pain and its treatment in advanced dementia and cognitively intact patients with hip fracture. J Pain Symptom Manage 2000;19:240–8.
60. American Geriatrics Society panel on persistent pain in older persons. The management of persistent pain in older persons. J Am Geriatr Soc 2002;50:S205–24.
61. Fuchs-Lacelle S, Hadjistavropoulos T. Development and preliminary validation of the Pain Assessment Checklist for Seniors with Limited Ability to Communicate (PACSLAC). Pain Manag Nurs 2004;5:37–49.

62. Hadjistavropoulos T, Herr K, Turk DC, et al. An interdisciplinary expert consensus statement on assessment of pain in older persons. Clin J Pain 2007;23:S1–43.
63. Zwakhalen SM, Hamers JP, Berger MP. The psychometric quality and clinical usefulness of three pain assessment tools for elderly people with dementia. Pain 2006;126:210–20.
64. Lussier D, Pickering G. Pharmacological considerations in older patients. In: Beaulieu P, Lussier D, Porreca F, Dickenson AH, editors. Pharmacology of pain. Seattle (WA): IASP Press; 2010. p. 547–65.
65. American Geriatrics Society Panel on Pharmacological Management of Persistent Pain in Older Persons. Pharmacological management of persistent pain in older persons. J Am Geriatr Soc 2009;57:1331–46.
66. Craig D, Mirakhur A, Hart DJ, et al. A cross-sectional study of neuropsychiatric symptoms in 435 patients with Alzheimer's disease. Am J Geriatr Psychiatry 2005;13:460–8.
67. Thompson C, Brodaty H, Trollor J, et al. Behavioral and psychological symptoms associated with dementia subtype and severity. Int Psychogeriatr 2010;22:300–5.
68. Gauthier S, Cummings J, Ballard C, et al. Management of behavioral problems in Alzheimer's disease. Int Psychogeriatr 2010;22:346–72.
69. Hurt C, Bhattacharyya S, Burns A, et al. Patient and caregiver perspectives of quality of life in dementia. An investigation of the relationship to behavioural and psychological symptoms in dementia. Dement Geriatr Cogn Disord 2008;26:138–46.
70. Kverno KS, Black BS, Blass DM, et al. Neuropsychiatric symptom patterns in hospice-eligible nursing home residents with advanced dementia. J Am Med Dir Assoc 2008;9:509–15.
71. Koopmans RT, van der Molen M, Raats M, et al. Neuropsychiatric symptoms and quality of life in patients in the final phase of dementia. Int J Geriatr Psychiatry 2009;24:25–32.
72. Volicer L, Van der Steen JT, Frijters DH. Modifiable factors related to abusive behaviors in nursing home residents with dementia. J Am Med Dir Assoc 2009; 10:617–22.
73. Kverno KS, Black BS, Nolan MT, et al. Research on treating neuropsychiatric symptoms of advanced dementia with non-pharmacological strategies, 1998–2008: a systematic literature review. Int Psychogeriatr 2009;21:825–43.
74. van Weert JC, van Dulmen AM, Spreeuwenberg PM, et al. Behavioral and mood effects of snoezelen integrated into 24-hour dementia care. J Am Geriatr Soc 2005;53:24–33.
75. Ballard C, Waite J. The effectiveness of atypical antipsychotics for the treatment of aggression and psychosis in Alzheimer's disease. Cochrane Database Syst Rev 2006;1:CD003476.
76. Mintzer JE, Tune LE, Breder CD, et al. Aripiprazole for the treatment of psychoses in institutionalized patients with Alzheimer dementia: a multicenter, randomized, double-blind, placebo-controlled assessment of three fixed doses. Am J Geriatr Psychiatry 2007;15:918–31.
77. McShane R, Areosa Sastre A, Minakaran N. Memantine for dementia. Cochrane Database Syst Rev 2006;2:CD003154.
78. Pollock BG, Mulsant BH, Rosen J, et al. A double-blind comparison of citalopram and risperidone for the treatment of behavioral and psychotic symptoms associated with dementia. Am J Geriatr Psychiatry 2007;15:942–52.
79. Lanctôt KL, Herrmann N, van Reekum R, et al. Gender, aggression and serotonergic function are associated with response to sertraline for behavioral disturbances in Alzheimer's disease. Int J Geriatr Psychiatry 2002;17:531–41.

80. Sultzer DL, Gray KF, Gunay I, et al. A double-blind comparison of trazodone and haloperidol for treatment of agitation in patients with dementia. Am J Geriatr Psychiatry 1997;5:60–9.

81. Tariot PN, Erb R, Podgorski CA, et al. Efficacy and tolerability of carbamazepine for agitation and aggression in dementia. Am J Psychiatry 1998;155:54–61.

82. Passmore MJ. The cannabinoid receptor agonist nabilone for the treatment of dementia-related agitation. Int J Geriatr Psychiatry 2008;23:116–7.

83. Mahlberg RK, Sutej I, Kühl KP, et al. Melatonin treatment of day-night rhythm disturbances and sundowning in Alzheimer disease: an open-label pilot study using actigraphy. J Clin Psychopharmacol 2004;24:456–9.

84. Chronic pain management in the long-term care setting: clinical practice guidelines. Columbia (MD): American Medical Directors Association; 1999.

85. Manfredi PL, Breuer B, Wallenstein S, et al. Opioid treatment for agitation in patients with advanced dementia. Int J Geriatr Psychiatry 2003;18:700–5.

86. Bielinski K, Lawlor B. Depression in severe dementia. In: Burns A, O'Brien J, Ames D, editors. Dementia. 3rd edition. London: Edward Arnold; 2005. p. 63–74.

87. Boyle PA, Malloy PF. Treating apathy in Alzheimer's disease. Dement Geriatr Cogn Disord 2004;17:91–9.

88. Magai C, Kennedy G, Cohen CI, et al. A controlled clinical trial of sertraline in the treatment of depression in nursing home patients with late-stage Alzheimer's disease. Am J Geriatr Psychiatry 2000;8:66–74.

# Management of End-Stage Heart Failure

Sandhya Murthy, MD[a], Hannah I. Lipman, MD, MS[b,c],*

**KEYWORDS**

• Heart failure • End stage • Management • Symptom burden

There are approximately 5.8 million Americans currently living with heart failure (HF), with more than 1.1 million hospitalized annually. HF is the only cardiac-related diagnosis that is increasing in prevalence. Increased incidence in the elderly population and improved survival contribute to the increase in prevalence. Despite modern advances in the treatment of HF, morbidity and mortality of the disease remain high. Overall 5-year mortality after hospitalization is 42%.[1] HF is the leading cause of hospital admissions in patients more than 65 years old. In this group, 1-year mortality for new HF admissions nears 60%.[2] Despite the wide array of advanced treatment options, HF remains an incurable disease in most cases. Nearly 300,000 are considered to have end-stage disease.[3] Many experience significant symptoms and frequent hospitalizations in the last year of life. Palliative care is comprehensive care aimed at relieving suffering and symptom distress for patients with serious illness and their families. There is a clear need for palliative care for the growing population of chronically ill patients with HF.

## CLASSIFICATION OF HF

The American College of Cardiology (ACC)/American Heart Association (AHA) classification system categorizes patients according to the presence of conditions that increase the risk of HF, structural heart disease, and symptoms. It emphasizes both the progression and preventability of the disease and identifies patients with modifiable risk factors. Patients with stage A disease are at high risk for developing HF, because of existing risk factors such as hypertension, diabetes, or coronary artery disease, but have no structural heart disease. Patients at stage B have structural heart disease, such as scar, valve lesions, or systolic dysfunction, but no symptoms of HF.

[a] Division of Cardiology, Montefiore Medical Center, Albert Einstein College of Medicine, 111 East 210th Street, Bronx, NY 10467, USA
[b] Department of Medicine, Divisions of Geriatrics and Cardiology, Montefiore Medical Center, Albert Einstein College of Medicine, 111 East 210th Street, Bronx, NY 10467, USA
[c] Montefiore-Einstein Center for Bioethics, Montefiore Medical Center, Albert Einstein College of Medicine, 111 East 210th Street, Bronx, NY 10467, USA
* Corresponding author. Montefiore-Einstein Center for Bioethics, Montefiore Medical Center, 111 East 210th Street, Bronx, NY 10467.
*E-mail address:* hlipman@montefiore.org

Prim Care Clin Office Pract 38 (2011) 265–276
doi:10.1016/j.pop.2011.03.007
0095-4543/11/$ – see front matter © 2011 Elsevier Inc. All rights reserved.

primarycare.theclinics.com

Patients at stage C have experienced typical HF symptoms: dyspnea, fatigue, or effort intolerance. Patients at stage D have refractory HF with symptoms at rest despite maximal therapy.[4]

The New York Heart Association (NYHA) classification is complementary to the ACC/AHA system and describes the functional capacity of patients with HF. The NYHA classification system reflects a subjective assessment by the provider and patient. Symptom class can vary, even in a short period.

| NYHA Functional Classification | |
| --- | --- |
| Class | Patient Symptoms |
| I | No functional limitation. No symptoms of HF (ie, dyspnea, fatigue) with ordinary physical activity |
| II | Some functional limitation with HF symptoms with ordinary physical activity. No symptoms at rest |
| III | Significant functional limitation with HF symptoms with less than ordinary activity. No symptoms at rest |
| IV | Severe functional limitation with symptoms with any physical activity. Symptoms even at rest |

## DEFINITION OF END-STAGE HF

There is no universally accepted definition of end-stage HF. Patients at stage D with refractory symptoms despite maximal medical therapy are end stage. Some may be candidates for advanced therapies such as transplant or left ventricular assist device (LVAD). The Heart Failure Society of America defines patients with end-stage HF as "those patients who have advanced, persistent HF with symptoms at rest despite repeated attempts to optimize pharmacologic and nonpharmacologic therapy," as evidenced by 1 or more of the following: frequent hospitalizations (3 or more per year), chronic poor quality of life with inability to accomplish activities of daily living, need for intermittent or continuous intravenous support, or consideration of assist devices as destination therapy.[5]

Because modern HF treatment modifies disease course and palliates symptoms, it is important to ensure that adequate attempts have been made to optimize therapy. However, patients may not be able to tolerate optimal medical therapy because of comorbid disease or side effects of treatment, and some may choose to forgo invasive treatments after careful consideration of their benefits and burdens. Palliative care is appropriate for any patient with serious illness and suffering, regardless of stage of disease or prognosis, and may be delivered concomitantly with life-prolonging or HF-directed therapy.

## REVIEW OF CHRONIC HF TREATMENT

To best individualize treatment by integrating HF-directed therapy and palliative care and to counsel each individual patient, it is important to be aware of the pharmacologic and mechanical options.

## MEDICAL THERAPY

Optimal medical therapy includes adequate treatment of underlying conditions that cause or exacerbate HF, including hypertension, ischemic heart disease, arrhythmias, and thyroid dysfunction. HF-specific medical therapy has evolved significantly in the past 30 years. Original trials of angiotensin-converting enzyme (ACE) inhibition showed a clear mortality benefit in patients with systolic dysfunction, both chronically and immediately after infarction, leading to a class I recommendation by the ACC/AHA.[4,6] ACE inhibitors have been tested in nearly 7000 patients with systolic HF in more than 30 clinical trials. ACE inhibitors reduce the risk of death and hospitalization in patients with mild, moderate, and severe disease.[7] Angiotensin receptor blockers (ARBs) also reduce morbidity and mortality and are an alternative for patients who cannot tolerate ACE inhibitors because of adverse reactions such as intractable cough.[8] Other treatment-limiting side effects of ACE inhibitors and ARBs include hypotension, hyperkalemia, and azotemia. The addition of ARBs to background ACE inhibitor therapy modestly decreases hospitalization without improving survival.[9]

β-Adrenergic receptor blockade is a cornerstone in the chronic care of patients with left ventricular dysfunction. There is evidence in more than 20,000 patients in 20 clinical trials of the benefits of β-blockade, including reduced mortality by 35%. This is well shown in patients with NYHA class II to III HF with carvedilol,[10] bisoprolol,[11] and extended-release metoprolol,[12] all class I recommendations by the ACC/AHA.[4] Patients with HF should be treated with one of these 3 agents with proven benefit in this population, because other β-blockers have not shown the same effect. Treatment-limiting side effects include hypotension, symptomatic bradycardia, and fatigue. Fluid retention may worsen with initiation or uptitration of β-blockers, and diuretics should be adjusted accordingly. Combination therapy with an ACE inhibitor, ARB, and β-blocker is not recommended.[13]

As shown in the Randomized Aldactone Evaluation Study (RALES), aldosterone antagonism leads to significant morbidity and mortality reduction in severely symptomatic patients with NYHA functional class III or IV. In addition, there was a 35% reduction in HF admissions with treatment. There is no evidence of benefit in less symptomatic patients with NYHA functional class I or II.[14] To avoid the main side effect of hyperkalemia, aldosterone blockers should be used with caution in patients with creatinine equal to or greater than 1.5 mg/dL, and should be avoided altogether in patients with worsening renal function or potassium more than 5 mEq/L.[4]

The combination of hydralazine and nitrates is recommended as part of standard therapy for African Americans with systolic dysfunction and NYHA functional classes II to IV, based on data from the African American Heart Failure Trial (A-HeFT),[15] which was terminated early because of the significantly higher mortality in the placebo group compared with the hydralazine/nitrate group. Currently, there are no published data to support its use in the non–African American population. However it is reasonable to consider this therapy in all patients who remain symptomatic despite other standard therapies or cannot tolerate ACE inhibitor or ARB because of renal dysfunction. Hypotension is the main short-term side effect. Patients may have difficulty with dosing 3 times a day.

Diuretic therapy is essential for maintaining euvolemia and improving congestive symptoms. Diuretics reduce the risk of death and worsening HF in patients with chronic HF[16] and are safe.[17] Digoxin improves symptoms, exercise tolerance, and quality of life, and reduces hospitalizations in patients with mild to moderate HF.[4,18,19]

## DEVICE AND SURGICAL THERAPY

There has been much progress in device therapies in the past few decades. When patients may be candidates for device therapy and such treatment is consistent with the goals of care, consider referral to a specialist for further evaluation. Implantable cardioverter-defibrillator therapy is recommended for the primary prevention of sudden cardiac death in patients with ischemic or nonischemic cardiomyopathy and ejection fraction (EF) less than 35%, who have a life expectancy greater than 1 year and NYHA class II or III symptoms. For patients with class I symptoms, an internal cardiac defibrillator (ICD) for primary prevention of sudden cardiac death is considered reasonable.[4] Major trials show a relative risk reduction of mortality of 20% to 30%. The decision to implant a device should be considered only after a period of optimal medical therapy and reevaluation for improvement in EF. Although ICD therapy decreases sudden death from ventricular arrhythmia, the mortality benefit was seen only after 2 years in the major trials.[20] This should be remembered when considering ICD therapy with significant comorbid disease or limited life expectancy.

Cardiac resynchronization therapy (CRT) restores ventricular synchrony by pacing both the right and left ventricles, thereby improving hemodynamic performance. It is indicated for patients with a wide QRS (at least 120 milliseconds) and NYHA class III or IV functional status. Recent data indicate a benefit for less symptomatic patients as well.[21] CRT reduces mortality, decreases hospitalizations, and improves quality of life and functional status.[22–24]

Surgical treatments for HF include coronary revascularization and valvular repair or replacement in appropriate patients. A small number of patients with HF may benefit from advanced therapies such as implantation of an LVAD or heart transplantation. Although great improvements have been made in the medical and surgical care of patients having heart transplants, the shortage of organs remains a significant barrier.

Select patients with severe, advanced HF may be candidates for an LVAD, an implanted battery powered pump that does the work of the left ventricle. First used only as a bridge to heart transplantation, the device is now approved for destination therapy for patients who are not transplant candidates and have EF less than 25%, NYHA class IV symptoms for at least 90 days despite medical therapy, and life expectancy of less than 2 years.[25] Complications of LVAD implantation include infection, stroke, and device malfunction. The burdens associated with LVAD therapy are high, including psychological, physical, and financial stress on recipients and caregivers. Taking care of an individual with an assist device can be especially challenging for families, and often requires intense social support. Continuity of palliative care support during LVAD therapy is essential to preserving quality of life, and to providing emotional and social support to families and patients.[26] Advance care planning is especially crucial in this population to clarify patients' values regarding treatment if significant complications occur.

## ACUTE DECOMPENSATED HF

During episodes of acute decompensation, patients may suffer severe symptoms and require invasive treatments and/or intensive care unit care. Acute decompensation confers a poor prognosis.[2] Questions of how best to integrate palliative care with HF-directed therapy often arise in the inpatient setting during an episode of acute decompensation. Although a comprehensive review of the management of acute decompensated HF is beyond the scope of this article, familiarity with the treatment options is imperative to counseling patients facing this phase of HF.

The goal of therapy is to provide symptom relief and hemodynamic support. Uncontrolled arrhythmia, ischemia, or hypertension, medication or diet change, use of nonsteroidal anti-inflammatory agents or thiazolidinedione, infection, anemia, and other possible precipitants should be sought and treated. Intravenous diuretics are the mainstay of treatment. Vasodilators such as nesiritide or nitroglycerin may be needed to decrease pulmonary capillary wedge pressures and pulmonary congestion.

Positive inotropic agents such as dobutamine or milrinone should be reserved for patients who require hemodynamic support because their routine use has not been shown to be of benefit.[27] Likewise, the routine use of intermittent inotropes is not recommended.[28,29] If inadequate diuresis is achieved through intravenous therapy, another option is mechanical fluid removal through ultrafiltration, which allows rapid diuresis at rates of up to 8 L per day, but requires specialized care.[30] In severe refractory cases, mechanical support with an intra-aortic balloon pump or LVAD may be considered.

## ESTIMATING PROGNOSIS

Several biochemical, hemodynamic, and functional markers have been identified as univariate predictors of poor prognosis. These markers include age, impaired renal function, cardiac cachexia, anemia, hypotension, hyponatremia, degree of systolic dysfunction, symptomatic arrhythmia, and recurrent hospitalizations.[4,5,31–33] NYHA class also correlates with prognosis: class I patients have 5% to 10% mortality per year, whereas class IV patients approach 40% to 50% per year.[12]

The Seattle Heart Failure Model is a multivariable model derived from clinical trials, registries, and observational studies, and is available in a web-based format. Clinical data, such as age, gender, systolic blood pressure, NYHA class, EF, presence of ischemic heart disease, and weight are used to estimate mean 1-year, 2-year, and 5-year survival. This model also predicts the benefit of adding medications and devices.[34] Recent studies have suggested that, in patients with more advanced disease, the model underestimates risk.[35] The OPTIMIZE-HF model uses data available at hospital admission, such as age, heart rate, serum sodium and creatinine, and systolic blood pressure, to predict in-hospital mortality.[36]

These models are useful for estimating outcomes for populations of patients. Because they provide only probability estimates, the data are difficult to apply to each specific individual. Therefore, treatment plans should be tailored to each patient by weighing the risks and benefits of each option in the context of the patient's prognosis and goals of care. Individual patients with significant symptoms, suffering or distress, regardless of prognosis, may benefit from palliative care supplementing disease-specific approaches.

## ADVANCE CARE PLANNING

HF is a chronic, progressive illness. Although most patients die of progressive pump failure, sudden cardiac death can occur in all stages of disease severity. Patients with NYHA functional class II have an annual mortality of 5% to 10%; however, up to 80% of these deaths are sudden. Conversely, functional class IV has a 50% mortality, but only 30% are sudden, and most are attributed to progressive pump failure.[12] A comprehensive HF treatment plan must integrate advance care planning throughout the disease course. Advance care planning is the process by which patients and families work with health care providers to clarify values and preferences in advance of worsening illness, crisis, or loss of decision-making capacity.[37] Specific advance directives, such as designating a health care proxy or delineating a living will, as well as stating resuscitation preferences, should be discussed when possible. However, the unpredictable disease trajectory of HF and provider and patient misperception of disease severity[38] are barriers to effective advance care planning. Both providers and patients overestimate prognosis.[39] In addition, patient preferences change with time.[40] Communication should be individualized to elicit each patient's values, and advance directives should be updated as the patient progresses through the course of the disease.

## TREATMENT OF COMMON SYMPTOMS: SPECIAL CONSIDERATIONS FOR PATIENTS WITH HF

### Dyspnea

Dyspnea is a hallmark symptom of HF. In the Study to Understand Prognoses and Preferences for Outcomes and Risks of Treatment (SUPPORT), 35% of patients reported severe dyspnea in the 3 to 6 months before death. In the last 3 days of life, 60% experienced severe dyspnea.[40,41] The perception of shortness of breath is multifaceted and not solely attributed to volume overload. Dyspnea may be a symptom of cardiac ischemia. Psychological factors also contribute to the severity of the sensation. Classic treatments include diuretics to relieve congestion, vasodilators to improve hemodynamics, and nitrates for ischemia. Mechanical fluid removal may benefit volume-overloaded patients who are refractory to diuretics. Opioids are beneficial in relieving the sensation of breathlessness.[42] Lower doses are used to treat dyspnea than are needed to treat pain. Dosing for specific patients depends on multiple factors, including renal and liver function and chronic opioid dose, if any.

### Pain

Pain is common in patients with HF. The SUPPORT data showed that 35% of patients who died in the index hospitalization reported severe pain.[40,41] Most physicians do not think of HF as a painful condition, but up to 78% of patients at end-stage report experiencing pain.[43] The cause of pain is multifactorial. Angina pectoris and bowel ischemia may contribute. Comorbid conditions such as osteoarthritis may also contribute. In addition to targeting the root cause of pain, therapy with opioids is often necessary. For more detailed guidance, please see the article by Shalini Dalal elsewhere in this issue. Nonsteroidal anti-inflammatory drugs should be avoided in patients with HF because they exacerbate the symptoms of HF by contributing to renal dysfunction and fluid retention.

### Depression

Estimates of the rate of depression in patients with HF range from 21% to more than 30%, with prevalence increasing with worsening functional class, and approaching nearly 70% in hospitalized patients with HF.[44,45] Patients with depression have an increased rate of cardiac events, hospitalization, and death.[45] Nearly 90% of depressed patients with HF do not receive adequate treatment.[46] The optimal treatment of depression for patients with HF is not known. A recent observational study confirmed the increased mortality risk for patients with HF with depression and also showed that concomitant use of selective serotonin uptake inhibitor (SSRI) with β-blockers was associated with a greater mortality than concomitant tricyclic antidepressant (TCA) and β-blocker use.[47] Further study is needed. SSRIs can cause hyponatremia because of water retention via antidiuretic hormone release. Their use near the end of life is limited by the long time to onset of therapeutic action. TCAs have significant anticholinergic side effects and may cause QT prolongation and arrhythmia.[48] Methylphenidate, which has rapid onset of treatment effect, has been used successfully in patients with cancer and human immunodeficiency virus to alleviate symptoms of depression and fatigue. Cardiac side effects, such as tachycardia, may limit its use in the HF population.[49]

### Sleep-disordered Breathing

Sleep-disordered breathing is increasingly recognized as a common phenomenon in patients with HF. Estimates of prevalence vary from 24% to 76%. Sleep-disordered breathing is implicated in progression of disease and worsening of symptoms and is associated with decreased exercise capacity, increased ventricular arrhythmias, and overall poorer prognosis. Central or obstructive sleep apnea may be present. It is important to distinguish, because the weight of evidence for benefit with treatment with continuous positive airway pressure (CPAP) is greater for obstructive sleep apnea compared with central sleep apnea. CPAP may improve systolic function as well as decrease the harmful neurohormonal activation associated with periods of nighttime apnea. There are insufficient data to conclude that it improves mortality. CPAP treatment can offer relief of fatigue, daytime somnolence, and improve quality of life in patients with HF. Formal sleep studies should be considered in patients complaining of excessive fatigue, somnolence, snoring, or nighttime apnea.[50–53]

## REFINING HF THERAPY AT END OF LIFE

Few specific data are available to guide discontinuation of HF medications as end of life approaches. Patients may become unable to take oral medications and experience more side effects of treatment without significant benefit. Patients with advanced HF may develop inability to tolerate HF medications because of hypotension or renal dysfunction. β-Blockers may provide palliation by controlling angina and tachycardia, but fatigue, volume overload, hypotension, or bradycardia should prompt consideration of their discontinuation. ACE inhibitors and ARBs improve hemodynamics, but should be discontinued in the setting of hypotension, renal failure, or hyperkalemia. Similarly, aldosterone receptor antagonists should be discontinued if renal failure or hyperkalemia develop. Digoxin is used to control the ventricular response in atrial fibrillation or flutter, but the risks of toxicity may outweigh the symptom benefit in patients with worsening renal function. Diuretic dose must be adjusted as the patient's oral intake and volume status fluctuate. Torsemide may be a better choice for patients with intestinal edema because it is better and more predictably absorbed after oral administration.[54] In end-stage disease, it is reasonable to withdraw digoxin therapy given the narrow therapeutic range and lack of mortality or symptom benefit in this sicker population. Statins provide short-term benefits for patients with active acute coronary syndromes but, because the primary benefits are with long-term use, they should be discontinued as end of life nears.[55] Although HF-directed therapy is symptom relieving, as the disease progresses treatments aimed solely at symptom relief may become necessary. The inability to tolerate ACE inhibitors and β-blockers carries a worse prognosis, and signals progression of disease.

## ICD DEACTIVATION

The burden of continued ICD therapy may outweigh the life-prolonging benefit in patients with progressive HF or other significant comorbid disease. Although ICD therapy is effective in reducing mortality caused by sudden cardiac death, as patients progress to end-stage disease and experience progressive pump failure, the frequency of shocks may increase. Shocks may be painful and anticipating them may cause significant anxiety. Avoiding sudden death may no longer be consistent with the goals and values of patients with advanced disease. Deactivation of ICD may be accomplished by reprogramming the device and does not require surgical explantation.[56] Deactivation prevents repetitive shocks, avoids prolonging dying, and provides relief of anticipatory anxiety. However, conversations about deactivating the ICD happen infrequently. Barriers to having effective conversations include discomfort discussing end-of-life issues, time constraints, and physicians' belief that ICD deactivation is a distinct topic from other, more common advance care planning discussions.[57] Patients often are misinformed about the implications of deactivating ICDs. Reassurance that reprogramming the device will not be painful should be provided.[58] The ACC/AHA guidelines include a class I recommendation to discuss with appropriate patients ICD deactivation at the end of life.[4] To ensure that care is given in accordance with patient preferences at the end of life, this is an important issue that should be raised while discussing other more traditional advanced directives.

The defibrillator function of an ICD, which treats fatal arrhythmias, is distinct from the pacing function. Pacing need not be disabled when the device is reprogrammed. Pacing to treat bradyarrhythmias and achieve cardiac resynchronization may provide symptomatic benefit for individual patients without associated discomfort. Therefore, the burdens and benefits of pacing should be considered separately from those associated with tachycardia therapy.

## CHRONIC INOTROPIC SUPPORT

Patients who cannot be successfully weaned from inotropes because of hemodynamic instability, refractory symptoms, or end-organ dysfunction are considered inotrope dependent. Continuous support with home inotropes, typically dobutamine or milrinone, may be considered. Both agents can be administered with a compact pump system. The benefit is that the patient can stay at home and avoid spending time in the hospital during the last stages of life. However, prolonged use carries a significant risk of arrhythmia, hypotension, and tachycardia and requires specialized home care. A recent analysis of Medicare data showed that 6-month mortality was 43% and 1-year mortality was 57%. However, this group included patients treated with intermittent as well as continuous inotrope infusion.[59] A small case series of continuous inotrope therapy for dependent patients showed 74% mortality at 6 months and 94% at 1 year.[60] Individual hospice programs vary in ability to provide this support at home because of the cost of the therapy. Both home dobutamine and milrinone may decrease recurrent hospitalizations, but only dobutamine is cost-effective.[59]

## HOSPICE

Hospice is one option for delivering palliative care. Hospice is interdisciplinary care focused on comfort for patients with an expected survival of 6 months or less, delivered in the home, acute-care, or long-term care settings. Patients and families are supported through the dying process. Services are also available to families through bereavement. Patients who are enrolled in palliative care programs or hospice report a higher level of satisfaction, reduced hospital stays, improved symptoms, and a greater likelihood of death at home.[61] Despite the high symptom burden and poor quality of life of patients with advanced HF[40] and significant burden on family caregivers, hospice is underused in this population.[62] Nationally, only about 10% of patients with HF die in a hospice setting, but the proportion of patients with HF referred to hospice is increasing. Patients with HF referred for hospice tend to be older and more likely to be female.[63–65] Patients referred during a hospitalization for acute decompensated HF are more likely to have had another HF hospitalization in the antecedent 6 months.[64]

Hospice referral should be considered for patients who have NYHA functional class IV symptoms despite maximally tolerated medical therapy, multiple markers of poor prognosis, progression of end-organ dysfunction, recent clinical decline without reversible cause, 2 or more admissions within 6 months, or who are dependent on inotropic support.[66] Barriers to hospice referral include difficulty in estimating prognosis and the fluctuating course of advanced HF. Both patients and health care providers overestimate survival.[40] In addition, once enrolled in hospice, patients with HF are more likely than patients who have cancer to remain on hospice for more than 6 months or to be discharged from hospice.[65] Coordination between HF and hospice providers helps ensure that patients continue HF-directed therapy as tolerated. Because HF-directed therapies are palliating, the oral regimen should be continued as long as tolerated. The HF physician can work closely with the hospice team to tailor therapy to the needs of each individual patient.

## SUMMARY

The prevalence of advanced HF is increasing because of advances in treatment of ischemic heart disease, prevention of sudden cardiac death, and growth of the geriatric population. Because modern HF treatment both modifies disease and palliates symptoms, ensuring adequate trial of HF-directed therapy is imperative. However, individual patients may not tolerate HF-directed therapy, may not be candidates for advanced therapies such as transplant or LVAD, or such treatments may not be consistent with patients' preferences. The symptom burden of advanced HF is high and worsens as death nears. Symptom-directed therapy should supplement HF-directed therapy when necessary. Communication between provider and patient is critical to ensure that treatment is individualized according to patient preferences. Advance care planning should occur early in the disease course, be updated with time, and include discussion of specific HF therapies, including deactivation of implantable defibrillators. Hospice referral should be considered for appropriate patients. Palliative care and HF-directed therapy should be delivered concurrently to provide comprehensive patient care.

## REFERENCES

1. Lloyd-Jones D, Adams RJ, Brown TM, et al. Heart disease and stroke statistics 2010 update: a report from the American Heart Association. Circulation 2010; 121:e46–215.
2. Jong P, Vowinckel E, Liu PP, et al. Prognosis and determinants of survival in patients newly diagnosed for heart failure. Arch Intern Med 2002;162:1689–94.
3. Adams KF, Zammad F, France N. Clinical definition and epidemiology of advanced heart failure. Am Heart J 1998;135:s204–15.
4. Jessup M, Abraham WT, Casey DE, et al. 2009 Focused update: ACCF/AHA guidelines for the diagnosis and management of heart failure in adults. Circulation 2009;119:1977–2016.
5. Heart Failure Society of America. Heart Failure Guidelines. Section 8: disease management in heart failure, education and counseling. J Card Fail 2006;12:e58–69.
6. The SOLVD Investigators. Effect of enalapril on survival in patients with reduced left ventricular ejection fractions and congestive heart failure. N Engl J Med 1991; 325:293–302.
7. Sharpe DN, Murphy J, Coxon R, et al. Enalapril in patients with chronic heart failure: a placebo-controlled, randomized, double-blind study. Circulation 1984;70:271–8.
8. Granger CB, McMurray JJ, Yusuf S, et al. Effects of candesartan in patients with chronic heart failure and reduced left-ventricular systolic function intolerant to angiotensin-converting-enzyme inhibitors: the CHARM-Alternative trial. Lancet 2003;362:772–6.
9. Cohn JN, Tognoni G. A randomized trial of the angiotensin receptor blocker valsartan in chronic heart failure. N Engl J Med 2001;345:1667–75.

10. Packer M, Coats AJ, Fowler MB, et al. Effect of carvedilol on survival in severe chronic heart failure. N Engl J Med 2001;334:1651.
11. CIBIS-II Investigators and Committees. The cardiac insufficiency bisoprolol study II (CIBIS-II): a randomised trial. Lancet 1999;353(9146):9–13.
12. MERIT-HF Study Group. Effect of metoprolol CR/XL in chronic heart failure: metoprolol CR/XL randomised intervention trial in congestive heart failure (MERIT-HF). Lancet 1999;353(9169):2001–7.
13. Ramani GV, Uber PA, Mehra MR. Chronic heart failure: contemporary diagnosis and management. Mayo Clin Proc 2010;85(2):180–95.
14. Pitt B, Zannad F, Remme WJ, et al. Randomized Aldactone Evaluation Study. N Engl J Med 1999;341:709.
15. Taylor AL, Ziesche S, Yancy C, et al. Combination of isosorbide dinitrate and hydralazine in blacks with heart failure. N Engl J Med 2004;351:2049–57.
16. Faris RF, Flather M, Purcell H, et al. Diuretics for heart failure. Cochrane Database Syst Rev 2006;1:CD003838.
17. Faris R, Flather M, Purcell H, et al. Current evidence supporting the role of diuretics in heart failure: a meta analysis of randomized controlled trials. Int J Cardiol 2002;82:149–58.
18. Guyatt GH, Sullivan MJ, Fallen EL, et al. A controlled trial of digoxin in congestive heart failure. Am J Cardiol 1988;61:371–5.
19. The Digitalis Investigation Group. The effect of digoxin on mortality and morbidity in patients with heart failure. N Engl J Med 1997;336:525–33.
20. Bardy GH, Lee KL, Mark DB, et al. Amiodarone or an implantable cardioverter-defibrillator for congestive heart failure. N Engl J Med 2005;352:225–37.
21. Moss AJ, Jackson Hall W, Cannom DS, et al. Cardiac-resynchronization therapy for the prevention of heart-failure events. N Engl J Med 2009;361:1329–38.
22. Higgins SL, Hummel JD, Niazi IK, et al. Cardiac resynchronization therapy for the treatment of heart failure in patients with intraventricular conduction delay and malignant ventricular tachyarrhythmias. J Am Coll Cardiol 2003;42(8):1454–9.
23. Young JB, Abraham WT, Smith AL, et al. Combined cardiac resynchronization and implantable cardioversion defibrillation in advanced chronic heart failure: the MIRACLE ICD Trial. JAMA 2003;289(20):2685–94.
24. McAlister F, Ezekowitz J, Wiebe N, et al. Cardiac resynchronization therapy for congestive heart failure. Summary, evidence report/technology assessment: Number 106. Rockville (MD): AHRQ Publication Number 05-E001-1; November 2004. July 12, 2009. Agency for Healthcare Research and Quality. Available at: http://www.ahrq.gov/clinic/epcsums/resynsum.htm. Accessed March 2, 2011.
25. Medicare National Coverage Determinations (NCD) manual, chapter 1, part 1 (sections 10-80.12) coverage determinations. Maryland: Centers for Medicare & Medicaid Services; 2005.
26. Rizzieri AG, Verheijde JL, Rady MY, et al. Ethical challenges with the left ventricular assist device as a destination therapy. Philos Ethics Humanit Med 2008;3:20.
27. Cuffe MS, Califf RM, Adams KF, et al. Short-term intravenous milrinone for acute exacerbation of chronic heart failure: a randomized controlled trial. JAMA 2002; 287:1541–7.
28. David S, Zaks JM. Arrhythmias associated with intermittent outpatient dobutamine infusion. Angiology 1986;37:86–91.
29. Elis A, Bental T, Kimchi O, et al. Intermittent dobutamine treatment in patients with chronic refractory congestive heart failure: a randomized, double-blind, placebo-controlled study. Clin Pharmacol Ther 1998;63:682–5.

30. Bart BA, Boyle A, Bank AJ, et al. Ultrafiltration versus usual care for hospitalized patients with heart failure: the relief for acutely fluid-overloaded patients with decompensated congestive heart failure (RAPID-CHF) trial. J Am Coll Cardiol 2005; 46(11):2043–6.
31. Eichhorn EJ. Prognosis determination in heart failure. Am J Med 2001;110(Suppl 7a):14S–36S.
32. Huynh BC, Rovner A, Rich MW. Identification of older patients with heart failure who may be candidates for hospice care: development of a simple four-item risk score. J Am Geriatr Soc 2008;56:1111–5.
33. Poole JE, Johnson GW, Hellkamp AS, et al. Prognostic importance of defibrillator shocks in patients with heart failure. N Engl J Med 2008;359:1009–17.
34. Levy WC, Mozaffarian D, Linker DT, et al. The Seattle Heart Failure Model: prediction of survival in heart failure. Circulation 2006;113:1424–33.
35. Kalogeropoulos AP, Georgiopoulou VV, Giamouzis G, et al. Utility of the Seattle Heart Failure Model in patients with advanced heart failure. J Am Coll Cardiol 2009;53:334–42.
36. Abraham WT, Fonarow GC, Albert NM, et al. Predictors of in-hospital mortality in patients hospitalized for heart failure: insights from the Organized Program to Initiate Lifesaving Treatment in Hospitalized Patients with Heart Failure (OPTIMIZE-HF). J Am Coll Cardiol 2008;52(5):347–56.
37. Adler E, Goldfinger J, Kalman J, et al. Palliative care in the treatment of advanced heart failure. Circulation 2009;120:2597–606.
38. Mccarthy M, Hall JA, Ley M. Communication and choice in dying from heart disease. J R Soc Med 1997;90:128–31.
39. Allen LA, Yager JE, Jonsson Funk M, et al. Discordance between patient-predicted and model-predicted life expectancy among ambulatory patients with heart failure. JAMA 2008;299(21):2533–42.
40. Krumholz HM, Phillips RS, Hamel MB, et al. Resuscitation preferences among patients with severe congestive heart failure: results from the SUPPORT project. Study to Understand Prognoses and Preferences for Outcomes and Risks of Treatments. Circulation 1998;98:648–55.
41. Levenson KW, McCarthy EP, Lynn J, et al. The last six months of life for patients with congestive heart failure. J Am Geriatr Soc 2000;48:S101–9.
42. Jennings AL, Davies AN, Higgins JP, et al. A systematic review of the use of opioids in the management of dyspnoea. Thorax 2002;57:939–44.
43. Stuart B. Palliative care and hospice in advanced heart failure. J Palliat Med 2007;10(1):210–28.
44. O'Connor CM, Joynt KE. Depression: are we ignoring an important comorbidity in heart failure? J Am Coll Cardiol 2004;43:1550–2.
45. Rutledge T, Reis VA, Linke SE, et al. Depression in heart failure. A meta-analytic review of prevalence, intervention effects, and associations with clinical outcomes. J Am Coll Cardiol 2006;46:1527–37.
46. Gottlieb SS, Khatta M, Friedmann E, et al. The influence of age, gender, and race on the prevalence of depression in heart failure patients. J Am Coll Cardiol 2004; 43:1542–9.
47. Fosbøl EL, Gislason GH, Poulsen HE, et al. Prognosis in heart failure and the value of beta blockers are altered by the use of antidepressants and depend on the type of antidepressants used. Circ Heart Fail 2009;2(6): 582–90.
48. Vieweg WV, Wood MA. Tricyclic antidepressants, QT interval prolongation, and torsade de pointes. Psychosomatics 2004;45(5):371–7.

49. Hardy SE. Methylphenidate for treatment of depressive symptoms, apathy, and fatigue in medically Ill older adults and terminally Ill adults. Am J Geriatr Pharmacother 2009;7(1):34–59.
50. Kohnlein T, Welte T, Tan LV, et al. Central sleep apnoea syndrome in patients with chronic heart disease: a critical review of the current literature. Thorax 2002;57: 547–54.
51. Chowdhury M, Adams S, Whellan DJ. Sleep-disordered breathing and heart failure: focus on obstructive sleep apnea and treatment with continuous positive airway pressure. J Card Fail 2010;16:164–74.
52. Bradley TD, Logan AG, Kimoff RJ, et al. Continuous positive airway pressure for central sleep apnea and heart failure. N Engl J Med 2005;353:2025–33.
53. Somers VK, White DP, Amin R, et al. Sleep apnea and cardiovascular disease: an American Heart Association/American College of Cardiology Foundation Scientific Statement From the American Heart Association Council for High Blood Pressure Research Professional Education Committee, Council on Clinical Cardiology, Stroke Council, and Council on Cardiovascular Nursing in collaboration with the National Heart, Lung, and Blood Institute National Center on Sleep Disorders Research (National Institutes of Health). J Am Coll Cardiol 2008;52:686–717.
54. Sica DA, Gehr TW, Frishman WH. Use of diuretics in the treatment of heart failure in the elderly. Clin Geriatr Med 2007;23:107–21.
55. Vollrath AM, Sinclair C, Hallenback J. Discontinuing cardiovascular medications at the end of life: lipid-lowering agents. J Palliat Med 2005;8:4.
56. Lampert R, Hayes DL, Annas GJ, et al. HRS expert consensus statement on the management of cardiovascular implantable electronic devices (CIEDs) in patients nearing end of life or requesting withdrawal of therapy. Heart Rhythm 2010;7(7):1008–26.
57. Goldstein NE, Mehta D, Siddiqui S, et al. "That's like an act of suicide." Patients' attitudes toward deactivation of implantable defibrillators. J Gen Intern Med 2008; 23:7–12.
58. Goldstein N, Carlson M, Livote E, et al. Brief communication: management of implantable cardioverter-defibrillators in hospice: a nationwide survey. Ann Intern Med 2010;152:296–9.
59. Hauptman PJ, Mikolajczak P, George A, et al. Chronic inotropic therapy in end-stage heart failure. Am Heart J 2006;152:1096.e1–8.
60. Hershberger RE, Nauman D, Walker TL, et al. Care processes and clinical outcomes of continuous outpatient support with inotropes (COSI) in patients with refractory endstage heart failure. J Card Fail 2003;9(3):180–7.
61. Morrison RS, Meier DE. Palliative care. N Engl J Med 2004;350:2582–90.
62. Usher BM, Cammarata K. Heart failure and family caregiver burden: an update. Prog Cardiovasc Nurs 2009;24(3):113–4.
63. Setoguchi S, Glynn RJ, Stedman M, et al. Hospice, opiates, and acute care service use among the elderly before death from heart failure or cancer. Am Heart J 2010;160:139–44.
64. Hauptman PJ, Goodlin SJ, Lopatin M, et al. Characteristics of patients hospitalized with acute decompensated heart failure who are referred for hospice care. Arch Intern Med 2007;167(18):1990–7.
65. Bain KT, Maxwell TL, Strassels SA, et al. Hospice use among patients with heart failure. Am Heart J 2009;158:118–25.
66. Stuart B, Alexander C, Arenella C, et al. Medical guidelines for determining prognosis in selected non-cancer diseases. 2nd edition. Arlington (VA): National Hospice Organization; 1996.

# Management of Patients with End-Stage Chronic Obstructive Pulmonary Disease

Andrew R. Berman, MD[a,b,*]

**KEYWORDS**

- Chronic obstructive pulmonary disease • Quality of life
- Prognosis • Mortality

Chronic obstructive pulmonary disease (COPD) is a disease characterized by airflow obstruction, which is not fully reversible and is usually progressive.[1] COPD is one of the most common diagnoses made during visits to a family physician,[2] though an equal number of patients with COPD are undiagnosed despite symptoms. As COPD progresses, patients experience significant disability and morbidity. COPD is currently the fourth most common cause of death in the United States, and is projected to be third by 2020.[3]

Severity of COPD is commonly assessed using the Global Initiative for Chronic Obstructive Lung Disease (GOLD) classification system. In this widely accepted system, patients are classified based on the forced expiratory volume in 1 second, or the $FEV_1$. Although the $FEV_1$ does not completely represent the complex clinical spectrum of COPD and the end points of this classification system have not been clinically validated,[1] the $FEV_1$ is reproducible and easy to measure. The GOLD system classifies patients as having mild, moderate, severe, or very severe COPD based on the $FEV_1$ percent predicted value (**Table 1**).

End-stage COPD refers to patients with GOLD Stage IV disease who have very severe airflow limitation and are breathless with minimal exertion. Though not specifically defined in the GOLD Executive Summary, such patients also often have gas

The author has nothing to disclose.
[a] Division of Pulmonary Medicine, Department of Medicine, Albert Einstein College of Medicine, Bronx, NY, USA
[b] Montefiore Medical Center, 111 East 210th Street, Bronx, NY 10467, USA
* Montefiore Medical Center, 111 East 210th Street, Bronx, NY 10467.
*E-mail address:* aberman@montefiore.org

Prim Care Clin Office Pract 38 (2011) 277–297
doi:10.1016/j.pop.2011.03.008
0095-4543/11/$ – see front matter © 2011 Elsevier Inc. All rights reserved.

Table 1
Classification of severity of COPD (all patients have an $FEV_1$/FVC ratio <70%)

| Stage | Characteristics |
|---|---|
| I: Mild COPD | $FEV_1 \geq 80\%$ predicted |
| II: Moderate COPD | $50\% \leq FEV_1 < 80\%$ predicted |
| III: Severe COPD | $30\% \leq FEV_1 < 50\%$ predicted |
| IV: Very severe COPD | $FEV_1 < 30\%$ predicted or $FEV_1 < 50\%$ predicted plus chronic respiratory failure |

Abbreviations: $FEV_1$, forced expiratory volume in 1 second; FVC, forced vital capacity; respiratory failure, arterial partial pressure of oxygen ($Pao_2$) less than 60 mm Hg with or without arterial partial pressure of $CO_2$ ($Paco_2$) greater than 50 mm Hg while breathing room air.

Data from Global initiative for Chronic Lung Obstructive Disease. Global strategy for the diagnosis, management, and prevention of chronic obstructive pulmonary disease, executive summary, Updated 2009. Available at: http://www.goldcopd.org. Accessed April 2, 2010.

exchange abnormalities (hypoxemia and/or hypercapnia) and right heart dysfunction (pulmonary hypertension). These patients have frequent exacerbations, which often result in hospitalizations and sometimes require assisted ventilation; they often have weight loss and/or a low body mass index (BMI; weight in kilograms divided by height in meters squared, ie, $kg/m^2$).

## QUALITY OF LIFE IN PATIENTS WITH END-STAGE COPD

Patients with end-stage COPD are breathless and have a poor quality of life. Such patients are often caught in a cycle of diminished mobility leading to further deconditioning and, in turn, worsening exertional tolerance. Patients become dependent on others for the routines of daily living and become socially isolated. In one study, 41% of patients who died of COPD left the house less than once per month or never in their last year of life.[4] In addition, anxiety and depression often accompany diminished quality of life and social isolation, and add a significant symptom burden.

Health-related quality of life can be measured using validated scales. The EuroQol 5-dimension (EQ-5D) questionnaire is measured by a validated scale consisting of 5 dimensions: mobility, self-care, usual activities, pain/discomfort, and anxiety/depression. Using a visual analog scale (VAS) modification to the EQ-5D, Rutten-van Mölken and colleagues[5] showed that increasing severity of COPD was associated with significant declines in EQ-5D VAS scores (Fig. 1). Patients with GOLD Stage IV (very severe) disease demonstrated worse health-related quality of life in all 5 dimensions, and these differences were maintained after correction for comorbidities. Similarly, using the validated Short Form 12 Health Survey Questionnaire (SF-12), which includes physical and mental component scales, Martin and colleagues[6] found that patients with advanced disease had worse scores on both scales. This result suggests that health-related quality of life is influenced by psychological symptoms as well as by physical limitations.

## DEPRESSION AND ANXIETY IN PATIENTS WITH SEVERE COPD
### Depression

Lung disease has a greater negative impact on life satisfaction than most systemic conditions,[7] and this is particularly true for patients with end-stage COPD. Depression is common in patients with advanced COPD, though it can be unrecognized[8] and undertreated. In a cross-sectional study of 109 patients with very severe COPD

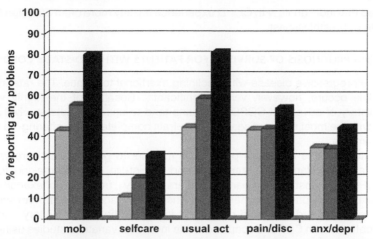

**Fig. 1.** Percentage of patients reporting any problems on the EuroQol 5-dimension questionnaire (collapsing data into 2 levels: no problems vs any problems). First bar, moderate COPD; second bar, severe COPD; third bar, very severe COPD. mob, mobility; act, activity; disc, discomfort; anx/dep, anxiety/depression. $P<.001$ (by $\chi^2$ test) for mobility, self-care, and usual activities; differences in pain/discomfort and anxiety/depression are not statistically significant. (*From* Rutten-van Mölken M, Oostenbrink J, Tashkin D, et al. Generic Euro-Qol five-dimension questionnaire differentiate between COPD severity stages? Chest 2006;130:1122; with permission.)

(median $FEV_1$ 34% predicted and most on long-term oxygen therapy for more than 1 year), 57% demonstrated significant depressive symptoms.[9] Nonetheless, only 6% of patients were taking an antidepressant medication. In a larger cross-sectional study of more than 1000 outpatients followed at a Veterans Administration, Kunik and colleagues[10] reported that only 31% of COPD patients with depression or anxiety were being treated with psychoactive drugs.

Depressive symptoms have been associated with higher rates of both COPD exacerbations and mortality.[11,12] This finding may be due to increased reporting of respiratory symptoms by depressed patients, more frequent interactions with health care providers by depressed patients and thus more potential opportunities to be diagnosed with a COPD exacerbation, or greater medical noncompliance in depressed patients, leading to diminished disease control. In general, depressed patients have been shown to be 3 times more likely to be noncompliant with medical treatment recommendations than nondepressed patients.[13] It is important to recognize and treat depression, as it has a direct and deleterious effect on both disease control and subsequent directions of care.

### Anxiety

Studies have documented that generalized anxiety disorder and panic disorder are more prevalent in patients with COPD than in the general population.[14] One study found that the prevalence of panic disorder in patients with COPD was up to 10 times greater than the overall population.[15] In addition, patients with COPD and anxiety have a higher longitudinal risk of COPD exacerbations.[16]

It may not be possible to ascertain whether anxiety is the cause of dyspnea or the result of it in patients with advanced COPD, though a small qualitative study of patients hospitalized with acute COPD exacerbations and extreme dyspnea suggested that individuals with COPD experience anxiety more often as a sign than as the cause of breathlessness.[17]

## PREDICTING PROGNOSIS OF SURVIVAL FOR PATIENTS WITH END-STAGE COPD

COPD is a progressive disease with declining exertional tolerance. The rate at which this decline occurs, however, varies significantly. Because of the highly variable natural history of advanced COPD, clinicians tend to underestimate survival among patients with the most severe disease,[18] or refrain completely from offering life expectancy estimates.

Many studies have examined prognostic markers to guide health care workers, patients, and their families in treatment and end-of-life decision making for end-stage COPD. The most studied parameters are the $FEV_1$, frequency of exacerbations, hypoxemia, hypercapnia, pulmonary hypertension, BMI, age, and symptom scores. In addition, genetics and comorbid conditions influence the natural history and prognosis of patients with COPD. Because of wide individual variation, studies using these parameters have had conflicting results, and it remains difficult to provide prognoses of survival to patients with end-stage COPD.

### $FEV_1$

The $FEV_1$ is the most frequently used parameter for assessing both disease severity and prognosis. In a study by Traver, 200 patients with COPD were followed for approximately 15 years.[19] After controlling for age, postbronchodilator percent predicted $FEV_1$ was the best predictor of prognosis. Patients whose postbronchodilator $FEV_1$ was 20%–29% predicted had a 5-year survival rate of 30% and a 10-year survival rate of 10%. In a second study by Anthonisen and colleagues,[20] nearly 1000 patients with a mean postbronchodilator $FEV_1$ of 36% predicted were shown to have an overall mortality of 23% after 3 years of follow up.

To improve the prognostic utility of the $FEV_1$, Celli and colleagues[21] developed a multidimensional assessment tool that incorporates 3 additional factors to predict the risk of hospitalization and death from COPD. This index, termed the BODE index, is based on: BMI (B), degree of airflow Obstruction using $FEV_1$ (O), Dyspnea (D), and Exercise capacity using a 6-minute walk test (E). To calculate the BODE index, either 0, 1, 2, or 3 points are assigned for each parameter, depending on its severity. Higher points indicate increasing severity for most parameters; for BMI 1 point is assigned if the BMI is 21 or less and 0 points are assigned if the BMI is greater than 21. Higher BODE indices are associated with greater risk of death, and this index has been shown to be more sensitive than $FEV_1$ alone.[21] As shown in **Fig. 2**, at 52 months patients in the highest quartile (ie, BODE score of 7–10) had a mortality rate of 80%.

### COPD Exacerbations

Frequency of COPD exacerbations has also been examined as a potential prognostic indicator. In a 3-year prospective study, Makris and colleagues[22] showed that frequent exacerbations were associated with a decline in $FEV_1$. The TORCH (Toward a Revolution in COPD Health) study, a multicenter, randomized, double-blind, placebo-controlled trial of more than 6000 patients with moderate to severe COPD, also showed that patients with frequent exacerbations had a faster decline in $FEV_1$.[23] Donaldson and colleagues,[24] studying patients with an $FEV_1$ ranging from 0.7 to 1.3 L/min, found that frequent exacerbations not only led to faster decline in $FEV_1$ but were also associated with increased hospital admissions and longer length of stay.

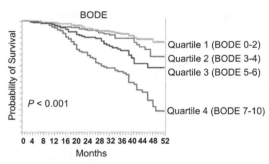

**Fig. 2.** BODE (Body mass index, airflow Obstruction, Dyspnea, and Exercise capacity) index and probability of survival. Survival differed significantly among the 4 groups (*P*<.001 by the log-rank test). (*Adapted from* Celli B, Cote C, Marin J, et al. The body-mass index, airflow obstruction, dyspnea, and exercise capacity index in chronic obstructive pulmonary disease. N Engl J Med 2004;350:1010; with permission.)

Despite these findings, frequent COPD exacerbations have not been consistently associated with survival. This inconsistency is partly due to heterogeneous methods for assessing COPD exacerbations, ranging from diary cards to active surveillance. In one study in which acute COPD exacerbations were defined based on change in symptoms and the need for hospitalization, SolerCataluña and colleagues[25] demonstrated that patients with 3 or more exacerbations during the year of the study had a survival rate of 30% after 5 years. This mortality rate was 4 times greater than for patients without acute exacerbations.

### Acute Respiratory Failure

Acute respiratory failure in and of itself has not been associated with diminished survival in COPD. In a study by Martin and colleagues,[26] 36 patients with severe airway obstruction and acute respiratory failure had comparable 2-year prognosis with control patients with similar lung function but without acute respiratory failure. Similarly, a multicenter prospective study by Senett and colleagues[27] of patients admitted to intensive care units for acute COPD exacerbations showed that, after controlling for severity of illness, mechanical ventilation was not associated with hospital mortality or 1-year survival. Finally, the SUPPORT investigators[28] (Study to Understand Prognoses and Preferences for Outcomes and Risks of Treatments) reported that, though hospitalized patients with acute COPD exacerbations and hypercapnia have high mortality, those with reversible hypercapnia had similar survival rates to eucapnic patients. In this study, poor prognosis was seen mainly in patients with chronic respiratory insufficiency.

### Pulmonary Hypertension

Pulmonary hypertension (PH) has been identified as a risk factor for shorter life expectancy. Although it is common among patients with advanced COPD it can occur at all stages, regardless of the degree of airflow obstruction or hypoxia.[29] Oswald-Mammosser and colleagues[30] investigated 84 patients with advanced COPD who underwent right heart catheterization before the initiation of long-term oxygen therapy. In this study, patients with mean pulmonary artery pressures of 25 mm Hg or greater, consistent with PH, demonstrated significantly shorter life expectancies (5-year survival of 36%) than COPD patients with normal right heart pressures (5-year survival of 62%, **Fig. 3**).

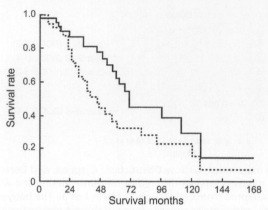

**Fig. 3.** Impact of pulmonary hypertension on survival in patients with advanced COPD. Solid line represents patients with normal right heart pressures, and dotted line represents those with pulmonary hypertension (PH). A significantly (P<.001) shorter life expectancy for patients with PH is demonstrated. (*From* Oswald-Mammosser M, Weitzenblum E, Quoix E, et al. Prognostic factors in COPD patients receiving long-term oxygen therapy: importance of pulmonary artery pressure. Chest 1995;107:1195; with permission.)

### Body Mass Index

Low body weight is an independent predictor of increased mortality in patients with COPD. Schols and colleagues[31] identified a threshold of 25, below which mortality was increased. Patients with the lowest BMIs, especially less than 20, were at greatest risk of death. In addition, weight loss in patients with advanced COPD is an independent risk factor for mortality, whereas weight gain can reverse the negative effect of low body weight.[31]

## PHARMACOLOGIC TREATMENT OF END-STAGE COPD
### Bronchodilators

Inhaled bronchodilators are the standard treatment to resolve symptoms in patients with COPD, but do not influence the natural rate of decline in lung function. Although many patients with end-stage COPD do not demonstrate significant changes in $FEV_1$ after bronchodilator administration, patients often report reduced dyspnea, which may be due to the effect of bronchodilators on reducing residual volume and dynamic hyperinflation.[32] In general, in more advanced stages of COPD, changes in lung volume are more important relative to changes in $FEV_1$.

Both short-acting β-agonists (eg, albuterol sulfate) and short-acting anticholinergics (eg, iprotropium bromide) are equipotent in improving dyspnea and exertional tolerance in patients with COPD. In general, albuterol is preferred because of its rapid onset. However, a meta-analysis of more than 15,000 patients suggested that anticholinergics were more effective than albuterol in severe exacerbations.[33] Combining both types of short-acting agents is common practice, though studies of combination therapies do not consistently show benefits of combination therapy over monotherapy. Nebulized delivery of bronchodilators offers no benefit over meter-dosed inhalers, except in patients who cannot effectively use inhalers.

In patients with severe (GOLD Stage III and IV) COPD, long-acting bronchodilators are indicated, in addition to short-acting bronchodilators.[1] Both long-acting β-agonists (eg, salmeterol and formoterol) and long-acting anticholinergics (eg, tiotropium) are effective, though tiotropium may be superior to long-acting β-agonists.[34]

Tiotropium has been shown to improve not only bronchodilation and dyspnea but also rates of COPD exacerbation and health-related quality of life.

Despite their benefits, long-acting agents have been associated with adverse effects in recent studies. Though now contraindicated as monotherapy in patients with asthma, the long-acting β-agonist salmeterol can be safely used in patients with stable moderate to severe COPD without risk of respiratory death.[35] Although some studies have also suggested cardiovascular complications of inhaled anticholinergics, tiotropium has not been shown to be associated with an increased risk of heart attack or stroke.[36]

## Inhaled Corticosteroids

GOLD guidelines recommend the use of inhaled corticosteroids (ICS) for Stage IV patients as additive treatment, and for Stage III patients with repeated exacerbations.[1] Common practice also includes ICS use when there are persistent symptoms despite long-acting bronchodilators, or if there is a demonstrated response in lung function to ICS. Despite these practices, data regarding clinical efficacy of ICS in COPD is inconclusive. Though lung function and mortality are not significantly altered, evidence suggests that ICS decrease the incidence of COPD exacerbations.[37] One study demonstrated that ICS use for 18 months would lead to one fewer exacerbation for every 12 patients with moderate to severe COPD.[38] Treatment with combined ICS and long-acting β-agonists reduces the rates of COPD exacerbation further when compared with either component agent alone.[35]

Although ICS are commonly used, meta-analyses of their effect on lung function and rate of decline of $FEV_1$ have yielded conflicting results.[39,40] In addition, a recent systematic review suggests that the benefits of ICS may be overstated.[41] In general, adverse effects of ICS tend to be local, though recent data suggest that there may be an increased risk of nonfatal pneumonia.[42] This association is currently being studied, and future results may influence the risk/benefit ratio of ICS.

Because there may be minimum airway inflammation in patients with end-stage COPD, some physicians contend that ICS use will not benefit such patients. Even if there is a significant alternative inflammatory process, most end-stage COPD patients cannot demonstrate an effective delivery of inhaled drugs to the sites of inflammation (eg, small distal airways), and may therefore not benefit fully from ICS.[43] Additional large-scale, placebo-controlled studies are needed to determine the role of ICS in patients with end-stage COPD.

## Systemic Steroids

It is generally accepted that the only role for systemic steroids in COPD is to manage acute exacerbations, and evidence in favor of chronic systemic steroid treatment in patients with stable severe COPD is unconvincing. A recent Cochrane review found no significant improvement in patient-oriented outcomes with long-term systemic steroids,[44] and further found that high steroid doses are associated with an unfavorable risk/benefit ratio. In other studies, long-term use of oral corticosteroids has been identified as a risk factor for higher mortality.[45] In one small study of previously steroid-dependent patients, half was continued on steroids and the other half was started on inhaled steroids and placed on a planned "taper to stop" regimen; no differences in exacerbations, dyspnea, or quality of life were then found between the two groups.[46] Although many clinicians still prescribe chronic systemic steroid regimens for patients with severe symptomatic COPD, attempts should be made to wean patients with advanced COPD off chronic steroids.

## Mucolytics and Expectorants

Most patients with advanced COPD describe a feeling of mucus in their upper airways that is difficult to cough up but, after doing so, there is transient relief of dyspnea. Because mucolytics decrease the viscosity of mucus and expectorants mobilize secretions, these agents may enhance clearing of respiratory secretions.

N-Actylcysteine (NAC) is the only mucolytic readily available in clinical practice, but there is inconclusive evidence for improvement following its use. A 2006 Cochrane systematic review reported an association between mucolytic use and decreased exacerbations (2.7 per year to 2.0 per year) in patients with moderate to severe COPD.[47] Conversely, the large Bronchitis Randomized on NAC Cost-Utility Study (BRONCUS) trial, published at about the same time, found that $FEV_1$ and number of COPD exacerbations were not significantly improved among patients taking NAC for 3 years, compared with patients taking placebo.[48]

The expectorant, guaifenesin, has not been studied in patients with COPD in randomized controlled trials. In practice, subjective responses are inconsistent, though medications containing guaifenesin are commonly purchased over the counter by patients. Randomized controlled studies are needed to determine the efficacy of guaifenesin in patients with advanced COPD.

## NONPHARMACOLOGIC TREATMENT OF SEVERE AND END-STAGE COPD
### Oxygen

Supplemental oxygen is one of the main treatment interventions for patients with advanced COPD. Long term oxygen therapy (LTOT) is indicated for patients with COPD who are hypoxemic at rest or with exertion. Results from the Nocturnal Oxygen Therapy Trial,[49] which compared nearly continuous oxygen therapy (18 hours a day) to nocturnal oxygen alone in patients with COPD and resting hypoxemia, showed a significant survival benefit for patients receiving continuous oxygen therapy. A systematic review of randomized trials found that continuous supplemental oxygen improved survival compared with either nocturnal oxygen or no oxygen, when used for 24 months in patients with an oxygen saturation of less than 88%.[50]

In more advanced COPD, the goal of oxygen therapy may not be long-term survival but rather increased endurance and improvement in other health-related outcomes. Bradley and O'Neill[51] showed that supplemental oxygen in patients with moderate to severe COPD and exertional desaturation was associated with greater distance walked and shorter recovery times after exertion, suggesting that oxygen treatment for such patients may break the dyspnea-deconditioning cycle. Long-term oxygen therapy in patients with COPD and severe resting arterial hypoxemia has been shown to improve exercise, sleep, and cognitive performance.[52]

Despite these benefits, compliance with home oxygen is suboptimal. Elkington and colleagues[4] found that in patients who died of COPD, the majority of patients who were prescribed home oxygen used it for less than 15 hours per day. Some physicians are reluctant to prescribe oxygen because of fears about inducing narcosis due to carbon dioxide retention, though this concern is often not realized. In general, supplemental oxygen is an underprescribed and underused but highly efficacious intervention.

Many patients with advanced COPD feel dyspneic but are not hypoxemic. Nonetheless, they may request supplemental oxygen. In patients who do not meet criteria for supplemental oxygen, improved quality of life has not been demonstrated with home oxygen treatment, suggesting that their shortness of breath may be due to factors independent of oxygenation. Although hospice patients may be prescribed oxygen without meeting approved guidelines, findings regarding the impact of oxygen on quality of life in this setting are inconsistent.[53]

## Pulmonary Rehabilitation

Pulmonary rehabilitation is a multidisciplinary intervention consisting of exercise training, educational support, and nutritional and psychological counseling. The goal is to improve quality of life by increasing exercise tolerance and reducing the perception of dyspnea. Although patients with advanced stages of COPD usually have limited exercise tolerance, pulmonary rehabilitation has still been shown to be effective in this group.[54] In a multicenter study of more than 1000 COPD patients, pulmonary rehabilitation was also found to be effective among patients with chronic respiratory failure.[55] Activities are tailored to the exercise tolerance of the participants, though rigorous rehabilitative training in patients with an $FEV_1$ of less than 1 liter has been tolerated.[56]

Pulmonary rehabilitation affects many aspects of COPD, but does so without affecting lung function. Pulmonary rehabilitation has been shown to reduce health care resource use and improve overall health status. In a study of patients with GOLD Stage IV disease (mean $FEV_1$ of approximately 30% predicted) receiving pulmonary rehabilitation, 71% of patients had an improved BODE index, due to decreased dyspnea (D) and improvement in exercise capacity (E).[54] In addition, patients with BODE quartile 4 also showed a survival advantage when compared with their counterparts not receiving pulmonary rehabilitation (**Fig. 4**).

## Noninvasive Positive Pressure Ventilation

Bilevel noninvasive positive pressure breathing is a form of assisted ventilation, delivered via a nasal or face mask, for patients with acute or chronic respiratory failure. In select patients with acute hypercapnic respiratory failure, noninvasive positive pressure ventilation (NIPPV) is used to support ventilation while the underlying condition is treated, with the overall goal of avoiding intubation and mechanical ventilation. Multiple randomized trials have shown that NIPPV reduces mortality and the need for intubation in patients with acute respiratory failure due to acute COPD exacerbation.[57]

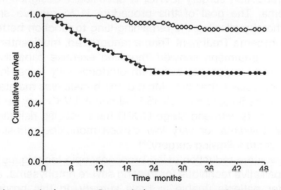

**Fig. 4.** Kaplan-Meier survival curves. Open circles represent patients participating in pulmonary rehabilitation; closed circles represent patients who declined participation in pulmonary rehabilitation. There is a significant survival advantage in the pulmonary rehabilitation group, $P<.0001$ by log-rank test. (*From* Cote C, Celli B. Pulmonary rehabilitation and the BODE index in COPD. Eur Resp J 2005;26:633; with permission.)

NIPPV is also used as a palliative measure for severe stable COPD patients with chronic respiratory failure and baseline hypercapnia. NIPPV rests respiratory muscles, allowing less work in breathing, and subsequently less breathlessness. In a systematic review of studies reporting on the use of NIPPV in patients who are chronically dyspneic from severe COPD, Kolodziej and colleagues[58] found that periods of regular NIPPV use led to significant improvement in exercise tolerance, dyspnea, and health-related quality of life. In addition, dyspnea relief has been demonstrated in patients with cancer.[59] Despite the benefits to symptom relief, there is inconsistent evidence regarding survival benefit of NIPPV in chronic stable COPD.[60,61]

In practice, many patients with severe COPD and hypercapnia prefer to wear NIPPV at night only, with the hope that resting the respiratory muscles at night will lead to increased exertional tolerance during the day. This practice has not been well studied, though nocturnal NIPPV may benefit patients with diminished sleep quality. Other factors leading to incomplete compliance with NIPPV use include excessive secretions, and patient intolerance to the mask and the pressure settings.

Treatment of chronic respiratory failure with NIPPV is not covered by most insurance carriers unless certain criteria are met. According to Medicare Part B, physicians prescribing NIPPV for patients with end-stage COPD must document: a partial pressure of carbon dioxide of greater than or equal to 52 mm Hg when the patient is awake and on their usual amount of supplemental oxygen, sleep oximetry revealing more than 5 minutes of oxygen desaturation of less than or equal to 88%, and absence of sleep apnea (though a sleep study is not required). Because of patient discomfort and insurance requirements, NIPPV is likely underprescribed by clinicians. Additional studies, advances in equipment, and health care provider education are therefore warranted.

### Surgical Treatment

Surgical interventions are not commonly considered for patients with end-stage COPD, though they should be for more functional patients with GOLD Stage IV disease. In practice, physicians often believe that patients are not appropriate surgical candidates, and patients with advanced lung disease are justifiably fearful of having lung surgery. Nonetheless, in selected patients improved outcomes have been demonstrated with surgical treatments.

Lung volume reduction surgery (LVRS) is specifically designed for patients with severe emphysema. The goal of this procedure is to remove small wedges of damaged lung, thereby allowing the remaining lung to function better. Results from the National Emphysema Treatment Trial, a randomized, multicenter trial comparing LVRS with medical treatment, showed improved exercise capacity, quality of life, and reduced mortality in patients with both predominantly upper-lobe emphysema and low baseline exercise capacity.[62] Most of the benefit was maintained for at least 2 years and as long as 5 years after LVRS.[63] Although LVRS may be helpful for some patients, many patients with end-stage COPD have specific risk factors (low $FEV_1$, homogeneous emphysema, or very low carbon monoxide diffusing capacity) for increased risk of death following surgery.[64]

Recently, lung volume reduction using bronchoscopic techniques has been introduced as a new palliative technique for treating severe emphysema, and is an attractive alternative for patients unable to have surgery. In this procedure, one-way endobronchial valves are placed into those lung segments most severely affected by emphysema, such that air and secretions can come out but no air can come in. This situation causes segmental collapse, effectively achieving the same result as LVRS. In contrast to LVRS, however, patients with heterogeneous emphysema or worse lung function may be candidates for an endobronchial valve. Endobronchial valve placement has been shown to be safe, with significant short-term improvements in functional status, quality of life, and relief of dyspnea in selected patients.[65]

Lung transplantation is also an option for selected patients with COPD and other advanced lung diseases.[66] Referral for lung transplantation should be considered for COPD patients with progressive deterioration despite optimal treatment. Appropriate patients have severe disease as defined by a low $FEV_1\%$ predicted (<25%), resting hypoxemia, hypercapnia, secondary PH, BODE index greater than 5, and an accelerated decline in $FEV_1$. Following lung transplantation, quality of life and functional capacity have been demonstrated to improve.[67] Lung transplant represents the only intervention that can substantially improve long-term outcomes in COPD patients with very advanced disease.[68] While surgical techniques are evolving and posttransplant survival is increasing, the number of available organs for transplant remains limited, and patients can die while waiting for a donor. This lack of organs creates a problematic situation whereby patients are concurrently waiting for curative-restorative care while needing palliative care.[69]

## TREATMENT OF CONDITIONS ASSOCIATED WITH END-STAGE COPD
### Osteoporosis

Osteoporosis, with resulting fractures, is a significant problem in patients with advanced COPD. The prevalence of osteoporosis in patients with COPD is 36% to 60%. Vertebral fractures have been found in 29% of patients with COPD.[70] As the disease progresses osteoporosis becomes more common, perhaps because of the immobility as a result of dyspnea and deconditioning. Other contributory causes of bone loss include smoking, vitamin D deficiency, low BMI, and the use of glucocorticoids, though osteoporosis can develop in patients not treated with steroids.

Patients with end-stage COPD should be treated for osteoporosis. Nonetheless, a Swedish study of GOLD Stage IV COPD patients showed that only 53% used either bisphosphonates or calcium supplementation.[71] A reasonable initial approach is to treat all patients with end-stage COPD with 400 to 800 IU vitamin D and 1000 to 1500 mg elemental calcium per day.

### Nutritional Depletion

Nutritional depletion is a common problem in end-stage COPD. As noted earlier, there is an inverse relationship between BMI and mortality in patients with COPD. Weight loss is also associated with a worse prognosis, and is more often seen in patients with advanced disease. Although nutritional guidelines for patients with advanced COPD recommend that patients eat many small meals (to avoid bloating) that are high in calories, to keep up with the high energy requirement from an increased workload for breathing, studies do not support these recommendations. In a meta-analysis of randomized controlled trials looking at nutritional support in COPD, Ferreira and colleagues[72] found no evidence that simple nutritional supplementation makes a significant difference to people with COPD. Further, in a prospective, double-blind, randomized controlled trial using the appetite stimulant megace acetate, underweight patients with COPD were able to gain weight, but did not improve respiratory muscle function or exercise tolerance.[73] These studies suggest that nutritional depletion in patients with end-stage COPD is multifactorial, and that consuming more calories to keep up with energy expenditure is an inadequate intervention.

Other mechanisms and therefore potential targets for intervention have been suggested to explain the cachexia seen in many patients with end-stage COPD. In addition to the imbalance of energy consumption and expenditure, patients with end-stage COPD have a preferential loss of muscle tissue over fat.[74] Nutritional supplementation combined with anabolic steroids to increase muscle mass may be one way of reversing the negative effects of weight loss. Schols and colleagues[31] demonstrated a decrease in mortality in patients referred to pulmonary rehabilitation who gained weight with this intervention. Inflammatory cytokines have also been offered as one possible explanation of weight loss in patients with advanced COPD.[75] A dietary supplement containing ω-3 polyunsaturated fatty acids, which has anti-inflammatory effects, has been shown to be safe in patients with COPD, and to improve exercise tolerance.[76] It is hoped that with greater understanding of the pathogenesis of cachexia in end-stage COPD, more effective treatments with multiple targets can be produced.

## Pulmonary Hypertension

COPD-associated PH contributes to functional limitation, resulting in worsening dyspnea on exertion. However, it may be difficult to determine whether worsening dyspnea reflects PH or COPD. Management of patients with COPD-associated PH starts with confirmation of the diagnosis. Doppler echocardiography is the best noninvasive test, but is prone to error. Once elevated pulmonary pressures are demonstrated by Doppler echocardiography, patients should undergo right-sided heart catheterization. After confirmation of elevated pulmonary pressures, other treatable causes of secondary pulmonary hypertension should be ruled out, such as chronic pulmonary emboli or sleep apnea. At the same time COPD medical therapy should be optimized, and the patient should be evaluated for supplemental oxygen and pulmonary rehabilitation.

The role of PH-specific medications in patients with COPD is not yet known. Treatment should be considered for patients who have persistent symptoms despite optimal COPD directed therapy, or when the degree of PH is disproportionate to the degree of airflow limitation. Systemic vasodilators, such as calcium channel blockers, are not recommended, as these agents can worsen ventilation-perfusion matching. Selective pulmonary vasculature vasodilators may be beneficial, though data are limited and studies with sildenafil and inhaled prostaglandin analogues are ongoing. Parenteral prostanoid analogues should not be used, as they may worsen ventilation-perfusion mismatch and hypoxia in patients with COPD. The endothelin receptor antagonist bosentan has been associated with decreases in arterial oxygen pressure, increases in the alveolar-arterial gradient, and deterioration in quality of life measurements.[77] At present, lung transplantation is considered the best long-term option for patients with COPD and PH.[78]

## Depression

The optimal regimen for treating depression in COPD has not been established. Low mood is common in patients during the last year of life, though most do not receive specific therapy for this.[4] Because depression is recognized as a risk factor for poor outcomes, early recognition may help identify patients at greater risk for exacerbations.

Most studies of pharmacotherapy for depression in COPD patients use older antidepressive drugs, such as nortriptyline, and show mixed results.[8] A placebo-controlled trial of the selective serotonin reuptake inhibitor, paroxetine, in patients with end-stage COPD and significant depressive symptoms found improvements in emotional function.[79] Because of a high drop-out rate in both groups, however, this finding was not statistically significant. Of note, paroxetine was not associated with any worsening of respiratory symptoms.[79] More studies are needed with newer antidepressants.

Nonpharmacologic interventions may also be beneficial. Pulmonary rehabilitation has been shown to improve depression in some patients. Conversely, the benefits of supplemental oxygen on mood in COPD are unproven.

### Anxiety

As with depression, treatment of anxiety in patients with advanced COPD should start with optimization of the management of COPD. Some of the medications used to achieve this, however, may mimic anxiety symptoms. β-Agonist bronchodilators, for example, can produce tachycardia and restlessness that can easily be misinterpreted for anxiety or, alternatively, provoke anxiety. Similarly, theophylline, though used much less often nowadays, can cause similar signs and symptoms when serum levels run high. Clinicians should keep in mind that anxiety in patients with end-stage COPD may reflect the underlying condition or its treatment.

If anxiety continues despite optimal treatment of COPD, psychotherapy and anxiolytic medical therapy should be introduced. Cognitive behavioral therapy (CBT) has been shown to be effective in patients with COPD. Livermore and colleagues[80] randomized 41 patients enrolled in pulmonary rehabilitation to CBT or routine care. After 18 months, no patients in the CBT group experienced panic attacks, compared with 60% in the routine care group. A recent meta-analysis, however, showed that the effects of CBT-based or psychotherapeutically based interventions on anxiety in patients with COPD were small.[81] Other nonpharmacologic interventions for anxiety include breathing exercises, such as purse-lip breathing, which reduces anxiety by promoting a slower and deeper breathing pattern, and has been shown to have a modest but significant effect on breathlessness.[82]

There are limited studies of pharmacotherapy for anxiety in patients with advanced COPD. Older studies using buspirone have demonstrated mixed results. In general, benzodiazepines are not recommended for patients with end-stage COPD because of the potential risk of respiratory depression, except when prescribed as part of an integrated palliative care plan.

## PALLIATIVE AND END-OF-LIFE CARE
### Breathlessness

Breathlessness is the most common symptom in end-stage COPD. Elkington and colleagues[4] reported that 98% of patients who died of COPD were breathless all the time or some of the time in their last year of life. If dyspnea persists despite optimal therapy with pharmacologic and nonpharmacologic interventions in patients with end-stage COPD, treatment with opiates should be considered to reduce ventilatory demand by decreasing central drive. In a systematic review, opiates were found to be a very effective treatment for breathlessness secondary to any cause.[83]

Opiates should be titrated to achieve relief of breathlessness and should be delivered parenterally. Although nebulized opiates have also been used, there is little evidence to support this form of delivery.[84] Common opiate side effects are drowsiness, nausea, vomiting, dizziness, and constipation, but there is no evidence indicating that opiate use is associated with deleterious effects on arterial blood gases or oxygen saturation in patients with COPD.[83] Despite this lack of evidence opiates are commonly withheld or underdosed in patients with advanced COPD, due to fear of reducing respiratory drive, promoting respiratory depression, and hastening death.[85] As a result, opiates, if prescribed at all, are given in relatively small doses, often without titration to achieve symptom relief, and usually with dosing intervals that are too long. As long as the intent of treatment is the relief of suffering, treatment with opiates is both ethically and legally sanctioned under the principle of double effect.[86] Each patient should be assessed individually and appropriate dose adjustments made based on the patient's current medical condition. There are no data to suggest that the use of opioids for management of breathlessness is associated with a reduction in a patient's life expectancy.[85]

### Discussion of Advance Directives

Patients with end-stage COPD are usually ill for a long time with significant limitations, and suffer periodic acute exacerbations that may result in death. As noted previously, decline in overall performance status is expected, but the rate at which this occurs is difficult to predict, as is time to death. When physicians have difficulty making a prognosis, they are less likely to initiate discussions regarding end-of-life care, and decisions regarding advance directives are deferred. In addition, while patients with advanced COPD experience poor quality of life, they often do not actively express their limitations because they have been ill for a long time and consider the numerous daily limitations they face as normal.[87] Most patients with moderate to severe COPD have not discussed advance care preferences with their physician.[88] Communication problems between patients and their health care providers lead to patients not receiving care to improve their quality of life or their quality of dying, and they may not be offered palliative and end-of-life care options.

An individualized integrated model of palliative care depends on good communication between patients, their families, and clinicians, and should begin once the patient becomes symptomatic despite maximal therapy.[89] At this point, some patients choose not to be intubated (DNI [do not intubate]) should respiratory failure occur, based on their view of the burden of treatment in relation to the likelihood of possible outcomes.[90] The ability of a physician to guide the patient in DNI decision making often rests on how well the physician knows the patient, as physicians may frame information to influence choice.[91] All health care providers should assist patients in thinking about their advance care during stable periods of health, before a life-threatening exacerbation. These discussions should prepare patients with advanced COPD for end-of-life care, as well as assisting them to have a reasonable quality of life.

### Depression and End-Of-Life Decision Making

Depression may influence end-of-life decision making, and should be considered in any advance care discussion. In a cross-sectional study of 101 patients with advanced COPD on long-term oxygen therapy, Stapleton and colleagues[92] found that depressed patients were twice as likely to refuse resuscitation as patients without depression. This finding is consistent with earlier ones from the SUPPORT study,[93] in which do-not-resuscitate status decisions were significantly associated with depressive symptoms in a cohort of 1590 seriously ill hospitalized patients. Further, these investigators noted that in those patients who demonstrated a reduction in depressive symptoms after 2 months of follow-up, there was a fivefold increase in the likelihood of patients changing preferences to desiring full cardiopulmonary resuscitation.[93]

### Transition to Palliative Care and Hospice Care

Palliative care should be available during the course of end-stage respiratory disease and critical illness. Palliative care can be provided in hospitals, intensive care units, nursing homes, outpatient clinics, and hospices. Hospice care is indicated for the majority of patients with end-stage COPD. Most patients nearing the end of life with

COPD require assistance, including home nursing care, help with transportation, homemaking services, and personal care. Families often end up assuming substantial responsibility and burden of care.[94] The patient's needs and preferences should determine the choice of the appropriate setting.

Whereas patients with advanced lung cancer often receive hospice care, patients with advanced COPD are less likely to receive this service,[52] even though patients with COPD have a worse quality of life than patients with lung cancer (**Fig. 5**).[95] Reasons for this difference include variations in patient and physician attitudes, and disease trajectories.[96] Without supportive end-of-life care, such as hospice care, patients suffer from continued symptoms and present with greater frequency to health care providers, which may lead to additional and perhaps unnecessary care.

The current Medicare Hospice benefit disease-specific criteria for patients with various forms of advanced pulmonary disease who eventually follow a final common pathway for end-stage pulmonary disease is outlined as follows.[97]

1. Severe chronic lung disease as documented by both:
   - Disabling dyspnea at rest, poorly responsive or unresponsive to bronchodilators, resulting in decreased functional capacity, for example, bed to chair existence, fatigue, and cough. Documentation of FEV$_1$ after bronchodilator $\leq$30% of predicted is objective evidence for disabling dyspnea, but is not necessary to obtain.
   - Progression of end-stage pulmonary disease, as evidenced by increasing visits to the emergency department or hospitalizations for pulmonary infections and/or respiratory failure or increasing physician home visits before initial certification.

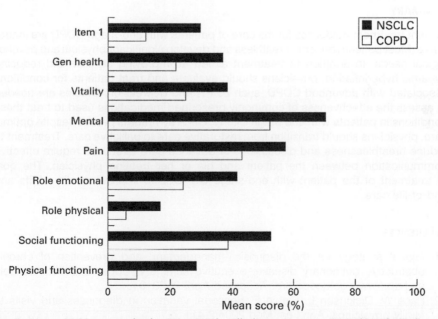

**Fig. 5.** Mean SF-36 scores (scale 0%–100%). All dimensions except roles physical and emotional are significantly different, $P\leq$.05 (Mann-Whitney $U$-test). Item 1 refers to how patients rate their general health; a higher score indicates a more favorable health status. (*From* Gore J, Brophy C, Greenstone M. How well do we care for patients with end stage chronic obstructive pulmonary disease (COPD)? A comparison of palliative care and quality of life in COPD and lung cancer. Thorax 2000;55:1002; with permission.)

Documentation of serial decrease of $FEV_1$ $\geq$40 mL/y is objective evidence for disease progression, but is not necessary to obtain.

2. Hypoxemia at rest on room air, as evidenced by $Po_2$ $\leq$55 mm Hg or oxygen saturation $\leq$88% on supplemental oxygen determined by either arterial blood gas levels or oxygen saturation monitors (these values may be obtained from recent hospital records) or hypercapnia, as evidenced by $Pco_2$ $\geq$50 mm Hg. This value may be obtained from recent (within 3 months) hospital records.
3. Right heart failure secondary to pulmonary disease (cor pulmonale), for example, not secondary to left heart disease or valvulopathy.
4. Unintentional progressive weight loss of $\geq$10% of body weight over the preceding 6 months.
5. Resting tachycardia $\geq$100 beats/min.

Documentation certifying terminal status must contain enough information to confirm terminal status on review. If the patient does not meet the above criteria yet is deemed appropriate for hospice care, sufficient documentation of the patient's condition that justifies terminal status would be necessary. Documentation might include comorbidities, rapid decline in physical and/or functional status despite appropriate treatment, or symptom severity that with reasonable reliability is consistent with a life span prognosis of 6 months or less.

Hospice care should be offered as a group of interdisciplinary services that are available for patients with end-stage COPD, to provide nursing care and symptom management as needed.

## SUMMARY

Current treatment guidelines for the care of patients with end-stage COPD are inadequate. Most patients become breathless and develop significant physical and psychological needs. In addition to treatment aimed at improving air flow and reducing dynamic hyperinflation, physicians should evaluate and treat patients for conditions associated with advanced COPD, such as PH and depression. Studies are needed to assess the effectiveness of commonly prescribed medications used to treat these conditions in patients with end-stage COPD. Once symptoms persist despite optimal care, physicians should transition from restorative care to palliative care. Treatment to reduce breathlessness and discussions of advance care directives require effective communication between the patient and his or her treating physician. The goal of treatment of the patient with end-stage COPD is to improve quality of life and end-of-life care.

## REFERENCES

1. Global strategy for the diagnosis, management, and prevention of chronic obstructive pulmonary disease, executive summary. Updated 2009. Available at: http://www.goldcopd.org. Accessed April 2, 2010.
2. Pace W, Dickinson L, Staton E. Seasonal variation in diagnoses and visits to family physicians. Ann Fam Med 2004;2:411–7.
3. Murray C, Lopez A. Alternative projections of mortality and disability by cause 1990-2020: global burden of disease Study. Lancet 1997;349:1498–504.
4. Elkington H, White P, Addington-Hall J, et al. The healthcare needs of chronic obstructive pulmonary disease patients in the last year of life. Palliat Med 2005; 19:485–91.

5. Rutten-van Mölken M, Oostenbrink J, Tashkin D, et al. Generic EuroQol five-dimension questionnaire differentiate between COPD severity stages? Chest 2006;130:1117–28.

6. Martin A, Rodriguez-Gonzalez J, Izquierdo J. Health-related quality of life in outpatients with COPD in daily practice: the VICE Spanish study. Int J Chron Obstruct Pulmon Dis 2008;3:683–92.

7. Singer H, Ruchinskas R, Riley K, et al. The psychological impact of end-stage lung disease. Chest 2001;120:1246–52.

8. Hill K, Geist R, Goldstein R, et al. Anxiety and depression in end-stage COPD. Eur Respir J 2008;31:667–77.

9. Lacasse Y, Rousseau L, Maltais F. Prevalence and impact of depression in patients with severe chronic obstructive pulmonary disease. J Cardiopulm Rehabil 2001;21:80–6.

10. Kunik M, Roundy K, Veazey C, et al. Surprisingly high prevalence of anxiety and depression in chronic breathing disorders. Chest 2005;127:1205–11.

11. Xu W, Collet J, Shapiro S, et al. Independent effect of depression and anxiety on chronic obstructive pulmonary disease exacerbations and hospitalizations. Am J Respir Crit Care Med 2008;178:913–20.

12. De Voogd J, Wempe J, Koeter G, et al. Depressive symptoms as predictors of mortality in patients with COPD. Chest 2009;135:619–25.

13. DiMatteo M, Lepper H, Croghan T. Depression is a risk factor for noncompliance with medical treatment. Meta-analysis of the effects of anxiety and depression on patient adherence. Arch Intern Med 2000;160:2101–7.

14. Brenes G. Anxiety and chronic obstructive pulmonary disease: prevalence, impact, and treatment. Psychosom Med 2003;65:963–70.

15. Livermore N, Sharpe L, McKenzie D. Panic attacks and panic disorder in chronic obstructive pulmonary disease: a cognitive behavioral perspective. Respir Med 2010;104:1246–53.

16. Eisner M, Blanc P, Yelin E, et al. Influence of anxiety on health outcomes in COPD. Thorax 2010;65:229–34.

17. Bailey PH. The dyspnea-anxiety-dyspnea cycle—COPD patients' stories of breathlessness: "It's scary when you can't breathe." Qual Health Res 2004;14: 760–78.

18. Lynn J, Ely E, Zhong Z, et al. Living and dying with chronic obstructive pulmonary disease. J Am Geriatr Soc 2000;48:S91–100.

19. Traver G, Cline M, Burrows B. Predictors of mortality in chronic obstructive pulmonary disease. A 15-year follow-up study. Am Rev Respir Dis 1979 Jun;119:895–902.

20. Anthonisen N, Wright E, Hodgkin J. Prognosis in chronic obstructive pulmonary disease. Am Rev Respir Dis 1986;133:14–20.

21. Celli B, Cote C, Marin J, et al. The body-mass index, airflow obstruction, dyspnea, and exercise capacity index in chronic obstructive pulmonary disease. N Engl J Med 2004;350:1005–12.

22. Makris D, Moschandreas J, Damianaki A, et al. Exacerbations and lung function decline in COPD: new insights in current and ex-smokers. Respir Med 2007;101: 1305–12.

23. Colli B, Thomas N, Anderson J, et al. Effect of pharmacotherapy on rate of decline of lung function in chronic obstructive pulmonary disease: results from the TORCH study. Am J Respir Crit Care Med 2008;178:332–8.

24. Donaldson G, Seemungal T, Bhowmik A, et al. Relationship between exacerbation frequency and lung function decline in chronic obstructive pulmonary disease. Thorax 2002;57:847–52.

25. SolerCataluña J, MartínezGarcia M, Roman Sanchez P, et al. Severe acute exacerbations and mortality in patients with chronic obstructive pulmonary disease. Thorax 2005;60:925–31.
26. Martin T, Lewis S, Albert R. The prognosis of patients with chronic obstructive pulmonary disease after hospitalization for acute respiratory failure. Chest 1982;82:310–4.
27. Seneff M, Wagner D, Wagner R, et al. Hospital and 1-year survival of patients admitted to intensive care units with acute exacerbation of chronic obstructive pulmonary disease. JAMA 1995;274(23):1852–7.
28. Connors A, Dawson N, Thomas C, et al. Outcomes following acute exacerbation of severe chronic obstructive lung disease. The SUPPORT investigators (Study to Understand Prognoses and Preferences for Outcomes and Risks of Treatments). Am J Respir Crit Care Med 1996;154:959–67.
29. Peinado V, Pizarro S, Barbera J. Pulmonary vascular involvement in COPD. Chest 2008;134:808–14.
30. Oswald-Mammosser M, Weitzenblum E, Quoix E, et al. Prognostic factors in COPD patients receiving long-term oxygen therapy: importance of pulmonary artery pressure. Chest 1995;107:1193–8.
31. Schols A, Slangen J, Volovics L, et al. Weight loss is a reversible factor in the prognosis of chronic obstructive pulmonary disease. Am J Respir Crit Care Med 1998;157:1791–7.
32. O'Donnell D. Hyperinflation, dyspnea, and exercise tolerance in chronic obstructive pulmonary disease. Proc Am Thorac Soc 2006;3:180–4.
33. Salpeter S, Buckley N, Salpeter E. Meta-analysis: anticholinergics, but not β-agonists, reduce severe exacerbations and respiratory mortality in COPD. J Gen Intern Med 2006;21:1011–9.
34. Brusasco V, Hodder R, Miravitlles M. Health outcomes following treatment for six months with once daily tiotropium compared with twice daily salmeterol in patients with COPD. Thorax 2003;58:399–404.
35. Calverley P, Anderson J, Celli B, et al. Salmeterol and fluticasone propionate and survival in chronic obstructive pulmonary disease. N Engl J Med 2007;356:775–89.
36. Tashkin D, Celli B, Senn S. A 4-year trial of tiotropium in chronic obstructive pulmonary disease. N Engl J Med 2008;359:1543–54.
37. Burge P, Calverely P, Jones P, et al. Randomised, double blind, placebo controlled study of fluticasone propionate in patients with moderate to severe chronic obstructive pulmonary disease: the ISOLDE trial. BMJ 2000;320:1297–303.
38. Gartlehner G, Hansen R, Carson S, et al. Efficacy and safety of inhaled corticosteroids in patients with COPD: a systematic review and meta-analysis of health outcomes. Ann Fam Med 2006;4:253–62.
39. Highland K, Strange C, Heffner J. Long-term effects of inhaled corticosteroids on $FEV_1$ in patients with chronic obstructive pulmonary disease a meta-analysis. Ann Intern Med 2003;138:969–73.
40. Sutherland E, Allmers H, Avas N, et al. Inhaled corticosteroids reduce the progression of airflow limitation in chronic obstructive pulmonary disease: a meta-analysis. Thorax 2003;58:937–41.
41. Agarwal R, Aggarwal A, Gupta D. Inhaled corticosteroids vs placebo for preventing COPD exacerbations: a systematic review and metaregression of randomized controlled trials. Chest 2010;137:318–25.
42. Ernst P, Gonzalez A, Brassard P, et al. Inhaled corticosteroid use in chronic obstructive pulmonary disease and the risk of hospitalization for pneumonia. Am J Respir Crit Care Med 2007;176:162–6.

43. Wilson A. Airway obstruction in severe COPD. Chest 2000;118:889–91.
44. Walters J, Walters E, Wood-Baker R. Oral corticosteroids for stable chronic obstructive pulmonary disease. Cochrane Database Syst Rev 2005;2:CD005374.
45. Groenewegen K, Schols A, Wouters E. Mortality and after hospitalization for acute exacerbation of COPD. Chest 2003;124:459–67.
46. Rice K, Rubins J, Lebahn F. Withdrawal of chronic systemic corticosteroids in patients with COPD. Am J Respir Crit Care Med 2000;162:174–8.
47. Poole P, Black P. Mucolytic agents for chronic bronchitis or chronic obstructive pulmonary disease. Cochrane Database Syst Rev 2010;2:CD001287.
48. Decramer M, Rutten-van Mölken M, Dekhuijzen P, et al. Effects of N-acetylcysteine on outcomes in chronic obstructive pulmonary disease (Bronchitis Randomized on NAC Cost-Utility Study, BRONCUS): a randomised placebo-controlled trial. Lancet 2005;365:1552060.
49. Continuous or nocturnal oxygen therapy in hypoxemic chronic obstructive lung disease: a clinical trial. Nocturnal Oxygen Therapy Trial Group. Ann Intern Med 1980;93:391–8.
50. Cranston J, Crockett A, Moss JR, et al. Domiciliary oxygen for chronic obstructive pulmonary disease. Cochrane Database Syst Rev 2005;4:CD001744.
51. Bradley J, O'Neill B. Short-term ambulatory oxygen for chronic obstructive pulmonary disease. Cochrane Database Syst Rev 2005;4:CD004356.
52. Celli B, MacNee W, Agusti A, et al. Standards for the diagnosis and treatment of patients with COPD: a summary of the ATS/ERS position paper. Eur Respir J 2004;23:932–46.
53. Yohannes A. Palliative care provision for patients with chronic obstructive pulmonary disease. Health Qual Life Outcomes 2007;5:17.
54. Cote C, Celli B. Pulmonary rehabilitation and the BODE index in COPD. Eur Respir J 2005;26:630–6.
55. Carone M, Patessio A, Ambrosino N, et al. Efficacy of pulmonary rehabilitation in chronic respiratory failure (CRF) due to chronic obstructive pulmonary disease (COPD): The Maugeri Study. Respir Med 2007;101:2447–53.
56. Casaburi R, Porszasz J, Burns M, et al. Physiologic benefits of exercise training in rehabilitation of patients with severe chronic obstructive pulmonary disease. Am J Respir Crit Care Med 1997;155:1541–51.
57. Brochard L, Mancebo J, Wysocki M, et al. Noninvasive ventilation for acute exacerbations of chronic pulmonary disease. N Engl J Med 1995;333:817–22.
58. Kolodziej M, Jensen L, Rowe B, et al. Systematic review of noninvasive positive pressure ventilation in severe stable COPD. Eur Respir J 2007;30:293–306.
59. Cuomo A, Delmastro M, Ceriana P, et al. Noninvasive mechanical ventilation as a palliative treatment of acute respiratory failure in patients with end-stage solid cancer. Palliat Med 2004;18:602–10.
60. Clini E, Sturani C, Rossi A, et al. The Italian multicentre study on noninvasive ventilation in chronic obstructive pulmonary disease patients. Eur Respir J 2002;20:529–38.
61. Budweiser S, Hitzl A, Jorres R, et al. Impact of noninvasive home ventilation on longterm survival in chronic hypercapnic COPD: a prospective observational study. Int J Clin Pract 2007;61:1516–22.
62. National Emphysema Treatment Trial Research Group. A randomized trial comparing lung-volume-reduction surgery with medical therapy for severe emphysema. N Engl J Med 2003;348:2059–73.
63. Yusen R, Lefrak S, Gierda D, et al. A prospective evaluation of lung volume reduction surgery in 200 consecutive patients. Chest 2003;123:1026–37.

64. National Emphysema Treatment Trial Research Group. Patients at high risk of death after lung volume reduction surgery. N Engl J Med 2001;345:1075–83.
65. Yim A, Hwong T, Lee T, et al. Early results of endoscopic lung volume reduction for emphysema. J Thorac Cardiovasc Surg 2004;127:1564–73.
66. Trulock E, Edwards L, Taylor D, et al. The Registry of the International Society for Heart and Lung Transplantation: twentieth official adult lung and heart-lung transplant report; 2003. J Heart Lung Transplant 2003;22:625–35.
67. Smeritschnig B, Jaksch P, Kocher A, et al. Quality of life after lung transplantation: a cross-sectional study. J Heart Lung Transplant 2005;24:474–80.
68. Todd JL, Palmer SM. Lung transplantation in advanced COPD: is it worth it? Semin Respir Crit Care Med 2010;31(3):365–72.
69. Janssen D, Spruit M, Does J, et al. End-of-life care in a COPD patient awaiting lung transplantation: a case report. BMC Palliat Care 2010;9:6.
70. Shane E, Silverberg S, Donovan D, et al. Osteoporosis in lung transplantation candidates with end-stage pulmonary disease. Am J Med 1996;101(3):262–9.
71. Stenfors N. Physician-diagnosed COPD global initiative for chronic obstructive lung disease stage IV in Östersund, Sweden: Patient characteristics and estimated prevalence. Chest 2006;130:666–71.
72. Ferreira I, Brooks D, Lacasse Y, et al. Nutritional support for individuals with COPD. A meta-analysis. Chest 2000;117:672–8.
73. Weisberg J, Wanger J, Olson J, et al. Megestrol acetate stimulates weight gain and ventilation in underweight COPD patients. Chest 2002;121:1070–8.
74. Debigare R, Cote H, Maltais F. Peripheral muscle wasting in chronic obstructive pulmonary disease. Clinical relevance and mechanisms. Am J Respir Crit Care Med 2001;164:1712–7.
75. Schols A, Buurman A, Staal-vd Brekel A, et al. Evidence for a relation between metabolic derangements and elevated inflammatory mediators in a subset of patients with chronic obstructive pulmonary disease. Thorax 1996;51:819–24.
76. Matsuyama W, Mitsuyama H, Watanabe M, et al. Effects of omega-3 polyunsaturated fatty acids on inflammatory markers in COPD. Chest 2005;128:3817–27.
77. Stolz D, Rasch H, Linka A, et al. A randomised, controlled trial of bosentan in severe COPD. Eur Respir J 2008;32:619–28.
78. Minai O, Chaouat A, Adnot S. Pulmonary hypertension in COPD: epidemiology, significance, and management: pulmonary vascular disease: the global perspective. Chest 2010;137:39S–51S.
79. Lacasse Y, Beaudoin L, Rousseau L, et al. Randomized trial of paroxetine in end-stage COPD. Monaldi Arch Chest Dis 2004;61:140–7.
80. Livermore N, Sharpe L, McKenzie D. Prevention of panic attacks and panic disorder in COPD. Eur Respir J 2010;35:557–63.
81. Baraniak A, Sheffield D. The efficacy of psychologically based interventions to improve anxiety, depression and quality of life in COPD: a systematic review and meta-analysis. Patient Educ Couns 2011;83(1):29–36.
82. Bianchi R, Gigliotti F, Romagnoli I, et al. Chest wall kinematics and breathlessness during pursed-lip breathing in patients with COPD. Chest 2004;125:459–65.
83. Jennings AL, Davies AN, Higgins JP, et al. A systematic review of the use of opioids in the management of dyspnoea. Thorax 2002;57:939–44.
84. Jennings A, Davies A, Higgins J, et al. Opioids for the palliation of breathlessness in terminal illness. Cochrane Database Syst Rev 2001;4:CD002066.
85. Mahler D, Selecky P, Harrod C, et al. American College of Chest Physicians consensus statement on the management of dyspnea in patients with advanced lung or heart disease. Chest 2010;137:674–91.

86. Luce J, Alpers A. Legal aspects of withholding and withdrawing life support from critically ill patients in the United States and providing palliative care to them. Am J Respir Crit Care Med 2000;162:2029–32.
87. Habraken J, Pols J, Bindels P, et al. The silence of patients with end-stage COPD: a qualitative study. Br J Gen Pract 2008;58:844–9.
88. Curtis J, Engelberg R, Nielson E, et al. D. Patient-physician communication about end-of-life care for patients with severe COPD. Eur Respir J 2004;24:200–5.
89. Lanken P, Terry P, DeLisser H, et al. American Thoracic Society. Official clinical policy statement: palliative care for patients with respiratory diseases and critical illnesses. Am J Respir Crit Care Med 2008;177(8):912–27.
90. Fried T, Bradley E, Towle V, et al. Understanding the treatment preferences of seriously ill patients. N Engl J Med 2002;346:1061–6.
91. Sullivan K, Hebert P, Logan J, et al. What do physicians tell patients with end-stage COPD about intubation and mechanical ventilation? Chest 1996;109: 258–64.
92. Stapleton R, Nielsen E, Engelberg R, et al. Association of depression and life-sustaining treatment preferences in patients with COPD. Chest 2005;127:328–34.
93. Rosenfeld K, Wenger N, Phillips R, et al. Factors associated with change in resuscitation preference of seriously ill patients. Arch Intern Med 1996;156:1558–64.
94. Emanuel E, Fairclough D, Slutsman J, et al. Assistance from family members, friends, paid care givers, and volunteers in the care of terminally ill patients. N Engl J Med 1999;341:956–63.
95. Gore J, Brophy C, Greenstone M. How well do we care for patients with end stage chronic obstructive pulmonary disease (COPD)? A comparison of palliative care and quality of life in COPD and lung cancer. Thorax 2000;55:1000–6.
96. Curtis J, Wenrich M, Carline J, et al. Patients' perspectives on physician skill in end-of-life care: differences between patients with COPD, Cancer, and AIDS. Chest 2002;122:356–62.
97. Determining terminal status in non-cancer diagnoses: pulmonary disease. The National Hospice Organization. Standards and accreditation committee medical guidelines task force. 1996. Appendix C. Available at: http://aspe.hhs.gov/daltcp/Reports. Accessed October 19, 2010.

# Palliative Care in the Treatment of End-Stage Renal Failure

Ronald Werb, MB, ChB, MRCP(UK), FRCP(C)[a,b,*]

## KEYWORDS

- Palliative care • Kidney failure • Renal failure

Palliative care services historically have focused on patients with incurable cancer. According to the current view, access to palliative care should be based on need and not diagnosis.[1] Palliative care begins with establishing goals of care based on estimated prognosis in end-stage renal disease (ESRD). A consensus statement from the US National Institutes of Health highlights the palliative care needs of patients with congestive heart failure, ESRD, liver failure, dementia, and chronic obstructive lung disease.[2] Patients with ESRD are increasingly characterized by older age and multiple comorbid illnesses,[3] and have a mortality rate 8 times higher than the general Medicare population.[4] Dialysis patients are appropriate for palliative care because of their high mortality rate and high symptom burden. More patients and families are choosing not to start or withdraw dialysis for multiple reasons, particularly in patients older than 60 years.

## PROGNOSIS IN END-STAGE RENAL DISEASE

The prognosis of patients receiving renal replacement therapies (excluding renal transplantation) is related to the age of the patients and especially whether the patients are also diabetic. Canadian data ending 1999 indicate a 5-year survival rate of 74.3% for patients aged 18 to 45 years, 60.5% for patients aged 45 to 54 years, 46.3% for the age group 55 to 64 years, 31.7% for the age group 64 to 74 years, and only 19.6% for patients older than 75 years. These older patients had a 37.5% 3 year survival rate.[5] More recent Canadian data ending 2007 indicate a 5-year survival of 72.3% for patients aged 18 to 64 years (49.3% if the patients are diabetic) and a 33.8% survival of patients older than 65 years (but only 29.7% if the patients are diabetic).[6]

This work was supported by the Carraresi Foundation.
The author has nothing to disclose.
[a] Division of Nephrology, Department of Medicine, University of British Columbia, Vancouver, British Columbia, Canada
[b] Providence Health Care, 1181 Burrard Street, Vancouver, British Columbia V6Z 1Y6, Canada
* Pacific Nephrology Group, Suite 602, 1160 Burrard Street, Vancouver V6Z 2E8, Canada.
E-mail address: rwerb@telus.net

Prim Care Clin Office Pract 38 (2011) 299–309
doi:10.1016/j.pop.2011.03.009
0095-4543/11/$ – see front matter © 2011 Elsevier Inc. All rights reserved.

primarycare.theclinics.com

The United States Renal Data System (USRDS) database confirms these statistics with analyses of mortality risks in the years 2003, 2005, and 2007. Age remains as a strong predictor of mortality. Comparing the relative risk for death in patients older than 85 years, using age 60 as the reference group, relative risk is 6.30 (2003), 6.43 (2005), and 6.34 (2007). In 2007 the risk for males was 13% higher than for females, and 15% higher for African Americans compared with Whites.

Even more dramatically, when one compares the outcome for patients receiving hemodialysis with age-matched controls, the differences are striking in the number of remaining years of life. A dialysis patient aged 15 to 19 years has 17.6 remaining life years, similar to a 65- to 69-year-old patient in the general population with 17.2 years remaining; a 75-year-old on dialysis can expect to live only 2.9 years compared with 10.8 years for a 75-year-old who does not need dialysis.[7] This finding is similar to those reported by Foley and colleagues[8] that demonstrated an annual cardiovascular mortality in 25- to 34-year-old hemodialysis patients to be the same as that of nondialysis patients aged 80 years and older. Adding diabetes and cardiovascular disease to kidney disease increases the relative risk of death to 4.07 compared with kidney failure patients without these comorbidities.

Cardiopulmonary resuscitation (CPR) in patients with renal failure is associated with very poor outcomes, with a reported survival of 0% to 8% patients alive to discharge.[9–11] A recent report from Canada[12] found that if CPR was required to treat an arrhythmia associated with an electrolyte imbalance, up to 79% survived 30 days after discharge.

## CAUSES OF DEATH

The reported causes of death in patients with renal failure are in the majority related to cardiovascular disease. Sudden death due to cardiac arrhythmias or cardiac arrest accounted for 50 deaths per 1000 patient-years, acute myocardial infarction another 9.1 deaths per 1000 patient-years. Septicemia accounted for 19.8 deaths per 1000 patient-years. Withdrawal from dialysis was associated with an overall death rate of 7.4 per 1000 patient-years; however, withdrawal from dialysis as a cause of death rose to 20.1 per 1000 patient-years for 65- to 74-year-old patients and as high as 47.3 per 1000 patient-years in the 75-plus age group.[13] The reasons for withdrawal ranged from failure to thrive in the total group at a rate of 20.6 per 1000 patient-years (but up to 86.6/100 patient-years in the 85-plus age group), request by a competent individual 14.6 per 1000 patient-years (but 44.9/1000 patient-years in the competent 85-plus age group), and only 0.7 per 1000 patient-years for access failure.[14] A preponderance of deaths from cardiovascular disease is also seen in matched peritoneal dialysis patients.[15,16]

Death from cerebrovascular disease is surprisingly documented at a relatively low overall rate of 8.8 per 1000 patient-years, even in the 75-plus age groups, whose rate was 14.0 per 1000 patient-years. The risk of stroke is 1.2 to 3.6 times higher in patients with chronic kidney disease (CKD), and the incidence of stroke is twice as common in patients with stage 5 CKD than in those with stage 3 CKD. The low observed rate is attributable to the fact that stroke incidence peaks in the 3 months before patients start dialysis and within 3 months after starting dialysis, effectively excluding these patients from the analysis of rates in dialysis patients in whom events in the first 90 days after starting renal replacement therapy (RRT) are censored out, to prevent the statistics from including patients with acute renal failure.[17]

Serum calcium $\times$ phosphorus ($Ca \times P$) product of more than 72 $mg^2/dL^2$ in patients on dialysis has been associated with an increase in all-cause mortality, cardiovascular mortality, and fracture-related hospitalizations, presumably through altered mineral metabolism and soft tissue calcification.[18,19] The incidence of hemodynamically significant heart valve calcification, especially aortic valve involvement, has also been linked to an elevated Ca×P product.[20] Coronary artery calcification (CAC) has been reported in association with aortic valve calcification in dialysis patients as young as 20 years. Compared with age-matched nondialysis patients, dialysis patients had a CAC score 2.5-fold higher, which worsened significantly over the next year.[21] Goodman and colleagues[22] reported similar findings using electron-beam computed tomography, with patient scores ranging from 2 to 7047. Ten percent of women and 25% of men between the ages of 40 and 49 years who have normal renal function have coronary artery calcification, whereas in this study of dialysis patients 88% of the women and 88% of the men aged 20 to 30 years had calcification. There is also confirmation in another report of progression over 20 ± 3 months, during which the scores doubled.[23] There was no significant difference in the death rate due to cardio-vascular disease whether patients were supported with hemodialysis or peritoneal dialysis.[24] Peritoneal dialysis patients have as many risk factors as hemodialysis patients for the development of cardiovascular disease.[15]

Septicemia as a cause of morbidity and mortality in hemodialysis patients can be directly associated with the presence of a central vein catheter, but is also seen in patients with arteriovenous grafts and arteriovenous fistulae as the hemodialysis access.[25] In this report by Ishani and colleagues, the occurrences of septicemia or bacteremia were associated with death (hazard ratio [HR] 2.33, 95% confidence interval [CI] 2.08–2.61) ($P<.0001$), congestive heart failure (HR 1.65, 95% CI 1.39–1.95) ($P<.0001$), myocardial infarction (HR 1.78, 95% CI 1.38–2.28) ($P<.0001$), peripheral vascular disease (HR 1.64, 95% CI 1.34–2.00) ($P<.0001$), and stroke (HR 2.04, 95% CI 1.27–3.28) ($P = .003$). Powe and colleagues[26] reported on an analysis over 7 years of 4005 hemodialysis patients in whom 11.7% had at least one episode of septicemia and 913 peritoneal patients in whom 9.4% had at least one episode of septicemia. Patients with septicemia had a doubling of their all-cause death rate and a fivefold to ninefold increased risk of death from sepsis.

Calciphylaxis/calcific uremic arteriolopathy (CUA) deserves special mention. First described by Selye in 1962 in an animal model, this condition is being recognized with increased frequency in dialysis patients, an incidence of between 1% and 4.1% being reported in the dialysis population.[27] CUA is characterized by the development of painful nodules, painful panniculitis, or livedo reticularis that is painful, exquisitely tender, and proceeds to ulcers of varying size with a dark or black eschar. The edges of the ulcers are slightly raised, extremely painful, and tender to touch. Original descriptions in the late 1960s and early 1970s noted that the lesions affected predominantly the distal aspects of the extremities. Whole digits may be affected. Over the last 10 years the descriptions are of more proximal lesions seen in obese patients. The lesions in these patients may be seen in the areas rich in adipose tissue, particularly in White females. The diagnosis is made on skin biopsy, which must include the deep adipose tissue. Histologically the lesions are characterized by calcification of the media of the small arteries and arterioles with infarctions of adjacent subcutis and skin. Predisposing factors include hypercalcemia, a high Ca×P product, and use of calcium-containing dietary phosphate binders and potent forms of vitamin D such as 1,25-dihydroxycholecalciferol. Hyperparathyroidism may be present and, if confirmed, patients may enjoy dramatic improvements in their skin lesions after parathyroidectomy.[28] There is no benefit to performing a parathyroidectomy in patients with normal or only slightly elevated parathyroid levels. The treatment is to withdraw calcium and vitamin D supplements, use of a low calcium dialysate, aggressive dialysis such as daily hemodialysis (patients on peritoneal dialysis need to change to hemodialysis), hyperbaric oxygen,[29] and parathyroidectomy[30] if indicated. Treatment with sodium thiosulfate has been shown to be beneficial. Sodium thiosulfate is administered intravenously at a dose of 25 g/1.73 $m^2$ after each dialysis.[31] Intraperitoneal dosing has also been described.[32] The prognosis for this condition varies from a 75% survival in distal lesions to a 26% survival in proximal CUA. Mortality is caused by secondary infections, sepsis, cardiovascular events, and withdrawal from dialysis secondary to intractable pain, suffering, and progressive frailty.

Surgical lower limb amputation is a serious complication of diabetic neuropathy and peripheral vascular disease, both conditions being common in the ESRD population and often coexistent in the same patient. Using the Health Care Financing Administration's ESRD program management and medical information system, Eggers and colleagues[33] reported an increasing rate of amputations, starting at 4.8 per 100 person-years in 1991 and rising to 6.4 per 100 person-years in 1994. Diabetic patients with ESRD had a rate 10 times that of diabetics without ESRD. A report from the Dialysis Outcomes and Practice Patterns Study (DOPPS) (an international database) by Combe and colleagues[34] found a high overall prevalence of 6% and an incidence of 2 per 100 patient-years in the 8877 patients studied. Diabetic patients had a ninefold greater incidence of amputations. Risk factors included age, peripheral vascular disease, smoking, and diabetes mellitus, as well as abnormalities of mineral metabolism and years of hemodialysis, as might be expected. Amputations are associated with a relative risk of death of 1.54, and mean survival after an amputation was 2 years versus 3.8 years in the matched cohort.

## THE SYMPTOM BURDEN

Once patients have progressed to ESRD their symptom burden increases with the advent of uremia.

There are also several comorbidities associated with significant kidney disease such as metabolic bone disease, vasculopathy, and anemia, all of which can alter the quality of life of these patients. Patients may suffer to varying degrees from nausea and vomiting, muscle cramping, neuropathy with dysesthesia, pain and numbness, anemia with dyspnea and weakness, volume overload, poor cognitive function, sexual dysfunction, itch, and a sensation of feeling constantly cold. With RRT, the hope is that patients will achieve resolution of their complaints, but this is unfortunately not always the case.[35,36] Dialysis is considered by patients and their families to be "life-saving" but the reality is that RRT is life-prolonging, allowing the patient the time to have worsening of preexisting comorbidities, or even experience an acceleration of vascular and cardiac diseases. Unfortunately, even patients who experience a significant improvement in symptoms are still living with the reality that the severity of their underlying condition is associated with a poor prognosis.

The literature suggests that 37% to 50% of hemodialysis patients experience chronic pain, and that for 82% of these patients pain is moderate to severe in intensity.[35,36] Recurrent pain may be caused by the vein punctures inherent in performing hemodialysis, muscle cramping during or separate from dialysis, and headaches (one cause being due to dialysis-induced urea disequilibrium). Musculoskeletal pain is the commonest cause of pain in patients with ESRD. The severity of musculoskeletal pain in these patients is ranked as high as neuropathic or ischemic pain.[36] Davison[36] states that there is a lack of recognition in the nephrology community regarding the prevalence and severity of pain in this population. The Dialysis Symptom Index developed by Weisbord and colleagues[37] has shown that dialysis patients average 9 symptoms, which is comparable to the number of symptoms reported in AIDS and cancer patients.[38] Again it was shown that approximately 50% of the patients complained of musculoskeletal pain. Tiredness, itch, neuropathic symptoms of numbness and tingling, decreased sexual desire and decreased arousal, and dry mouth were the other most frequently reported symptoms.[38] Pain management is complicated by the altered pharmacokinetics and pharmacodynamics in renal failure of some commonly prescribed medications.[36] Morphine must be avoided in ESRD because of the accumulation in the central nervous system of morphine-6-glucuronide, which is normally excreted by the kidneys and is neurotoxic. Patients may manifest myoclonus and prolonged coma lasting 4 to 7 days, which is not improved with dialysis.[39–41] Hydromorphone is not associated with the same problem.[42]

Gabapentin dosing must be adjusted for renal function, as outlined in the following table, to prevent toxicity.[43]

| Creatinine Clearance (ml/min) | Total Daily Dose Range (mg/d) | Dose Regimen (mg) (Titrate every 3 days, to 7 days if renal failure) |
|---|---|---|
| >60 | 900–3600 | 300 thrice a day (TID), 400 TID, 600 TID, 800 TID, 1200 TID |
| >30–59 | 400–1400 | 200 twice a day (BID), 300 BID, 400 BID, 500 BID, 700 BID |
| >15–29 | 200–700 | 200 every day (QD), 300 QD, 400 QD, 500 QD, 700 QD |
| 15 or less | 100–300 | 100 QD, 125 QD, 150 QD, 200 QD, 300 QD |

## DECISION MAKING AND COMMUNICATION IN END-STAGE RENAL DISEASE

The challenge for all practitioners dealing with renal failure patients is the delicate task of balancing the hope of the patients that RRT will bring symptomatic improvement and be a life-saving therapy, with the realities of the prognosis and the morbidity and mortality yet to come. Most staff in dialysis units are unaware of the prognosis of the patients with whom they are dealing. Family physicians often believe that the attending nephrologist will be informing the patient of the good news that RRT will likely make the patient feel better, and the bad news about the prognosis of the illness. Unfortunately, kidney specialists are generally uncomfortable having these discussions with patients and their families, which is not surprising in view of the fact that only 1% of nephrology trainees have had palliative care training compared with, for example, 71% of geriatrics trainees.[44]

Nephrology fellows reported less training in end-of-life care than in managing distal renal tubular acidosis or hemodialysis therapy.[45] Talking to patients and families about their prognosis is a skill that can be learned and should have more emphasis in the training of specialists in this field. Twenty-six percent of family meetings occurred without a nephrologist being present.[45]

Patients generally want to have these discussions. A survey by the National Kidney Foundation found that 54% of patient respondents had never talked about their prognosis and end-of-life care with a dialysis team member; however, 76% wanted to have such a discussion. Only 14% expressed discomfort at the thought of such a discussion, and 5% did not want to speak about these matters. Another survey of 100 patients with CKD indicated that 97% wanted prognostic information and 95% did so because they wanted to be better prepared for the future. Ninety-two percent wanted the nephrologist to provide life expectancy information without having to be prompted.[46,47] All dialysis patients are aware that their lives are dependent on technology and that problems may arise that will interfere with their treatment. Patients are more informed than ever, and show little surprise when the information regarding prognosis is given. This information is best given before the patients actually commence RRT. The prognostic information and advance care planning should be part of the care of CKD patients, just as is the treatment of metabolic bone disease.

If 50% of patients survive 5 years or less after starting RRT, the other patients must be doing relatively well. The task at hand is to identify which patients need a palliative care approach to their care. Approaches to this include the use of the Edmonton Symptom Assessment Scale, modified for patients on dialysis, and validated in this population,[38] the "Surprise Question" (would you be surprised if this patient died within 1 year?) (odds ratio 3.507, 95% CI 1.356–9.067, $P = .01$),[48] and the Charlson Comorbidity Score.[49] A low serum albumin level, both at baseline and during the course of dialysis treatment, is a consistent and strong predictor of death. For example, the 1-year and 2-year survival of patients with an albumin level of greater than 3.5 g/dL is 86% and 76%, respectively, compared with 50% and 17% if the albumin level is less than 3.5 g/dL.[50] In a study by Miskulin and colleagues,[51] the serum albumin level contributed most to the prediction of mortality.

Cohen and colleagues[52] recently reported on a short-term (6 month) prognostic model in a derivation cohort of 512 hemodialysis patients, which was tested against a validation cohort of 514 patients. The 5 variables independently associated with mortality were older age (HR for a 10-year increase 1.36; 95% CI 1.17–1.57), dementia (HR 2.24; 95% CI 1.11–4.48), peripheral vascular disease (HR 1.88; 95% CI 1.24–2.84), decreased albumin (HR for a 1-U increase 0.27; 95% CI 0.15–0.50), and the Surprise Question (HR 2.71; 95% CI 1.76–4.17). This model has yet to be validated in practice.

## ADVANCE DIRECTIVES

Knowledge of the outcome of ESRD treated with RRT should enable the medical team to discuss appropriate and focused goals of care with patients. Nephrologists should explicitly include in their advance care planning with patients/surrogates information about the outcomes of cardiopulmonary resuscitation for patients with ESRD, and a discussion of patients' preferences regarding cardiopulmonary resuscitation if cardiac arrest were to occur while patients are undergoing a dialysis treatment.

Honest, thoughtful, and compassionate discussions about prognosis actually tend to empower patients, maintain hope that the patient's wishes will be respected, and stay consistent with their underlying values. This approach leads to a reinforcement of trust with the medical team.[53]

The concern that introducing the topics of advance directives and resuscitation directives will destroy all hope in patients with renal failure has been shown to be false. Davison and Simpson[54] have reported that patients in their survey identified hope as central to the process of advance care planning. Hope helped them to determine future goals of care and provided insight into the perceived benefits of advance care planning, and influenced their willingness to engage in end-of-life discussions. Patients were able to imagine future scenarios that were consistent with their values and hopes. The reliance on health care professionals to initiate these discussions was seen as a barrier to advanced care planning. Facilitated and early discussion about prognosis and allowing the patient to plan for future interventions enhances, rather than diminishes, hope in these patients.[54] In a recent Australian article by Detering and colleagues,[55] end-of-life wishes were more likely to be known and followed in 86% of the patients if they had participated in advance care planning, as compared with only 30% of patients who were in a control group and who had not had these discussions. Anxiety, stress, depression, and patient and family satisfaction were all positively affected by the process and completion of advance care plans.

### Withdrawal from Dialysis

The most recent USRDS database documents a rate of 47.3 per 1000 patient-years in the 75-plus age group who withdraw from dialysis.[13] In 1993 Mailloux and colleagues[56] reported on an analysis of 340 deceased patients over a 20-year period from 1970 to 1989, 18.5% of whom died after withdrawal from dialysis; of note, 65% of these patients were older than 61 years. Withdrawal deaths were doubled in patients older than 60 years compared with those who were younger. A review in 2006 found that the time to death after withdrawal from dialysis was 8 to 10 days, with a few patients surviving upwards of 1 month. For patients who choose never to start RRT, the causes of death and time to death are more variable. Chater and colleagues[57] reported that unfortunately, following withdrawal, patients do experience distressing symptoms, the most common of which were confusion, agitation, pain, and dyspnea. Seventeen percent had suffering during the withdrawal period, 24% had unrelieved symptoms, and 19% psychological distress. A third of patients died alone. Appropriate symptom management with opioids and benzodiazepines was associated with a reduction in the number and severity of symptoms in the last 24 hours of life. These investigators emphasized that dialysis patients who withdraw from RRT should have full support from a palliative care team.

### Clinical Practice Guideline in Withdrawal of Dialysis

The Renal Physicians Association (RPA) and American Society of Nephrology (ASN) established a multidisciplinary working group including representatives from kidney patients, family members, and public policy experts. The Clinical Practice Guideline on Shared Decision Making in the Appropriate Initiation of and Withdrawal of Dialysis includes recommendations regarding ongoing discussions with patients and families about prognosis, treatment options, advance directives, a systematic approach for conflict resolution, and the statement that all members of the renal health care team including nephrologists, nephrology nurses, nephrology social workers, and renal dietitians should obtain education and skills in the principles of palliative care to ensure that ESRD patients and families receive multidimensional, compassionate, and competent care at the end of life.[58,59]

In responding to a patient's decision to forgo dialysis, the provider is obliged to determine, if possible, why the patient has made this decision in order to be sure that the patient correctly understands the information that has been presented to him or her as well as the consequences of the decision. Once the provider is satisfied that the patient's decision to forgo dialysis is informed and uncoerced, the physician should respect the wishes of the patient. If a patient lacks decision-making capacity, decisions should involve a legal agent. Shared decision making may involve family members with the patient's consent. Nephrologists and primary care physicians should obtain education and skills in advance care planning so that they are comfortable addressing end-of-life issues with their patients.

After a decision is made to forgo dialysis, the renal team may refer the patient to a hospice or adopt a palliative care approach to patient care. In either case, the nephrologist or primary care physician may remain active in the patient's care to maintain continuity of relationships and treatment. Hospice and palliative care programs should be involved in managing the physical and psychosocial aspects of end-of-life care. Bereavement support should be offered to families of patients.

The RPA/ASN encourages dialysis facilities to develop policies and procedures for respecting the wishes of dialysis patients with regard to cardiopulmonary resuscitation in all settings, including in the dialysis unit.

The guideline also states that it is appropriate to withhold or withdraw dialysis for patients with either acute renal failure or ESRD in the following situations:

- Patients with decision-making capacity, who being fully informed and making voluntary choices, refuse dialysis or request dialysis be discontinued
- Patients who no longer possess decision-making capacity who have previously indicated refusal of dialysis in an oral or written advance directive
- Patients who no longer possess decision-making capacity and whose properly appointed legal agents refuse dialysis or request that it be discontinued
- Patients with irreversible, profound neurologic impairment such that they lack signs of thought, sensation, purposeful behavior, and awareness of self and environment.

### Dialysis in the Elderly

The "very" elderly (75 years or older) have been reported to have a very poor prognosis in the first year after starting dialysis, if there is inclusion of all deaths in the first 3 months after starting RRT. The reported survival rates are 53.5% at 1 year and 2.4% at 5 years. The surviving patients spent 20% of their time in hospital. In this age group, withdrawal from dialysis was reported to be the most common cause of death (38%), followed by cardiovascular disease (24%) and infections (22%). Dialysis patients with dementia have a particularly poor prognosis. In a retrospective study of 272,024 Medicare/Medicaid patients in the USRDS who started RRT between April 1, 1995 and December 31, 1999, patients with dementia had a 2-year survival rate of only 24%. The average time to death was 1.09 years versus 2.7 years in the cohort of patients without dementia ($P<.001$). Furthermore, the odds ratio for dementia in the group older than 76.4 years in this study was reported to be 19.65 (95% CI 14.48–26.67; $P<.05$).[60]

Age itself is not a contraindication for dialysis, but when advanced age is associated with other comorbidities, especially dementia, there is a need to examine the goals of care and to be clear about the expected outcomes of the treatments being offered. Whenever possible, efforts must be made to have advance directives in place before RRT is started.

### SUMMARY

Patients with severe renal failure reaching the stage of requiring RRT experience a symptom burden equivalent to patients with AIDS or advanced cancer, and have a prognosis worse than most malignancies. Understanding the severity and complications of the illness, even in younger patients, should enable attending physicians to be more comfortable and willing to discuss palliative therapies with these patients. Advance directives and resuscitation directives are important to ensure compassionate and goal-directed care of these long-suffering people. Drug toxicities are avoidable by using appropriate drugs at the correct doses and dosing intervals.

## APPENDIX

Resources:
Kidney End of Life Coalition (www.kidneyeol.org)
Gundersen Lutheran Medical Foundation. Respecting Choices. (Advance care planning) (www.respectingchoices.org)
British Columbia Provincial Renal Agency. End of Life Resources. (http://www.bcrenalagency.ca/professionals/default.htm)
Recommendations for Addressing End-of-Life Care in ESRD Mid-Atlantic Renal Coalition (marc@nw5.esrd.net)
Hemodialysis Mortality Predictor—Surprise Question. (www.nephron.com)

## REFERENCES

1. Addington-Hall J. Reaching out: specialist palliative care for adults with non-malignant disease. London: National Council for Hospices and Specialist Palliative Care Services; 1995.
2. National Institutes of Health. NIH State of the Science conference on improving end of life care. December 6–8, 2004. Available at: http://consensus.nih.gov/ta/024/024EndOfLifepostINTRO.htm. Accessed March 2, 2011.
3. Moss AH. Kidney failure. In: Emanuel LL, Librach SL, editors. Palliative care: core skills and clinical competencies. Philadelphia: Saunders Elsevier; 2007. p. 355–69.
4. US Renal Data System. USRDS. Annual report: atlas of end-stage renal disease in the United States. Bethesda (MD): National Institute of Diabetes and Digestive and Kidney Diseases; 2006: 136.
5. Canadian Organ Replacement Registry. Annual Report 2006.
6. Canadian Organ Replacement Registry Annual Report 2009.
7. United States Renal Data System April 2009. Table H31.
8. Foley RN, Parfrey PS, Sarnak MJ. Clinical epidemiology of cardiovascular disease in chronic renal disease. Am J Kidney Dis 1998;32:S112–9.
9. Lefevre F, Yarnold PR, Cohn EB, et al. Predicting survival from in-hospital CPR: meta-analysis and validation of a prediction model. J Gen Intern Med 1993;8(7):347–53.
10. Lai MN, Hung KY, Huang JW, et al. Findings and outcomes of intra-hemodialysis cardiopulmonary resuscitation. Am J Nephrol 1999;19:468–73.
11. Moss AH, Holley JL, Upton MB. Outcomes of cardiopulmonary resuscitation in dialysis patients. J Am Soc Nephrol 1992;3:1238–43.
12. Lafrance J-P, Nolin L, Senecal L, et al. Predictors and outcome of cardiopulmonary resuscitation (CPR) calls in a large haemodialysis unit over a seven-year period. Nephrol Dial Transplant 2006;21(4):1006–12.
13. United States Renal Data System April 2009. Table H29.
14. United States Renal Data System April 2009. Table 30.
15. García–López E, Carrero JJ, Suliman ME, et al. Risk factors for cardiovascular disease in patients undergoing peritoneal dialysis. Perit Dial Int 2007;27 (Suppl 2):205–9.
16. Locatelli F, Marcelli D, Conte F, et al. Survival and development of cardiovascular disease by modality of treatment in patients with end-stage renal disease. J Am Soc Nephrol 2001;12:2411–7.
17. United States Renal Data System; April 2009. p. 9–10.
18. Block GA, Hulbert-Shearon TE, Levin NW. Association of serum phosphorus and calcium x phosphate product with mortality risk in chronic hemodialysis patients: a national study. Am J Kidney Dis 1998;31(4):607–17.

19. Block GA, Klassen PS, Ofsthun N, et al. Mineral metabolism mortality, and morbidity in maintenance hemodialysis. J Am Soc Nephrol 2004;15(8):2208–18.
20. Rufino M, García S, Jiménez A, et al. Heart valve calcification and calcium x phosphorus product in hemodialysis patients: analysis of optimum values for its prevention. Kidney Int Suppl 2003;63:S115–8, 1523–755. 63.
21. Agatston AS, Janowitz WR, Hildner FJ, et al. Quantification of coronary artery calcium using ultrafast computed tomography. J Am Coll Cardiol 1990;15:827–32.
22. Goodman WG, Goldin J, Kuizon BD, et al. Coronary artery calcification in young adults with end-stage renal disease who are undergoing dialysis. N Engl J Med 2000;342(20):1478–83.
23. London GM, Pannier B, Marchais SJ, et al. Calcification of the aortic valve in the dialyzed patient. J Am Soc Nephrol 2000;11:778–83.
24. Locatelli F, Marcelli D, Conte F, et al. Survival and development of cardiovascular disease by modality of treatment in patients with end-stage renal disease. J Am Soc Nephrol 2000;12:2411–7.
25. Ishani A, Collins AJ, Herzog CA, et al. Septicemia, access and cardiovascular disease in dialysis patients: The USRDSWave 2 Study1. Kidney Int 2005;68:311–8.
26. Powe NR, Jaar B, Firth SL, et al. Septicemia in dialysis patients: incidence, risk factors, and prognosis. Kidney Int 1999;55:1081–90.
27. Budisavljevic MN, Cheek D, Ploth DW. Calciphylaxis in chronic renal failure. J Am Soc Nephrol 1996;7(7):978–82.
28. Llach F. The evolving clinical features of calciphylaxis. Kidney Int Suppl 2003; 63(Suppl 85):S122–4.
29. Vassa N, Twardowsky ZJ, Campbell J. Hyperbaric oxygen therapy in calciphylaxis induced necrosis in a peritoneal dialysis patient. Am J Kidney Dis 1994;23:878–82.
30. Hafner J, Keusch G, Wahl C, et al. Uremic small artery disease with medial calcification and intimal hypertrophy (so-called calciphylaxis): a complication of chronic renal failure and benefit from parathyroidectomy. J Am Acad Dermatol 1995;33:954–62.
31. Araya CE, Fennell RS, Neilberger RE, et al. Sodium thiosulphate treatment for calcific uremic areteriolopathy in children and young adults. Clin J Am Soc Nephrol 2006;1:1161–6.
32. Mataic D, Bastani B. Intraperitoneal sodium thiosulfate for the treatment of calciphylaxis. Ren Fail 2006;28(4):361–3.
33. Eggers PW, Gohdes D, Pugh J. Non-traumatic lower extremity amputations in the Medicare end stage renal disease population. Kidney Int 1999;56:1524–33.
34. Combe C, Albert JM, Bragg-Gresham JL, et al. The burden of amputation among hemodialysis patients in the Dialysis Outcomes and Practice Patterns Study (DOPPS). Am J Kidney Dis 2009;54(4):680–92.
35. Davison SN. Pain in hemodialysis patients: prevalence, cause, severity, and management. Am J Kidney Dis 2003;42(6):1239–47. Top of Form.
36. Davison SN. Chronic pain in end-stage renal disease. Am J Kidney Dis 2005; 12(3):326–34.
37. Weisbord SD, Fried LF, Arnold RM, et al. Development of a symptom assessment instrument for chronic hemodialysis patients: the Dialysis Symptom Index. J Pain Symptom Manage 2004;27(3):226–40.
38. Davison SN, Jhangri GS, Johnson JA. Longitudinal validation of a modified Edmonton symptom assessment system (ESAS) in haemodialysis patients. Nephrol Dial Transplant 2006;21:3189–95.
39. Aitkenhead AR, Vater M, Achola K, et al. Pharmacokinetics of single-dose i.v. Morphine in normal volunteers and patients with end-stage renal failure. Br J Anaesth 1984;56:813–9.

40. Sawe J, Odar-Cederlof I. Kinetics of morphine in patients with renal failure. Eur J Clin Pharmacol 1987;32:377–82.
41. Wolff J, Bigler D, Christensen CB, et al. Influence of renal function on the elimination of morphine and morphine glucuronides. Eur J Clin Pharmacol 1988;34:353–7.
42. Lee MA, Leng ME, Tiernan EJ. Retrospective study of the use of hydromorphone in palliative care patients with normal and abnormal urea and creatinine. Palliat Med 2001;15(1):26–34.
43. FDA Approved Labeling Text; Feb 2005. p. 1–29.
44. Sullivan AM, Lakoma MD, Block SD. The status of medical education in end-of-life care. A National Report. J Gen Intern Med 2003;18(9):685–95.
45. Holley JL, Carmody SS, Moss AH, et al. The need for end-of-life care training in nephrology (National survey results of nephrology fellows). Am J Kidney Dis 2003;42(4):813–20.
46. Wittenberg SM, Cohen LM. Estimating prognosis in end-stage renal disease. Progr Palliat Care 2009;17(4):165–9.
47. Fine A, Fontaine B, Kraushar MM, et al. Nephrologists should voluntarily divulge survival data to potential dialysis patients: a questionnaire study. Perit Dial Int 2005;25(3):269–73.
48. Moss AH, Ganjoo J, Sharma S, et al. Utility of the "Surprise" question to identify dialysis patients with high mortality. Clin J Am Soc Nephrol 2008;3:1379–84.
49. Charlson ME, Pompei P, Ales KL, et al. A new method of classifying prognostic comorbidity in longitudinal studies: development and validation. J Chronic Dis 1987;40(5):373–83.
50. Owen WF, Lew NL, Yiu Y, et al. The urea reduction ratio and serum albumin concentration as predictors of mortality in patients undergoing hemodialysis. N Engl J Med 1993;329(14):1001–6.
51. Miskulin DC, Martin AA, Brown R, et al. Predicting 1 year mortality in an outpatient haemodialysis population: a comparison of comorbidity instrument. Nephrol Dial Transplant 2004;19:413–20.
52. Cohen LM, Ruthazer R, Moss AH, et al. Predicting six-month mortality for patients who are on maintenance hemodialysis. Clin J Am Soc Nephrol 2010;5:72–9.
53. Miyaji NT, Holcombe RF. Letters to the editor. N Engl J Med 1994;331(12):810.
54. Davison SN, Simpson C. Hope and advance care planning in patients with end stage renal disease: qualitative interview study. BMJ 2006;333:886.
55. Detering KM, Hancock AD, Reade MC, et al. The impact of advance care planning on end of life care in elderly patients: a randomised controlled trial. BMJ 2010;340:c1345.
56. Mailloux LU, Bellucci AG, Napolitano B, et al. Death by withdrawal from dialysis: a 20 year clinical experience. J Am Soc Nephrol 1993;3:1631–7.
57. Chater S, Davison SN, Germain MJ, et al. Withdrawal from dialysis: a palliative care perspective. Clin Nephrol 2006;66(5):364–72.
58. Clinical practice guideline on shared decision-making in the appropriate initiation of and withdrawal from dialysis. Renal Physicians Association and American Society of Nephrology. Number 2, Washington, DC: Clinical Practice Guideline; 1999.
59. Moss AH, Renal Physicians Association, American Society of Nephrology Working Group. A new clinical practice guideline for the initiation and withdrawal of dialysis that makes explicit the role of palliative care medicine. J Palliat Med 2000;3(3):253–60.
60. Rakowski DA, Caillard S, Agodoa LY, et al. Dementia as a predictor of mortality in dialysis patients. Clin J Am Soc Nephrol 2006;1:1000–5.

# Palliative Care in the Management of Advanced HIV/AIDS

James A. Fausto Jr, MD[a],*, Peter A. Selwyn, MD, MPH[b]

**KEYWORDS**

• End of Life • AIDS • AIDS-defining illnesses • Prognosis

In the early days of the HIV and AIDS, patients and clinicians came to know the infection as a terminal condition. At that time, high-quality care of patients with AIDS required that clinicians learn palliative care. By the mid-1990s, AIDS care was transformed by highly active antiretroviral therapy (HAART), and the disease trajectory for many patients with AIDS transitioned from a terminal disease model to a chronic disease model. Over time the one clinician who cared for patients with AIDS in the early days diverged into several providers: primary care provider, HIV specialist, and palliative care provider, if a patient became terminal. This division of care increasingly dismissed the importance of comprehensive primary care and palliative care for patients with HIV.[1] In time, HIV as a chronic disease will return to the primary care provider, and the primary care clinicians who can integrate basic elements of palliative care, HIV care, and the coordination of complex case management will render the highest quality care to patients with HIV and AIDS.

This issue reviews many of the basic elements found in the various domains of palliative care. Many of the basic elements of symptom management (pain, dyspnea, fatigue, and so forth) are covered in depth in articles throughout this issue. These basic elements can and should be translated into practice for patients with HIV/AIDS. Additionally, more than half of clinical events and deaths occurring among patients on HAART are now classified as non-AIDS illnesses.[2] Thus, end-of-life care for patients with late-stage AIDS needs to broadly include any palliative measures that are used for patients without AIDS. Covering all of the possible non–AIDS-defining conditions and AIDS-defining conditions that patients with AIDS may suffer or die from is, however, beyond the scope of this article. Therefore, this article narrows its focus to

The authors have nothing to disclose.

[a] Palliative Care Program, Department of Family and Social Medicine, Montefiore Medical Center, Albert Einstein College of Medicine, 3347 Steuben Avenue, 2nd floor, Bronx, NY 10467, USA

[b] Department of Family and Social Medicine, Montefiore Medical Center, Albert Einstein College of Medicine, 3544 Jerome Avenue, Bronx, NY 10467, USA

* Corresponding author.

*E-mail address:* JFausto@montefiore.org

Prim Care Clin Office Pract 38 (2011) 311–326

doi:10.1016/j.pop.2011.03.010

0095-4543/11/$ – see front matter © 2011 Elsevier Inc. All rights reserved.

the unique elements of late-stage AIDS due to AIDS-defining illnesses. There has been a dramatic decline in the rates of AIDS-defining opportunistic illnesses among HIV-infected patients, but opportunistic illnesses remain a leading cause of hospitalization and death among HIV-infected individuals.[3] Therefore, this topic deserves review of the unique elements of late-stage AIDS due to AIDS-defining illnesses. In an effort to meet this need, the article reviews the epidemiology of HIV/AIDS, prognostic indicators, opportunistic infections (OIs), specific AIDS-defining malignancies and non–AIDS-defining malignancies, substance abuse/liver disease, and, finally, HAART and comfort measures for late-stage AIDS patients due to an AIDS-defining illness.

## EPIDEMIOLOGY

In the three decades since the first cases to become known as AIDS were identified, the epidemiology of HIV/AIDS has metamorphosed in many ways. As discussed previously, in the early days, HIV infection was essentially a terminal diagnosis, but with the advent of HAART in the mid-1990s and continued updates, HIV/AIDS is now more correctly considered a chronic illness for most.

The most recent Centers for Disease Control and Prevention (CDC) HIV/AIDS Surveillance Report[4] shows the highest prevalence of HIV/AIDS infection in the United States since its identified onset in 1981. The report currently estimates 1.1 million people living with HIV/AIDS, of which 468,000 are living with AIDS.[4] In total, approximately 1.7 million people have been infected with HIV in the United States, and approximately 580,000 have died from AIDS. Currently, approximately 15,000 people die in the United States from AIDS-related causes yearly, and the yearly incidence of new HIV infection is 56,000. One-fifth of people living with HIV do not know they are infected.[5]

HIV/AIDS infection has a disproportionate impact on people depending on race, gender, socioeconomic status, age, and sexual practices. The latest data continue to show that some racial and ethnic minorities (specifically, blacks and Latinos) disproportionately carry the burden of new AIDS cases (71%), new HIV infection (67%), and AIDS deaths (70%). Alternatively, declines in HIV rates among gay and bisexual men have declined but they continue to be high risk for HIV with a new infection rate of 53%. Younger gay and bisexual men of color are at particularly high risk for infection. Currently, women represent a larger share of new and total number of infections compared with the early days of the epidemic. Close to 280,000 women live with HIV and AIDS in the United States. New infections are disproportionately high among black non-Hispanic women, at 65% of new infections in women, and young women (ages 13–29) in this group fall into the highest risk for new infection.[4,5]

The trajectory of HIV infection to AIDS and death has changed in the past 30 years. One model of this trajectory categorizes the first decade (1981–1991) as the OI era, when people died secondary to OIs; followed by the antiviral era (1991–2001), when patients and the disease were medicalized; and the current era—the chronic disease era. In this era, HIV/AIDS can be managed with HAART, but many patients experience the acceleration of early-onset diabetes, lipid disorders, cancer, and overall debility.[6,7]

## PROGNOSTIC INDICATORS

Prognosticating or the ability to predict the course of a disease is critical to the care of patients with HIV/AIDS. In the pre-HAART era, a patient's prognosis could largely be predicted based on viral load and CD4 cell count.[8] The introduction of HAART in the mid-1990s has altered the survival of patients with AIDS who respond to HAART. Several studies have reviewed survival data in industrialized countries for patients with HIV/AIDS pre-HAART and post-HAART. In the pre-HAART era, estimates of life expectancy were reduced by 17 years and now, post-HAART mortality rates for persons infected sexually with HIV are much closer to those of the general population in the first 5 years after infection. Mortality excesses begin to show, however, as duration of HIV infection lengthens.[9,10] HAART has drastically changed the landscape of prognostication for patients HIV/AIDS. The traditional model of CD4 cell count and viral load has been supplanted by a more complex model that should incorporate multiple factors, such as age, HAART exposure, OIs, non–AIDS-defining illnesses, functional status, CD4 cell count, and viral load once on HAART.[8,10–12] As Tarwater and colleagues[12] state, "...no patient with AIDS should be considered late-stage until a physician with expertise in the treatment of patients with HIV has completed a thorough evaluation of the patient's condition."

Therefore, primary care providers are advised to seek the counsel of expert HIV physicians and palliative care physicians for patients presenting with findings consistent with late-stage HIV. In addition to expert evaluation, the factors repeatedly shown to correlate with a poor prognosis are impaired functional status (eg, Karnofsky performance status scale score), impairments in activities of daily living, age older then 65 years, 6-month CD4 count and HIV-1 RNA level on HAART, infection through intravenous drug use, diarrhea for greater than 1 month, and advanced liver disease.[8,10–13] Additionally, certain malignancies and OIs purport a poor prognosis (discussed later). Lastly, the Antiretroviral Therapy Cohort Collaboration (ATCC) has created a risk calculator for HIV+ patients starting antiretroviral therapy that can help with prognosis at the start of HAART and 6 months into HAART. The calculator can be found at http://www.art-cohort-collaboration.org.[8]

If a patient is determined to have a poor prognosis and the addition of hospice is warranted, the Centers for Medicare & Medicaid systems local coverage determinations (LCDs) assist with the identification of a Medicare beneficiary whose clinical status and anticipated change in disease is more likely than not to result in a life expectancy of 6 months or less. The LCDs help guide life expectancy prognosis both by clinical status changes and at times by disease-specific criteria. The LCDs are guidelines and not strict criteria; therefore, an awareness of their content is helpful, but assessment by a hospice and palliative medicine consultant is also important. The contents in **Table 1** are a partial extraction of the HIV/AIDS-related LCDs current as of this article's publication.

## OPPORTUNISTIC INFECTIONS

On June 5, 1981, the CDC reported 5 cases of *Pneumocystis carinii* pneumonia (PCP), later renamed *Pneumocystis jirovecii* pneumonia, among previously healthy young men in Los Angeles.[14] These 5 cases would later be the first documented cases of AIDS in the United States and PCP would be labeled an OI and become known as one of the 26 AIDS-defining illnesses. For years, OIs led to the diagnosis of AIDS and caused premature morbidity and mortality for many infected with HIV. The advent of HAART in the mid-1990s slowed the ravaging effects of OIs as HAART helped restore patients' immune status. In a 2010 publication, Buchacz and colleagues[13] reviewed more current rates of opportunistic illnesses (both OIs and opportunistic malignancies) in a cohort study of more than 8000 patients from the years 1994 to 2007. This group found significant declines in OIs from the years 1994 to 2007 with a trend toward stabilization of low rates instead of further declines in the latter years of the study. Specific data on the decline of OIs show the following rates of OIs: 89.0 per 1000 person years (1994–1997), 25.2 per 1000 person years (1998–2002), and 13.3 per 1000 person years

**Table 1**
**The Centers for Medicare & Medicaid Services disease-specific LCD guidelines for HIV/AIDS**

The disease-specific guidelines are to be used in conjunction with the *Part II. Non–disease-specific baseline guidelines* (both of these should be met)
1. Physiologic impairment of functional status as demonstrated by Karnofsky performance status scale score or palliative performance score <70%. Note that 2 of the disease-specific guidelines (HIV disease, stroke, and coma) establish a lower qualifying Karnofsky performance status scale score or palliative performance score.
2. Dependence on assistance for 2 or more activities of daily living
   A. Feeding
   B. Ambulation
   C. Continence
   D. Transfer
   E. Bathing
   F. Dressing

If patients have findings consistent with the *Part II. Non–disease-specific baseline guidelines* and the HIV/AIDS findings, as noted below, then they could be considered in the terminal stage of their illness (life expectancy of 6 months or less). However, they should meet the following criteria
(1 and 2 should be present; factors from 3 add supporting documentation):
1. CD4+ count <25 cells/μL or persistent (2 or more assays at least 1 month apart) viral load >100,000 copies/mL, plus one of the following:
   Central nervous system lymphoma
   Untreated, or persistent despite treatment, wasting (loss of at least 10% lean body mass)
   MAC bacteremia, untreated, unresponsive to treatment, or treatment refused
   PML
   Systemic lymphoma, with advanced HIV disease and partial response to chemotherapy
   Visceral KS unresponsive to therapy
   Renal failure in the absence of dialysis
   Cryptosporidium infection
   Toxoplasmosis, unresponsive to therapy
2. Decreased performance status, as measured by the Karnofsky performance status scale, of ≤50%
3. Documentation of the following factors support eligibility for hospice care:
   Chronic persistent diarrhea for 1 year
   Persistent serum albumin <2.5
   Concomitant, active substance abuse
   Age >50 years
   Absence of, or resistance to, effective antiretroviral, chemotherapeutic, and prophylactic drug therapy related specifically to HIV disease
   Advanced AIDS dementia complex
   Toxoplasmosis
   Congestive heart failure, symptomatic at rest
   Advanced liver disease

*Data from* CMS. LCD for hospice determining terminal status (L13653). Available at: www.cms.gov.

(2003–2007). These authors trend the latest rates of the most frequent OIs as esophageal candidiasis (5.2 per 1000 person years), PCP (3.9 per 1000 person years), *Mycobacterium avium* complex (MAC) (2.5 per 1000 person years), cytomegalovirus (CMV) disease (all) (1.8 per 1000 person years), HIV encephalopathy (1.4 per 1000 person years), *Mycobacterium tuberculosis* (TB) (0.8 per 1000 person years), *Cryptococcus* infection (0.8 per 1000 person years), progressive multifocal leukoencephalopathy (PML) (0.7 per 1000 person years), and toxoplasmosis (0.5 per 1000 person years). Alternatively, a publication from the ATCC examined AIDS-defining illnesses based not on frequency but instead on variable impact on patients. They categorized both OIs and opportunistic malignancies as severe, moderate, and mild based on adjusted mortality hazards ratios (aMHRs) after 6 months of HAART. This method of categorization is significant given the varying impact of these OIs. For example, esophageal candidiasis may be the most frequent OI found in the Buchacz and colleagues[13] study versus PML as one of the more rare OIs. The ATCC study, however, found the aMHRs for PML to be 9.41 versus 1.84 for esophageal candidiasis, demonstrating that although PML is rare, its impact on patients is severe and significantly changes their prognosis. In light of the frequency and severity of various OIs, the following sections highlight a few of the OIs that are most likely to categorize patients as having late-stage AIDS with an AIDS-defining illness.

### Pneumocysti Carinii Pneumonia

PCP remains a leading cause of morbidity and mortality in HIV-infected persons. Radhi and colleagues[15] published a retrospective cohort study of patients admitted to Los Angeles County University Hospital with PCP and death as the main outcome measures. With 262 patient cases reviewed, they found hospital mortality to be 11%. Patients who required admissions to an ICU had 29% mortality. Factors they found as independent predictors of increased mortality were the need for mechanical ventilation, the development of a pneumothorax, and low serum albumin. Earlier studies of patients with PCP in ICUs during the early days of HAART showed mortality ranging from 53% to 62%.[16–18] One of these studies showed improved mortality for patients receiving HAART during hospitalization.[17] The Radhi and colleagues[15] study and one other study[19] done more recently showed that use of HAART during admission did not have an association with decreased mortality, and both conclude that improved outcomes in ICU-level treatment of PCP in the HAART-era are likely due to improvements in ICU medical management. In their concluding remarks, Radhi and colleagues comment that PCP diagnoses in patients on HAART likely represented a failing HAART regimen or noncompliance. The rates of PCP in the current era may have decreased significantly, but of those patients who become hospitalized for it, the rate of mortality can be high. Therefore, a medical provider for a patient with PCP should recognize that a low albumin, a pneumothorax, and/or a need for mechanical ventilation purport a poor prognosis may help guide the care and discussion of prognosis with a patient's family.

### Disseminated Mycobacterium Avium Complex

Disseminated MAC infections typically appear late in the course of HIV disease and have been shown an independent predictor of mortality, even after adjustment for CD4 lymphocyte count. The clinical presentation of MAC often involves fever, weight loss, night sweats, fatigue, diarrhea, lymphadenopathy, hepatosplenomegaly, anemia, and elevated values of liver tests. This constellation of symptoms mimics many other conditions, making the diagnosis of MAC challenging. Once diagnosed, patients with MAC in the pre-HAART era had a survival of approximately 3 to 4 months. In the HAART era, patients off HAART or actively taking HAART who present with MAC still have a poor prognosis. Karakousis and Colleagues[20] report on data from the Johns Hopkins HIV Clinical Cohort, that show patients on HAART after 1996 with MAC had a median survival of 319 days. Although, HAART more than doubles a patient's survival time, prognosis with optimal HAART and antibiotic regimen still purports a prognosis of 10 months. Karakousis and colleagues[20] note that the major effect of HAART on MAC has been primary prevention rather than in survival after diagnosis. This observation is evident in Buchacz and colleagues'[3] finding that MAC incidence in 1994 to 1997 was 26.9 per 1000 person years and 2.5 per 1000 person years by 2003 to 2007, representing a 10-fold decrease in incidence. In summary, HAART has significantly reduced the incidence of MAC infection for patients with HIV, but the diagnosis of MAC in patients taking HAART purports a poor prognosis.

## Cytomegalovirus

The ATCC categorizes CMV infection as a mild type of AIDS-defining illness. Buchacz and colleagues[3] found a 15-fold decrease incidence of all CMV disease from 31 per 1000 person years (1994–1997) to 1.8 per 1000 person years (2003–2007). HAART has been shown to significantly improve survival and outcomes in patients diagnosed with CMV disease. A relatively recent retrospective cohort study of 154 AIDS patients with organ involvement of CMV disease, including the retina, central nervous system, lungs, and/or gastrointestinal tract, reported that 29% of patients died during the 32-month follow-up period.Those taking HAART, however, had a significantly improved survival of greater than 116 months versus 22 months for patients not taking HAART.[21] Thus, CMV can present a potentially high mortality condition, but the effective use of HAART can improve a patient's prognosis.

## Mycobacterium Tuberculosis

In non–HIV-infected patients, the lifetime risk of active TB infection is approximately 10% to 20%. In contrast, patients coinfected with HIV/TB have an annual risk of active TB infection in excess of 10%.[22–24] Fortunately, the use of HAART significantly reduces the incidence of active TB infection in patients with HIV infection (0.9/1000 person years).[3] Additionally, for HIV-infected patients who acquire active TB while not on HAART, studies have shown dramatic improvements in 3-year survival for patients who initiate HAART when diagnosed with TB (HAART+ group 3-year survival 87.7% and HAART− group 3-year survival 9.3%).[24,25] Therefore, TB in HIV+ patients not on HAART should initiate HAART if nothing precludes this option, and for patients who have acquired TB while on HAART, the regimen and/or compliance should be reviewed.

## Cryptococcus Infection

Cryptococcus infection incidence is low in the current HAART era, at approximately 0.8 per 1000 person years.[3] The ATCC found that its aMHR among OIs is second, however, only to PML, purporting a high impact factor for patients effected by cryptococcal infection.[26] A 2006 French retrospective, multicenter, cohort study of 389 patients during pre-HAART and post-HAART eras found that the average mortality per 100 person years was significantly different, at 63.8 per 100 person years and 15.3 per 100 person years, respectively, and that the probability of death at 3 months was 18% and 21%, respectively. Patients in the post-HAART era with cryptococcal infections tend to be older and have higher CD4 counts, greater dissemination of disease, and more severe meningitis.[27] This infection remains rare likely due to effective HAART, but when it presents, 3-month survival can be relatively high.

## Progressive Multifocal Leukoencephalopathy

The ATCC found the highest aMHR of 9.4 (the second highest was Cryptococcus at aMHR 4.3) for PML among the OIs.[26] This demyelinating disease of the central nervous system is caused by the JC virus and generally occurs in patients with severe immunodeficiency. In HIV-infected patients, the disease typically presents with progressive neurologic deficits, leading to death after a median of 4 to 6 months, and represents an important cause of morbidity and mortality.[28–30] Many studies have found that HAART has improved patient prognosis in a statistically significant manner.[31,32] Drake and colleagues[32] report an improved survival from median survival increase from 14 to 64 weeks, from the pre-HAART era to the post-HAART era. This diagnosis still purports a poor prognosis with a median survival near 1 year, however, with 50% case fatality rates and with survivors experiencing severe chronic disability.[33] Thus far, the best observed indicators for better prognosis with PML are higher CD4 cell counts and better Karnofsky performance status scale score.[30,34]

### Toxoplasmosis Encephalitis

Buchacz and colleagues[3] report an 8-fold decrease of incidence for pre-HAART era and post-HAART era toxoplasmosis infections (4.1 per 1000 person years to 0.5 per 1000 person years). Similar dramatic declines have been reported in other studies, although more patients in the post-HAART era are developing toxoplasmosis encephalitis as their first AIDS-defining illness. Additionally, these patients are typically not receiving HAART or toxoplasmosis prophylaxis. If treated quickly, data suggest a near 90% survival in the current era; however, several patients persist with neurologic deficits. Also, variables shown consistent with a better prognosis included no previous AIDS-defining illness, age less than 45 years, and LDH level less than 300 U/L.[35]

In summary, the incidence of OIs has been significantly reduced given the advent of HAART; however, when present, several of these OIs purport a poor prognosis, whereas other OIs should alert a medical provider to actively pursue treatment of the infection, HAART initiation or optimization, and OI prophylaxis when appropriate.

## HIV/AIDS AND MALIGNANCY

In the early 1980s, the CDC designated a list of diseases that defined AIDS. This list of AIDS-defining conditions always included certain malignancies as AIDS-defining malignancies. Its latest revision in 2008 designates Kaposi sarcoma (KS), non-Hodgkin lymphomas (NHLs) (diffuse large B-cell lymphoma [DLBCL], Burkitt lymphoma, primary central nervous system lymphoma, and other more rare immunoblastic lymphomas), and invasive cervical cancer as AIDS-defining malignancies.[36] These cancers gained this distinction due to their increased frequency in AIDS. The advent of HAART has produced declines in the frequency, morbidity, and morality of most of these cancers relative to the pre-HAART era. Additionally, HAART has transformed HIV infection into a chronic illness with fewer deaths due to OIs leading to malignancy as an increasing cause of death in late-stage AIDS.[37–39] The HAART era has also revealed that HIV-infected people are predisposed to earlier onset and higher rates of non–AIDS-defining cancers (eg, Hodgkin lymphoma, invasive anal carcinoma, multiple myeloma, leukemia, lung cancer, prostate cancer, and colon cancer).[37,40] Therefore, understanding pre-HAART era incidence and prognosis relative to HAART era prognosis and treatment options informs the care of AIDS patients with malignancies.

## AIDS-DEFINING MALIGNANCIES
### Kaposi Sarcoma

KS is a hypervascular neoplastic disease that commonly affects the skin, intestinal tracts, and lungs. In the general population, it is a rare cancer, but in HIV-infected people, it is the most common AIDS-associated malignancy.[41] HAART has reduced the incidence of KS[37]; HAART era data show increased rates of 2-year survival from diagnosis (30% pre-HAART vs 58% HAART era),[6] but the natural history of KS continues to create significant morbidity and mortality. Stebbing and colleagues[41] developed a prognostic index that attempts to categorize patients into prognostic tiers of best, intermediate, and worst prognosis on a 15-point scale. The scoring system is too detailed to explain in this article, but in brief, this index scores patients according to age, occurrence of KS at or after AIDS onset, presence of comorbid conditions, and CD4 cell count. Once categorized, the index purports to advise on treatment strategies. For patients with the best prognostic score, treatment of choice is HAART alone. Patients with the worst prognostic score should be treated with HAART and systemic chemotherapy and reportedly have a median survival of 242 days. The group was unable to draw conclusions on treatment of choice for patients with an intermediate prognostic score.

## Non-Hodgkin Lymphoma

The 1980s revealed that HIV-infected people had a 100-fold increased risk of developing NHL relative to noninfected people.[42,43]

HAART has reduced the incidence of NHL, but it still remains the second most common AIDS-associated malignancy worldwide. One of the longest and largest studies on the effects of HAART on the incidence of this AIDS-defining cancer identified 429 cases of NHL between 1984 and 2006. In the pre-HAART era, the incidence of NHL was 13.6 per 1000 person years and HAART-era incidence declined to 1.6 per 1000 person years. This decline in NHL seems profound, but it is dwarfed by the declines seen in OIs, resulting in a relative increase in AIDS-related lymphoma (ARL) as a presenting AIDS-defining illness.[42] NHLs consist of an array of lymphocyte blood tumors; however, in the case of ARLs, greater than 95% are derived from B cells. Comparing NHL encountered in the HIV-infected populations with noninfected populations. HIV-infected patients present with advanced disease, B symptoms, extranodal disease, leptomeningeal disease, and disease in unusual locations.[37] This article focuses on the NHLs that are most common or carry the worst prognosis: DLBCL, Burkitt lymphoma, and primary central nervous system lymphoma (PCNSL).

## Diffuse Large B-Cell Lymphoma

DLBCL is a heterogeneous group of intermediate to high-grade mature B-cell neoplasms. Several studies have reviewed survival and prognostic indicators of DLBCL in HIV-infected patients both pre-HAART and post-HAART. Lim and colleagues,[44] in a retrospective review of 192 HIV-DLBCL patients (1982–2003), report an improved complete response rate to treatment from 32% pre-HAART to 57% post-HAART ($P = .0006$) and a median survival change from 8.2 to 43.2 months ($P = .0005$). Alternatively, Bower and colleagues[45] attempt to validate the use of the International Prognostic Index (derived from age, tumor stage, lactate dehydrogenase level, *Eastern Cooperative Oncology Group* performance status, and number of extranodal sites) in post-HAART era HIV-DLBCL patients who receive chemotherapeutic treatment. They note 2-year survival outcomes that do not significantly differ compared with non–HIV-infected patients in low-risk, low to intermediate risk, and intermediate to high-risk groups. They did observe, however, significantly worse 2-year survival in the International Prognostic Index HIV-DLBCL (7%) high-risk group versus 20% in the non–HIV-DLBCL high-risk group, therefore concluding that patients in the first 3 categories should undergo standard chemotherapeutic treatment as prescribed for non–HIV-DLBCL patients but groups in the high-risk category might best be considered for clinical trials or newer approaches. In summary, DLBCL combined with Burkitt lymphoma comprises greater than 90% of all ARL NHLs.[42] DLBCL, in contrast to Burkitt lymphoma, has seen significant improvements in survival outcomes in the post-HAART era of AIDS.

## Burkitt Lymphoma

Before HAART, distinguishing DLBCL from Burkitt lymphoma was relatively unimportant because both had median survival of 6 months or less. As discussed previously, however, DLBCL now approaches treatment outcomes seen in non–HIV-infected people. This turn in survival has not occurred widely with Burkitt lymphoma. Despite the addition of HAART and standard chemotherapy, median survival of Burkitt lymphoma remains at 5 to 7 months.[46] Small trials, however, of intensive chemotherapy with cyclophosphamide, doxorubicin, high-dose methotrexate–ifosfamide, etoposide, and high-dose cytarabine (CODOX-M/IVA) have begun to show near-equivalent 2-year survival data between HIV-infected and non–HIV-infected patients.[46,47] Larger trials of this method of treatment are needed. Therefore, at this time Burkitt lymphoma remains as an ARL NHL that connotes a poor prognosis.

## Primary Central Nervous System Lymphoma

PCNSL accounts for 15% of ARL NHLs compared with less than 1% of NHLs in non–HIV-infected populations.[42,48] The clinical features of PCNSL are variable and can include change in mental status, hemiparesis, aphasia, focal neurologic deficits, seizures, fever, and B symptoms. PCNSL is the second most common cause of focal brain disease in AIDS (toxoplasmosis is the most common),[49] and differentiating between these two is important. MRI has high diagnostic yield and CT scan can also be effective. Alternatively, single-photon emission CT scanning combined with Epstein-Barr virus DNA in the cerebrospinal fluid by polymerase chain reaction has a sensitivity of 100% and specificity of 97% in one case series.[42,50] Median survival in untreated patients is 1 to 3 months. HAART combined with whole brain radiation therapy (WBRT) showed significant improved median survival to 170 days.[49] Additionally, studies involving high-dose methotrexate therapy combined with other chemotherapeutic agents with and without WBRT are showing increases in median survival from months to years.[51] PCNSL when left untreated purports a poor prognosis and when treated with HAART, chemotherapy, and WBRT likely results in improved outcomes if patients are not overwhelmed with chemotherapeutic toxicity or radiation-related necrosis.

## Invasive Cervical Cancer

Of the AIDS-defining cancers, the least is known about the pre-HAART and post-HAART incidence and prognosis of invasive cervical cancer. The dramatic changes witnessed in KS and NHL have not been evident in invasive cervical cancer. On the contrary, in Chaturvedi and colleagues'[52] study of nearly 500,000 individuals diagnosed with AIDS from 1980 to 2004, a nonsignificant increase in cervical cancer was witnessed. Although the result was not a significant increase, it denotes that no decrease was observed. This finding is speculated to be due to people surviving longer with AIDS and being effected by the natural history of HPV-associated cancers. Greater surveillance and treatment of these types of cancers are needed, especially given that women with HIV are known to have a 5-times higher risk of cervical cancer relative to the general population.

## NON–AIDS-DEFINING CANCERS

HIV-infected people have been known to be at risk for AIDS-defining cancers, but in addition to these cancers, people with HIV infection have had increased incidence and decreased survival with non–AIDS-defining cancers (NADCs). Biggar and colleagues[6] set out to determine 24-month survival of 8 NADCs (lung, larynx, colorectum, anus, Hodgkin lymphoma, breast, prostate, and testis) in the pre-HAART and post-HAART eras relative to the general population. A review of New York City adults, ages 15 to 69 years, from 1980 to 2000, with AIDS and invasive cancer revealed that in the post-HAART era, greater than 50% of persons with AIDS survived 24 months with 6 of the 8 cancers; the exceptions were lung and laryngeal cancer. There was a trend toward lower percentage of 24-month survival for all persons with AIDS compared with the general population at large with equivalent cancers.

### Lung Cancer

For persons with AIDS and lung cancer, pre-HAART 24-month survival was 5% and post-HAART 10% and for the general population without AIDS, 24-month survival for lung cancer was 31%. These findings were not statistically significant.[6]

### Laryngeal Cancer

For persons with AIDS and laryngeal cancer, pre-HAART 24-month survival was 63% and post-HAART 31% and for the general population without AIDS, 24-month survival for laryngeal cancer was 70%. These pre-HAART and post-HAART findings seemed to become worse for persons with AIDS, but the findings were not significant.[6]

### Colorectal Cancer

For persons with AIDS and colorectal cancer, pre-HAART 24-month survival was 9% and post-HAART 63% and for the general population without AIDS, 24-month survival for colorectal cancer was 73%. These pre-HAART and post-HAART findings were significant and show a trend toward HAART improving survival in persons with AIDS and colorectal cancer toward that of the general population.[6]

### Hodgkin Lymphoma

For persons with AIDS and Hodgkin lymphoma, pre-HAART 24-month survival was 19% and post-HAART 55% and for the general population without AIDS, 24-month survival for Hodgkin lymphoma was 89%. These findings were not statistically significant.[6]

### Prostate Cancer

For persons with AIDS and prostate cancer, pre-HAART 24-month survival was 44% and post-HAART 67% and for the general population without AIDS, 24-month survival for prostate cancer was 95%. These findings were not statistically significant but show a marked discrepancy between those with and those without AIDS.[6]

### Squamous Cell Cancer of the Anus

For persons with AIDS and squamous cell caner of the anus, pre-HAART 24-month survival was 32% and post-HAART 76% and for the general population without AIDS, 24-month survival for squamous cell cancer of the anus was 78%. These findings display the equivalent rates of survival for persons with and without AIDS[6]; therefore, suggesting treatment should not be withheld or restrained based on HIV status.[53]

## SUBSTANCE ABUSE AND LIVER DISEASE
### Injection Drug Use

Injection drug use (IDU) is the second most common mode of HIV transmission in the United States.[54] The use of noninjection illicit drugs may also aid in sexual transmission of HIV due to compromised decision making secondary to intoxication. Methamphetamine and amyl nitrate have been strongly associated with high-risk sexual behavior in men who have sex with men. The use of illicit substances has been linked with increased risk of HAART failure or noninitiation of HAART due to the daily dysfunction of routine activities associated with illicit drug abuse.[54]

Illicit drug dependence has been associated with several comorbid conditions, ranging from mental health disorders to exposure to infectious pathogens to end-organ damage. Illicit drug use has been associated with high rates of depression and anxiety, and depression in HIV-infected patients has been highly correlated with poor adherence and poor treatment outcomes.[54] Therefore, evaluation and treatment of depression in patients with illicit drug use should be a priority. The specific subgroup of HIV-infected patients with past history or active IDU is a group that experiences high rates of morbidity and mortality. Patients with HIV and active IDU can present special treatment challenges, including medical and comorbid conditions, limited access to HIV care, inadequate adherence to therapy, medication side effects and toxicities, need for substance abuse treatment, and drug interactions that complicate HIV treatment.[54] Additionally, factors associated with lower rates of HAART use in IDU patients include active drug use, younger age, female gender, suboptimal health care, lack of access to drug treatment programs, recent incarceration, and lack of expertise among health care providers.[54] Efficacy of HAART has been shown, however, similar to non-IDU when patients are not actively using drugs. Therefore, treatment of IDU is often essential for treatment of HIV infection in IDU patients. Additionally, common pharmacologic methods of opioid maintenance therapies (eg, methadone or buprenorphine) present some challenges with HAART and require attention to the hepatic metabolism HAART and certain long-acting opioids. Referencing the *Guidelines for the Use of Antiretroviral Agents in HIV-1-Infected adults and Adolescents*[54] or seeking expert counsel on the management of such patients is advised.

The use of nonsterile needles poses significant risk of skin and soft tissue infections, recurrent bacterial pneumonia, endocarditis, neurologic disease, renal disease and hepatitis, most commonly, hepatitis B and/or hepatitis C (HCV). HCV coinfection with HIV has been seen at rates of up to 75% in substance abusers. Patients coinfected with HIV and HCV have been shown to more rapidly progress to cirrhosis and death when compared with HIV or HCV infection alone.[1]

### End-Stage Liver Disease in HIV and Hepatitis C Coinfected Patients

As discussed previously, in IDU, infection with both HIV and HCV is high. A French prospective study comparing pre-HAART era and post-HAART era deaths from end-stage liver disease (ESLD) observed that among 25,178 HIV-infected patients followed in a 5-year period, 265 deaths were observed and 38 of these deaths were attributed to ESLD. Thirty-six of the 38 patients who died of ESLD were coinfected with HIV and HCV. The pre-HAART and post-HAART trends of death due to ESLD were 1995, 1.5% (P<.01), versus 1997, 6.6% (P<.01). Additionally, death rates due to hepatocellular carcinoma in this population significantly increased from 1996 to 2001 (1995, 4.7%; 1997, 11%; and 2001, 25% [P<.05]), displaying a trend consistent with increasing rates of mortality due to co-occurring disease as opposed to AIDS-defining illnesses.[55]

### HAART IN THE PATIENT DYING OF LATE-STAGE AIDS

Discontinuation of HAART may result in a variety of clinical outcomes that would typically be considered undesirable, such as viral rebound, immune decompensation, and disease advancement. Therefore, in patients who are clinically stable with good immune status and adequate viral load suppression, discontinuation of HAART is not recommended. This section addresses some of the issues faced by caregivers and by patients who are at the end of life despite the use of HAART. A common belief in both hospice and palliative medicine is that the unit of care involves the patient and the family or caregivers. In one qualitative study of 144 patients exploring feelings about HAART therapy in patients with advanced HIV/AIDS that included family/caregivers, it was found that patient-caregiver dyads had more positive feelings of health care experiences when the patient-caregiver dyads had greater concordant perceptions about treatment with HAART relative to discordant perceptions. This finding suggests that including caregivers in discussions of HAART and decisions about HAART seems to improve the patient-caregiver experience.[56] Therefore, it is likely that in patients at the end of life on HAART, inclusion of caregivers and family in decisions about withdrawal of HAART would be important in most cases. An additional study of patient-caregiver dyads at the end of life, however, found that relying solely on caregivers for decision making at the end of life contributed to both unmet care and the delivery of unnecessary or unwanted care.[57] Clinical criteria for the withdrawal of HAART at the end of life do not exist. End-of-life decision making about continuing, decreasing, or the withdrawal of life-prolonging measures is often emotionally charged and difficult for patients, caregivers, and medical providers. The advent of HAART and the staggering changes of mortality pre-HAART and post-HAART have had a profound impacted on patients' and caregivers' beliefs about HAART in both expected and unexpected ways. Therefore, it can be difficult to guide patients and caregivers about the continuation or the withdrawal of HAART at the end of life and at times intensive focus on this discussion may act as a distraction to other end-of-life issues. Additionally, the continued use of OI prophylaxis or suppression deserves serious consideration given that several these medications may be the best modality of controlling symptoms due to OIs. In the following sentences a listing of risk and benefits of continued HAART and OI prophylaxis at the end of life may help a medical provider guide patients and caregivers faced with these decisions at the end of life. The potential theoretic benefits of continuing HAART include suppression of more pathogenic virus, protection against HIV encephalopathy/dementia, relief of constitutional symptoms associated with high viral load, and the psychological comfort of combating the disease felt by some patients on HAART. Alternatively, potential risks or certain reasons to consider stopping HAART include toxicity or pharmacologic interactions with comfort medication, diminished quality-of-life return versus treatment burden, therapeutic confusion (curative treatment vs comfort treatment), and distraction from end-of-life or advanced care planning.[1] As discussed previously, before a patient with HIV/AIDS is deemed at end of life, an evaluation by an HIV expert is crucial because the appropriate implementation of HAART can result in improved prognosis.

## LATE-STAGE AIDS AND SYMPTOMS

Symptom and comfort measures at the end of life for HIV-infected patients share many of the features seen in non–HIV-infected patients at the end of life, because a large percentage of late-stage AIDS patients are now dying of non–AIDS-defining illnesses. Therefore, translation of basic principles in pain and symptom management should be used for HIV-infected patients at the end of life.

Given the large number of both pre-HAART era and post-HAART era symptoms in AIDS, it is worth a review of the prevalent symptoms. The 5 most prevalent symptoms reported among AIDS patients are fatigue, weight loss, pain, anorexia, and anxiety. Other less prevalent symptoms include insomnia, cough, nausea/vomiting, dyspnea, depression, diarrhea, and constipation.[1]

Many of these symptoms can be palliated with the appropriate mix of interventions. Covering this broad topic is beyond the scope of this article. Fatigue, experienced by up to 85% of patients with AIDS, is therapeutically challenging to treat. A large review of published studies and abstracts on HIV, AIDS, fatigue, exhaustion, tiredness, weariness, antiretroviral treatment, and therapy found high rates of fatigue in both patients with HIV and with AIDS. Data on treatment and treatment outcomes, however, were limited. The review concluded that the evidence for medication interventions was not strong. The best evidence was found for cognitive behavioral therapy and graded exercise therapy in patients with HIV, but no commentary was given for patients at the end of life. The study supported the use of standard tools for measuring fatigue, screening for depression and anxiety, and using a multidisciplinary approach for treating HIV-infected patients experience fatigue.[58]

## SUMMARY

HIV/AIDS has metamorphosized in the 30 years since the first cases were diagnosed. It has transformed from a terminal condition to a disease that can be managed with HAART. Patients continue to suffer morbidity and mortality, however, from chronic infection with HIV, other coinfections, and the accelerated onset of other disease processes. Additionally, there is still a subset of patients who suffer morbidity and mortality from AIDS-defining illnesses. This article has reviewed prognostic indicators of late-stage AIDS, trends in OI, trends of AIDS-defining malignancies and non–AIDS-defining malignancies, and substance abuse/liver disease in an effort to help primary care providers identify when patients could be considered end stage due to an AIDS-defining illness. Once identified, providing high-quality care for patients at the end of life with AIDS requires the coordination of a multidisciplinary team that is likely inclusive of but not limited to an HIV specialist, palliative care provider, and primary medical care.

## REFERENCES

1. Selwyn P. Palliative care for patient with human immunodeficiency virus/acquired immune deficiency syndrome. J Palliat Med 2005;8:1248–68.
2. Justice A. HIV and aging: time for a new paradigm. Curr HIV/AIDS Rep 2010;7: 69–76.
3. Buchacz K, Baker RK, Palella FJ Jr, et al. AIDS-defining opportunistic illnesses in US patients 1994–2007: a cohort study. AIDS 2010;24:1549–59.
4. Centers for Disease Control and Prevention. HIV/AIDS Surveillance Report, 2007, vol. 19. Atlanta: US Department of Health and Human Services, Centers for Disease Control and Prevention; 2009. p. 1–64. Available at: http://www.cdc. gov/hiv/topics/surveillance/resources/reports/. Accessed March 2, 2011.
5. HIV/AIDS Fact sheet. The Kaiser Family Foundation's; 2009. Available at: http:// www.kff.org/hivaids/upload3029-10.pdf. Accessed March 2, 2011.
6. Biggar RJ, Engles EA, Ly S, et al. Survival after cancer diagnosis in persons with AIDS. J Acquir Immune Defic Syndr 2005;39:293–9.
7. Schambelan M, Benson CA, Carr A, et al. Management of metabolic complications associated with antiretroviral therapy for HIV-1 Infection: recommendations of an International AIDS Society-USA Panel. J Acquir Immune Defic Syndr 2002; 31(3):257–75.
8. May M, Sterne JA, Sabin C, et al, The Antiretroviral Therapy (ART) Cohort Collaboration. Prognosis of HIV-1-infected patients up to 5 years after initiation of HAART: collaborative analysis of prospective studies. AIDS 2007;21:1185–97.

9. Lohse N, Hansen AB, Pedersen G, et al. Survival of persons with and without HIV infection in Denmark, 1995–2005. Ann Intern Med 2007;146(2):87–95.

10. Bhaskaran K, Hamouda O, Sannes M, et al. Changes in the risk of death after HIV seroconversion compared with mortality in the general population. JAMA 2008; 300(1):51–9.

11. Shen JM, Blank A, Selwyn PA. Predictors of mortality for patients with Advanced Disease in an HIV palliative care program. J Acquir Immune Defic Syndr 2005;40: 445–7.

12. Tarwater PM, Gallant JE, Mellors JW, et al. Prognostic value of plasma HIV RNA among highly active antiretroviral therapy users. AIDS 2004;18:2419–23.

13. Smit C, Geskus R, Walker S, et al, The CASCADE Collaboration. Effective therapy has altered the spectrum of cause-specific mortality following HIV-seroconversion. AIDS 2006;20:741–9. Mortality due to hepatitis C-related liver disease in HIV-infected patients in France (Mortavic 2001 study).

14. CDC. Pneumocystis pneumonia—Los Angeles. MMWR Morb Mortal Wkly Rep 1981;30:250–2.

15. Radhi S, Alexander T, Ukwu M, et al. Outcome of HIV-associated Pneumocystis pneumonia in hospitalized patients from 2000 through 2003. BMC Infect Dis 2008;8:118.

16. Curtis RJ, Yarnold PR, Schwartz DN, et al. Improvements in outcomes of acute respiratory failure for patients with human immunodeficiency virus-related Pneumocystis carinii pneumonia. Am J Respir Crit Care Med 2000; 162:393–8.

17. Morris A, Wachter RM, Luce J, et al. Improved survival with highly active antiretroviral therapy in HIV-infected patients with severe Pneumocystis carinii pneumonia. AIDS 2003;17:73–80.

18. Khouli H, Afrasiabi A, Shibli M, et al. Outcome of critically ill human immunodeficiency virus-infected patients in the era of highly active antiretroviral therapy. J Intensive Care Med 2005;20:327–33.

19. Miller RF, Allen E, Copas A, et al. Improved survival for HIV infected patients with severe Pneumocystis jirovecii pneumonia is independent of highly active antiretroviral therapy. Thorax 2006;61:716–21.

20. Karakousis PC, Moore RD, Chaisson RE. Mycobacterium avium complex in patients with HIV infection in the era of highly active antiretroviral therapy. Lancet Infect Dis 2004;4:557–65.

21. Sungkanuparph S, Chakriyanuyok T, Butthum B. Antiretroviral therapy in AIDS patients with CMV disease: impact on the survival and long-term treatment outcome. J Infect 2008;56:40–3.

22. Selwyn PA, Hartel D, Lewis VA, et al. A prospective study of the risk of tuberculosis among intravenous drug users with human immunodeficiency virus infection. N Engl J Med 1989;320:545–50.

23. Jon F. Tuberculosis. In: Jonathan C. Willium P, editors. Infectious diseases, vol. 1. 2nd edition. Spain. Mosby; 2004. p. 401–18.

24. Manosuthi W, Chottanapand S, Thongyen S, et al. Survival rate and risk factors of mortality among HIV/Tuberculosis-Coinfected patients with and without antiretroviral therapy. J Acquir Immune Defic Syndr 2006;43:42–6.

25. Velasco M, Castilla V, Sanz J, et al. Effect of simultaneous use of highly active antiretroviral therapy of survival of HIV patients with tuberculosis. J Acquir Immune Defic Syndr 2009;50:148–52.

26. Mocroft A, Sterne JA, Egger M, et al. Antiretroviral Therapy Cohort Collaboration. Variable impact on mortality of AIDS-defining events diagnosed during

combinatino antiretxroviral therapy: not all AIDS-defining conditionsare created equal. Clin Infect Dis 2009;48:1138–51.

27. Lortholary O, Poizat G, Zeller V, et al. Long-term outcome of AIDS-associated cryptococcosis in the era of combination antiretroviral therapy. AIDS 2006;20: 2183–91.

28. Berger JR, Kaszovitz B, Post MJ, et al. Progressive multifocal leukoencephalopathy associated with human immunodeficiency virus infection. A review of the literature with a report of sixteen cases. Ann Intern Med 1987;107:78–87.

29. Fong IW, Toma E. The natural history of progressive multifocal leukoencephalopathy in patients with AIDS. Canadian PML Study Group. Clin Infect Dis 1995;20:1305–10.

30. De Luca A, Ammassari A, Pezzotti P, et al. Cidofovir in addition to antiretroviral treatment is not effective for AIDS-associated progressive multifocal leukoencephalopathy: a multicohort analysis. AIDS 2008;22:1759–67.

31. Palella FJ Jr, Delaney KM, Moorman AC, et al. Declining morbidity and mortality among patients with advanced human immunodeficiency virus infection. HIV Outpatient Study Investigators. N Engl J Med 1998;338:853–60.

32. Drake AK, Loy CT, Brew BJ, et al. Human immunodeficiency virus-associated progressive multifocal leucoencephalopathy: epidemiology and predictive factors for prolonged survival. Eur J Neurol 2007;14:418–23.

33. Gasnault J, Taoufik Y, Goujard C, et al. Prolonged survival without neurological improvement in patients with AIDS-related progressive multifocal leukoencephalopathy on potent combined antiretroviral therapy. J Neurovirol 1999;5:421–9.

34. De Luca A, Giancola ML, Ammassari A, et al. The effect of potent antiretroviral therapy and JC virus load in cerebrospinal fluid on clinical outcome of patients with AIDS-associated progressive multifocal leukoencephalopathy. J Infect Dis 2000;182:1077–83.

35. Hoffmann C, Ernst M, Meyer P, et al. Evolving characteristics of toxoplasmosis in patients infected with human immunodeficiency virus-1: clinical course and Toxoplasma gondii-specific immune responses. Clin Microbiol Infect 2007;13: 510–5.

36. Centers for Disease Control and Prevention. Revised Surveillance Case Definitions for HIV Infection among adults, adolescents, and children aged <18 months and for HIV infection and AIDS among children aged 18 months to <13 years – United States, 2008. MMWR 2008;57(No. RR-10):1–16.

37. Cheung MC, Pantanowitz L, Dezube BJ. AIDS related malignancies: emerging challenges in the era of highly active antiretroviral therapy. Oncologist 2005;10: 412–26.

38. Bonnet F, Lewden C, May T, et al. Malignancy-related causes of death in human immunodeficiency virus-infected patients in the era of highly active antiretroviral therapy. Cancer 2004;101:317–24.

39. Louie JK, Hsu LC, Osmond DH, et al. Trends in causes of death among persons with acquired immunodeficiency syndrome in the era of highly active antiretroviral therapy, San Francisco, 1994–1998. J Infect Dis 2002;186:1023–7.

40. Gachupin-Garcia A, Selwyn PA, Budner NS. Population-based study of malignancies and HIV infection amoung injecting drug users in a New York City methadone treatment program, 1985–1991. AIDS 1992;6:843–8.

41. Stebbing J, Sanitt A, Nelson M, et al. A prognostic index for AIDS-associated Kaposi's sarcoma in the era of highly active antiretroviral therapy. Lancet 2006; 367:1495–502.

42. Hull A. Does ARV therapy reduce incidence of non-Hodgkin lymphoma? HIV Clin 2009;21(4):6–8.

43. Goedert JJ, Coté TR, Virgo P, et al. Spectrum of AIDS associated malignant disorders. Lancet 1998;351:1833–9.

44. Lim ST, Karim R, Tulpule A, et al. Prognostic factors in HIV-related diffuse large-cell lymphoma: before versus after highly active antiretroviral therapy. J Clin Oncol 2005;23:8477–82.

45. Bower M, Gazzard B, Mandalia S, et al. A prognostic index for systemic AIDS-related non-Hodgkin lymphoma treated in the era of highly active antiretroviral therapy. Ann Intern Med 2005;143:265–73.

46. Mounier N, Spina M, Gisselbreght C. Modern management of non-Hodgkin lymphoma in HIV-infected patients. Br J Haematol 2007;136:685–98.

47. Wang ES, Straus DJ, Teruya-Feldstein J, et al. Intensive chemotherapy with cyclophosphamide, doxorubicin, high-dose methotrexate/ifosfamide, etoposide, and highdose cytarabine (CODOX-M/IVAC) for human immunodeficiency virus-associated Burkitt lymphoma. Cancer 2003;98:1196–205.

48. Coté TR, Biggar RJ, Rosenberg PS, et al. NHL among people with AIDS. Int J Cancer 1997;73:645.

49. Skiest DJ, Crosby C. Survival is prolonged by highly active antiretroviral therapy in AIDS patients with primary central nervous system lymphoma. AIDS 2003;17:1787–93.

50. Antinori A, Ammassari A, De Luca A, et al. Diagnosis of AIDS-related focal brain lesion: a decision-making analysis based on clinical and neuroradiologic characteristics combined with polymerase chain reaction assays in CSF. Neurology 1997;48:687.

51. Ansell SM, Rajkumar SV. Hematology: trials and tribulations in primary CNS lymphoma. Nat Rev Clin Oncol 2010;7:125–6.

52. Chaturvedi AK, Madeleine MM, Biggar RJ, et al. Risk of human papillomavirus–associated cancers among persons with AIDS. J Natl Cancer Inst 2009;101:1120–30.

53. Chiao EY, Giordano TP, Richardson P, et al. Human immunodeficiency virus-associated squamous cell cancer of the anus: epidemiology and outcomes in the highly active antiretroviral therpy era. J Clin Oncol 2008;26:474–9.

54. Panel on Antiretroviral Guidelines for Adults and Adolescents. Guidelines for the use of antiretroviral agents in HIV-1-infected adults and adolescents. Department of Health and Human Services; 2009. p. 1–161. Available at: http://www.aidsinfo.nih.gov/ContentFiles/AdultandAdolescentGL.pdf. Accessed March 2, 2011.

55. Rosenthal E, Poiree M, Pradier C, et al. Mortality due to hepatitis C-related liver disease in HIV-infected patients in France (Mortavic 2001 study). AIDS 2003;17:1803–9.

56. Sacajiu G, Raveis VH, Selwyn P. Patients and family care givers' experiences around highly active antiretroviral therapy (HAART). AIDS Care 2009;21(12):1528–36.

57. Krug R, Karus D, Selwyn PA, et al. Late-stage HIV/AIDS patients' and their familial caregivers agreement on the palliative care outcome scale. J Pain Symptom Manage 2010;39(1):23–32.

58. Jong E, Oudhoff LA, Epskamp C, et al. Predictors and treatment of strategies of HIV-related fatigue in the combined antiretroviral therapy era. AIDS 2010;24:1387–485.

# Pediatric Palliative Care

Karen Moody, MD, MS[a],*, Linda Siegel, MD[b],
Kathryn Scharbach, MD[c], Leslie Cunningham, PhD[a],
Rabbi Mollie Cantor, BCC[d]

**KEYWORDS**

- Palliative care • Pediatric palliative care
- Advanced care planning • End-of-life care

Pediatric palliative care has lagged significantly behind the strides made in hospice and palliative care for adults with terminal illness. However, since the World Health Organization, the American Academy of Pediatrics, and the Institute of Medicine called attention to the unmet needs of dying children,[1–3] forward progress in pediatric palliative care has gained momentum. Nevertheless, there remain significant barriers to the appropriate provision of palliative care to ill and dying children in the United States, including the lack of properly trained health care professionals, resources to finance such care, and scientific research in this area, as well as a continued cultural denial of death in children.[4,5] In this article, the authors review from available literature and their own experience: the epidemiology of pediatric palliative care, special communication concerns, decision making, ethical and legal considerations, symptom assessment and management, psychosocial issues, provision of care across settings, end-of-life care, and bereavement. Educational and supportive resources for health care practitioners and families, respectively, are included at the end of the article. It is the authors' intention to facilitate the health care practitioner's ability to provide palliative and end-of-life care to children so as to minimize their suffering and maximize their quality of life.

The authors have nothing to disclose.
[a] Division of Pediatric Hematology/Oncology, Albert Einstein College of Medicine, Children's Hospital at Montefiore, 3415 Bainbridge Avenue, 111 East 210th Street, Rosenthal 3, Bronx, NY 10463, USA
[b] Division of Pediatric Critical Care, Albert Einstein College of Medicine, Children's Hospital at Montefiore, 3415 Bainbridge Avenue, 111 East 210th Street, Rosenthal 4, Bronx, NY 10463, USA
[c] Division of Social Pediatrics, Albert Einstein College of Medicine, Children's Hospital at Montefiore, 3415 Bainbridge Avenue, 111 East 210th Street, Rosenthal 4, Bronx, NY 10463, USA
[d] Center for Pastoral Education, Jewish Theological Seminary, 3080 Broadway, New York, NY 10027, USA
* Corresponding author.
*E-mail address:* kmoody@montefiore.org

Prim Care Clin Office Pract 38 (2011) 327–361
doi:10.1016/j.pop.2011.03.011
0095-4543/11/$ – see front matter © 2011 Elsevier Inc. All rights reserved.

primarycare.theclinics.com

## EPIDEMIOLOGY OF PEDIATRIC PALLIATIVE CARE

Identifying which children would benefit from palliative care can be challenging, and palliative care should not be limited to children at the end-of-life. Approximately 53,000 children die in the United States each year, nearly 55% of whom are younger than 1 year.[6] **Fig. 1** highlights the leading causes of death in infants, children, and adolescents younger than 19 years.[6]

Nearly 450,000 noninstitutionalized children live with chronic, life-threatening conditions that render them unable to engage in age-appropriate activities, and over 2 million more are limited in the kind or amount of age-appropriate activities in which they participate because of a chronic illness.[7] At a minimum, the estimated 16,000 children whose deaths are attributable to a complex chronic condition (more than 10,000 infants and more than 5000 children aged 1–18 years), should be considered amenable to palliative care.[6,8] Though there are no criteria, per se, for palliative care in children, general categories of conditions apposite for palliative care include conditions for which curative treatment is possible but may fail, conditions requiring intensive long-term treatment aimed at maintaining the quality of life even though premature death is anticipated, progressive conditions in which treatment is exclusively palliative after diagnosis, and conditions involving severe, nonprogressive disability, causing extreme vulnerability to health complications (**Box 1**).[4,9]

At present, only about 5000 of the 53,000 children dying each year receive hospice services,[9] indicating that the vast majority of children who might benefit from palliative care and hospice services are not being reached.

### Developmental Considerations

Complex medical conditions and their treatments often have a profound effect on a child's growth as well as their emotional and social development. An understanding

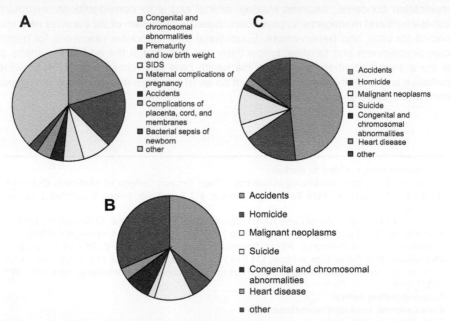

**Fig. 1.** (*A*) Leading causes of infant death in the United States, 2006. SIDS, sudden infant death syndrome. (*B*) Leading causes of childhood death (1–14 years) in the United States, 2006. (*C*) Leading causes of adolescent death (15–19 years) in the United States, 2006.

---

**Box 1**
**Conditions appropriate for pediatric palliative care**

Conditions for which curative treatment is possible but may fail

    Advanced or progressive cancer or cancer with a poor prognosis

    Complex and severe congenital or acquired heart disease

    Complex and severe congenital or acquired airway anomalies

    Organ failure with potential for transplantation

Conditions requiring intensive long-term treatment aimed at maintaining the quality of life

    Human immunodeficiency virus infection

    Cystic fibrosis

    Sickle cell disease

    Severe gastrointestinal disorders or malformations such as gastroschisis

    Severe epidermolysis bullosa

    Severe immunodeficiencies

    Renal failure in cases in which dialysis, transplantation, or both are not available or indicated

    Chronic or severe respiratory failure

    Muscular dystrophy and other muscle disorders

    Posttransplantation (eg, solid organ, bone marrow)

Progressive conditions in which treatment is exclusively palliative after diagnosis

    Progressive metabolic disorders

    Certain chromosomal abnormalities, such as trisomy 13 or trisomy 18

    Severe forms of osteogenesis imperfecta

Conditions involving severe, nonprogressive disability, causing extreme vulnerability to health complications

    Severe cerebral palsy with recurrent infection or difficult-to-control symptoms

    Extreme prematurity

    Severe neurologic sequelae of infectious disease

    Hypoxic or anoxic brain injury

    Traumatic brain injury

    Holoprosencephaly or other severe brain malformations

*Data from* Himelstein B, Hilden JM, Boldt AM, et al. Pediatric palliative care. N Engl J Med 2004;350(17):1752–62.

---

of cognitive development can provide valuable insight into how to best communicate with pediatric patients with a life-limiting or life-threatening illness. Although Piaget has been criticized for creating a schema that is too rigid,[10] his stages of cognitive development continue to be referred to and afford a useful framework for considering how infants, children, and adolescents understand their illness and future. Although it is clear from the literature on pediatric palliative care that awareness of the developmental level of the pediatric patient is critical to effective communication,[11,12] little is written regarding children's concepts of illness and death, and specifically how to communicate with them and their families (**Table 1**).[4,10,13]

Maximizing development in all realms is of paramount importance in providing an optimal quality of life. Physical, occupational, and speech therapies can aid in the timely achievement of developmental milestones and in the maintenance of function in patients whose condition is worsening. In addition, these therapies can improve function and quality of life in children with physical disabilities or treatment-related symptoms.

## COMMUNICATION

The communication needs of pediatric palliative care patients and families can be categorized into cognitive needs and affective needs. Cognitive needs include the need to know and understand the diagnosis, treatment plan, and prognosis while affective needs describe an emotional need to feel known and understood.[14] To meet these needs, pediatric palliative care providers must have knowledge of the patient's illness, develop a relationship with the patient and family, and learn about the culture of the family. Educating children and their families about the patient's illness is an iterative process that requires discussion of the patient's and family's personal and cultural understanding of the illness and treatment, and its impact on each person's life. Sufficient time is needed to build rapport and to understand the family in order to gain trust.[14] Communication must be responsive to the changing needs of the patient in the context of his or her family dynamics.

Studies have shown that patients, parents, family members, and health care providers identify similar skills and approaches when asked what is most important in the communication between providers, pediatric patients, and families in the palliative care setting. The important components of communication that can be facilitated by the health care team are outlined in **Table 2**. In addition, parents cite care coordination as an important domain in communication in the pediatric palliative care setting.[15] The best approach to communication is flexibility.[16] Health care providers must accommodate existing needs of diverse patient-family units, strengthen clinical relationships, and foster the personal growth of the infant, child, or adolescent through his or her experience with illness.[16]

### Barriers to Palliative Care for Children

In a 2008 study of perceptions of end-of-life care, approximately half of the nurse and physician participants reported that the following barriers occurred frequently or almost always: uncertain prognosis (55%), family not ready to acknowledge incurable condition (51%), language barriers (47%), and time constraints (47%).[17] These issues clearly are not unique to pediatrics. Cultural barriers exist in all health care settings and addressing these cultural differences, including language barriers, is an important role that a palliative care team must fulfill. Palliative care providers must recognize and put aside their own cultural expectations and biases, learn the culture of the family, and bridge the cultures of medicine and the family.[18] In a study that spoke with parents of deceased children, Spanish-speaking parents conveyed feelings of isolation, confusion, and distrust of the hospital system.[19]

### Talking with Parents

A specific issue that should be addressed when speaking with parents regards the information that will be conveyed to the child. This aspect includes who will deliver the information, what will be told to the child, and how medical information will be

**Table 1**
**Children's concept of illness and death**

| Stage | Characteristics | Concept of Illness | Concept of Death |
|---|---|---|---|
| Sensorimotor 0–2 years | Has sensory and motor relationships with environment<br>Recognizes self as agent of action and begins to act intentionally<br>Achieves object permanence<br>Has limited language skills | None | None |
| Preoperational 2–6 years | Developing language skills<br>Has egocentric thinking and difficulty taking viewpoint of others. Learns to represent objects by images and words, engages in symbolic play<br>Uses magical thinking | Illness may be perceived as caused by external concrete phenomena that coincided with the onset of the illness<br>Child cannot explain how an illness occurs | Believes death is like sleep (temporary and reversible) and can be caused by thoughts[4] |
| Concrete operational 6–12 years | Can think logically about objects and events<br>Can differentiate between self and others and between internal and external phenomena | Sickness often perceived as an action, object, or a person separate from child that is capable of causing injury<br>Later in this stage, child might be able to understand that an illness resides internally but may have been caused by something external | May be aware of brevity of time left though may not fully comprehend irreversibility of death[21] |
| Formal operational >12 years | Can think logically about abstract concepts and test hypotheses systematically<br>Becomes concerned with the hypothetical, the future, and ideological problems<br>Capable of self-reflection<br>Body image and self-esteem paramount | Begins to recognize differences between physiologic and psychological symptoms and conditions. Can often differentiate thoughts and feelings and understand how those thoughts and feelings may impact on their body and its function | Understands irreversibility of death[21]<br>May be focused on the future and limited amount of time left[21]<br>Explores nonphysical explanations of death[4] |

**Table 2**
**Important components of communication that can be facilitated by the health care team**

| Communication Domain | Attributes of Healthcare Team |
|---|---|
| Relationship building | 1. Continuity<br>2. Spends time with patient and family to get to know each other and build rapport<br>3. Builds a personal relationship<br>4. Shows compassion, caring, and "humanness"<br>5. Discusses psychosocial issues in addition to physical issues |
| Effort & availability | 6. Shows interest and determination to help<br>7. Is accessible to patient and family |
| Competence | 8. Demonstrates knowledge and capacity to help |
| Information exchange | 9. Listens attentively with patient and family<br>10. Uses straightforward and nontechnical language<br>11. Prepares patient and family for bad news<br>12. Gathers information from the patient, family, and other health care providers |
| Parent & child involvement | 13. Recognizes and is responsive to patient and family's desired level of involvement in communicating with health care professionals and decision making<br>14. Engages parents in deciding how to communicate information to child<br>15. Engages patient in care and decision making<br>16. Gives patient control over treatment when possible<br>17. Provides opportunities for patient to speak with provider alone |

Data from Refs.[1,2,4-6]

discussed. At the time of initial diagnosis, health care providers should discuss with parents the importance of being truthful and forthcoming in their communication with the child as well as the importance of including the child in such discussions in a developmentally appropriate manner.[16]

A 2001 Swedish study interviewed parents of children who died of malignant disease 4 to 9 years earlier. Of the 147 parents who had spoken with their child about death, none regretted it, whereas 27% of parents who had not spoken with their child about death regretted that they had not.[20] Parents were more likely to talk to their child about death if they sensed that the child was aware that he or she was dying. Among parents who did not speak with their child about death, they were more likely to regret not having talked about death if the child was older or if they sensed that the child was aware of his or her imminent death.

### Talking with Children and Adolescents

An understanding of a pediatric patient's cognitive potential (as highlighted in the section Developmental Considerations) provides insight into how members of the health care team may effectively approach children and adolescents regarding treatment plans and psychosocial concerns. In addition, in speaking with adolescents it is important to remember the specific emotional and social developments that occur during adolescence. During early adolescence (10–14 years) there is a shift of attachment from parents to peers. Following this, during middle adolescence (15–17 years), consolidation of self-image occurs with the development of feelings of achievement and power, increased experimentation, and the advancement of logical thought with capacity for abstract reasoning. In late adolescence (18 years and older), individuals develop an increased sense of comfort with oneself, awareness of others, and appreciation for meaningful relationships.[16]

### Talking with Health Care Staff

Severe illness and death of a child can evoke powerful emotions in the health care team such as feelings of failure, personal helplessness, sadness, and anticipatory grief.[21] Open communication among health care providers on an ongoing basis is important. However, meetings specifically arranged to discuss personal and professional reflections on patients' illness and how they affect providers can help staff cope with strong emotions that often arise in caring for sick children. In allowing health care providers to vent and process their feelings, they may be more open to the perspectives of the patients. Health care staff should be encouraged to regard the opinions of patients seriously, and to allow the patient and family to have some control over the patient's care and the details concerning their care environment, such as who may visit and when.[16]

### DECISION MAKING IN PEDIATRIC PALLIATIVE CARE
### Establishing Goals of Care

When a child is first diagnosed with a life-threatening disease, families will be overwhelmed and unable to focus on long-term decision-making. As the family has time to digest the information and come to terms with the diagnosis, the physician should begin to address goals of care with them. Initially, cure will be the number one priority for families. Although parents may not be willing or able to discuss end-of-life issues initially, approaching them about what is important to them and to their child will allow them to share their values, hopes, and dreams in a safe setting. Goals may change over time as a child responds or does not respond to treatment. Even when the prognosis is relatively favorable, palliative care can play an important role in helping the child and family to cope. Care plans should include an assessment of physical, emotional, and spiritual suffering of the child and family, and attempt to minimize or alleviate that suffering, no matter what the goal or the prognosis.[22,23] The goal should be to "add life to the child's years, not simply years to the child's life."[12]

To set goals of care, the parents and, sometimes if developmentally appropriate, the patient, should be invited to a team meeting to discuss the child's condition and realistic outcomes. The decision to include the patient up-front in these discussions will depend on the age and developmental stage of the child as well as his or her preferences and the families' desires. Most often, discussions are first held with parents and/or key family decision makers, then the child is brought into the meeting later after there is clarity regarding what will be communicated. Alternatively, parents may wish to convey information to the child privately or with the assistance of one or a few selected members of the team. Overall team members may include a social worker, nurse practitioner, child life specialist, and chaplain. It is important to have many disciplines present but also to be cognizant that families may be overwhelmed by meeting with too many people. Parents should be asked if there are other family members or friends who they would like to be present. Some teams will have someone take notes for the family so they can focus on listening; some teams will allow families to record the meeting so they can review it later.[24]

The medical staff should meet together first, without the family present, so that the team can discuss, identify, and agree about the diagnosis and prognosis of the child, and the goals of the meeting. One person should be chosen to initiate and lead the discussion. The meeting should take place in a comfortable, private location, with as few interruptions as possible. Beepers and cell phones should be off or turned to vibrate mode to minimize distractions. Tissues should be available. While having this and any discussion, the team must be sensitive to the family's culture and language. If a translator is needed for the family meeting, a proper, certified translator should be used because family members, especially children, may not convey information reliably, which places an undue burden on the person translating.

When the family joins the meeting, it is useful to ask the family to describe their understanding of their child's illness and current condition. By doing so, the team can assess not only the parents' understanding of what is happening, but also how well the parents are managing the information they have been given and how ready they are to have a realistic discussion about goals of care. This preliminary conversation allows the physician to affirm the parents' knowledge and to correct any misconceptions. It can then be helpful to explore the parents' hopes and dreams for the future and what they think the child is hoping for, so that the team obtain direction for the conversation about the goal of care.

Once what the family understands is clear and it is determined how well they are coping with and assimilating the information given to them, the team can start to talk about the medical facts regarding prognosis. The physician is obligated to tell the family the truth so that they can make well-informed decisions. As the conversation proceeds, it is possible to gauge the parents' reaction and tailor the discussion to what they seem able to hear. To maintain clarity, the use of euphemisms or medical jargon must be avoided. In an attempt to be gentle with families, the physician might use phrases such as "things are not going well" or "it's not looking good," which leaves room for misunderstanding because parents can easily misinterpret vague comments. Because families do not want to hear that their child might die, they might not catch subtle hints alluding to this fact. In addition, when families are not given full, clear information, they cannot make appropriate decisions about treatment and about other life issues such as what to do about vacations, jobs, or school. Families cannot ask for help from others if they do not know what they are dealing with. The health care team should tell families to hope for the best, but to also prepare for the worst.[4,23,24]

Some of the goals that are discussed are clear, with cure being the ultimate goal for everyone in the beginning. Other goals may include minimizing physical, emotional, and spiritual pain and suffering; being able to go to school; leaving a legacy; having a peaceful death; and being able to decide where to die and who should be there. When such goals are first addressed with families, it does not require the family to acknowledge that the child might die. If a palliative care team is introduced at time of diagnosis or early in the child's course of illness, the team members can learn about the family and help them define goals in the beginning. If there comes a time when cure is not possible, they can help families transition to other, more realistic goals. In this way the transition to palliative care is not an abrupt switch away from people they know and feel comfortable with to the palliative care team.[4,12,23]

Once the goals of care are stated, the team can make recommendations about each treatment option offered. For each treatment option, consideration must be given to the benefit to burden ratio. Treatments that are clearly not beneficial should not be offered, especially if they are potentially burdensome or harmful. The benefits must take into account not only the short-term effectiveness but also the long-term overall prognosis for the child and his or her expected quality of life. For treatments that are of uncertain benefit, parents must be given a broad range of decision-making authority, while the health care team makes recommendations based on the family's stated goals for the child and family. At times, goals may be conflicting (ie, prolong life and vs limit suffering), and over time goals will change. Regardless, parents should be supported in their decisions and reassured that they are making the best choices for their child, and did not cause unnecessary pain or deny the child a chance to recover, so that they can have as uncomplicated a bereavement process as possible.[4,23,25]

### Advanced Care Planning

Advance care planning is becoming more the norm in adult patients. When an adult with decision-making capacity fills out an advanced care plan, it allows him or her to make choices about how to spend the end of their life. It also allows families to decide how to spend remaining time together, and may prevent unwanted interventions. It is also possible for a minor to fill out an advanced care document. This document will not be legally binding, but can give an older child the opportunity to express what he is thinking and feeling, and can help parents and caregivers when they are making decisions. It can also be a useful way to start talking about the fact that the child might not survive.[4] "Five wishes" is one example of a form designed for children.[26] It not only addresses issues surrounding resuscitation but also how the child wants to be treated, and who and what is important to him or her. More and more pediatric teams are using these kinds of forms to allow children to have a voice in their medical care and, if necessary, the dying process.

### Ethical and Legal Considerations in Pediatric Palliative Care

Respect for patient autonomy is a fundamental ethical principle in all disciplines of medicine. The standard application of this principle for those younger than 18 years (the usual age of legal competency in the United States) designates parents or legal guardians as surrogate decision makers for children with respect to most aspects of life. Children are considered to have diminished decision-making capacity and generally, their parents are the persons best able to act in the child's best interest. The challenge arises when children or adolescents are partially or completely competent to make decisions regarding their care. Two issues may arise in this context: (1) a legal minor disagrees with the parent on a care decision, or (2) a parent wishes to keep medical information from the minor patient.

Functional competence or decision-making capacity requires the ability to reason, to understand, to choose voluntarily, and to appreciate the nature of the decision.[16] Many children have developed such functional competence before the age of 18 years. Freyer[16] asserts that there is a consensus among pediatric health professionals, developmental psychologists, ethicists, and lawyers that adolescents 14 years of age or older should be presumed, unless demonstrated otherwise, to have the functional capacity to make medical decisions for themselves (including decisions related to end-of-life issues). However, in practice there exists some controversy regarding the age at which decision-making capacity should be presumed, and suggestions range between 10 and 18 years of age. A series of interviews of patients aged 10 to 20 years conducted within 1 week of participating in an end-of-life decision (enrollment in a phase 1 trial, adoption of a DNR [do not resuscitate] order, initiation of terminal care) supports the notion that individuals younger than 18 years may have decision-making capacity.[11] Eighteen of the 20 patients interviewed accurately recalled their treatment options and were able to identify the likely outcome of each; they understood that they were participating in a decision about the end of their own life, and recognized the consequences of their decision.[11] These patients negotiated a complex decision process pertaining to the end of their own life (including short-term, intermediate-term, and long-term possible outcomes and the impact of decisions on others) by integrating diverse elements into the decision.[11]

Although more than half of the states in the United States have no statutes specifically addressing end-of-life decisions by minors and there exists no federal mandate on the issue, some states recognize "emancipated minors" or have "minor treatment" statutes that provide for legal competency to be recognized in specific individuals younger than 18 years and/or in certain situations for patients younger than 18. "Emancipated minors" statutes recognize the autonomy of individuals on the basis of marriage, parenthood, financial independence, and other circumstances. "Minor treatment" statutes permit minors to authorize treatment for medical conditions they might not attend to if their parents were to know about them (sexually transmitted infections, pregnancy, and substance abuse). Under the "mature minor doctrine" some states have authorized judicial hearings in specific situations to grant capable adolescents the authority to decide for themselves about recommended medical therapy, sometimes against their parents' views.[16]

Children and younger adolescents may be able to engage in mature decision making only in certain situations or with support and guidance. Such persons should be given meaningful decisional opportunities and their preferences should be considered seriously, while maintaining final authority with an adult caregiver.[11,16] Autonomy of action may not be appropriate for children and young adolescents; however, their autonomy of thought and feeling must be respected by diligent communication regarding diagnosis, treatment, and prognosis.[16] Mindful communication with caregivers and early involvement of pediatric patients in decision making will foster the ability of the palliative care team to resolve disagreements between a patient and his or her caregiver regarding the treatment plan. Early and open communication with caregivers must take place regarding the health care provider's responsibility to the pediatric patient (ie, physicians are obligated to tell the truth to the child or adolescent if directly asked about dying) and the fact that nondisclosure can interfere with a child's or adolescent's preparatory work before dying, in order to avoid situations in which important information is kept from the patient.

## PEDIATRIC PAIN ASSESSMENT

Similar to adults, pain in children can be nociceptive or neuropathic. Nociceptive pain includes visceral (spleen, liver, gallbladder, ascites, intestinal cramps) and somatic pain (mucous membranes, bone, muscle, skin). Neuropathic pain can be centrally or peripherally mediated. Although it was once thought that neonates do not feel pain intensely, research has shown that they do in fact feel pain and may experience pain more strongly than adults, due to their immature inhibitory pathways.[27] Nevertheless, pain is a subjective experience and ideally, the assessment of pain relies heavily on self-report.

Pediatric pain assessment differs from adult pain assessment in that it must take into consideration the developmental stage of the child. As in adults, the gold standard for pain assessment is self-report for a child who is able to report his or her pain. In addition, and also similar to adults, children with chronic pain often do not exhibit changes in vital signs, or common behavioral changes associated with pain such as withdrawing from the environment or crying. Children with chronic pain can learn to sleep or play as they have come to adapt to their chronic pain. Accurate assessment of pain is necessary to adequately treat pain, and there are many developmentally appropriate pain assessment tools available.

Young infants and newborns may show pain by crying, stiffening their bodies, withdrawing to painful stimuli, or with facial grimace (brow bulge, eyes squeezed shut, mouth open, exaggerated nasolabial furrow). Toward the latter half of their first year, infants will begin to exhibit stranger anxiety and are best assessed while in a comfortable environment such as in their caregiver's arms. When assessing babies, information must be gathered from a caregiver in addition to that obtained from the use of an objective tool. Babies have a small range of activities and states such as feeding, sleeping, and periods of alertness that can all be affected by an illness. Primary caregivers such as parents or grandparents generally know their children best, and great attention must be given to their concerns and observations, even if findings during the clinical examination are subtle. Therefore, the caregiver report is used in conjunction with an objective tool, and there are many such tools available. The CRIES scale uses a pneumonic to cue 5 pain indicators: crying, requirement of oxygen, increased blood pressure and/or heart rate, expression on face, and sleeplessness.[28] Each factor is given 0 to 2 points and then the points are summed (10 is the maximum). Scores of 6 or greater suggest the need for analgesia. The PIPP (Premature Infant Pain Profile) is appropriate for premature neonates and includes gestational age, behavioral state, heart rate, oxygen saturation, and facial expression.[29] Two additional scales include the Neonatal Infant Pain Scale[30] and the Neonatal Pain, Agitation and Sedation Scale (N-PASS). The N-PASS can also be adjusted for gestational age.[31]

Similar to older infants, toddlers (age 1–3 years) can exhibit significant stranger anxiety and are often best evaluated initially by simple observation while allowing them to be free to roam within a safe space equipped with developmentally appropriate props (toys, colorful pictures, puppets, and so forth). If the child is verbal, it is helpful to first identify what terms are used for pain in his or her household before questioning the child directly about it. Children can be asked a variety of questions to elucidate their experience of pain. For example, they can show you where it is, describe what it feels like, explain what they would or would not like you to do about it, and report how it affects other things they like to do such as play. Caregiver reports should be incorporated into the assessment as well, and an objective tool can be used to help track responses to interventions. For nonverbal children, because of either cognitive impairment or regression, caregiver reports, clinician observation, and especially objective tools can be effectively used together. The Faces, Legs, Activity, Cry and Consolability Scale (FLACC) can be used from infancy to age 7 years and does not require the child to be verbal. Each of the 5 subcategories can be given a score of 0 to 2 points and summed, therefore a score of 0 is no pain and a score of 10 is worst pain ever.[32] The Douleur Enfant Gustav-Roussy scale is used to measure chronic pain in children aged 2 to 6 years and incorporates pain items, anxiety questions, and psychomotor behaviors. There are 15 items that are scored from 0 to 4, with a score of 60 being worst pain.[33]

Preschoolers, aged 3 to 6 years, also may exhibit stranger anxiety but can be reasonable self-reporters of pain if they are verbal, have a trusting relationship with the provider, and are not afraid they will derive an unpleasant consequence of reporting their pain. Occasionally at this age children may be uncooperative with self-reporting for other reasons, and the clinician must fall back to observation, caregiver reports, and scales for nonverbal children. The FACES pain-rating scale is a self-report scale for use in children 3 years old and upward. This scale includes 6 faces that start with a happy face and progress to a crying face. Clinicians explain to the child that the first face has no pain, the second face has a little pain, the third face has a little more pain, the fourth has more pain still, the fifth face has a lot of pain, and the sixth face is the worst pain ever, but that the child need not be crying to experience the worst pain ever. Then the child is asked which face best describes how they feel. The faces are anchored with even numbers from 0 to 10 for a concomitant numerical score. The

FACES can also be used with the numbers 0 to 5.[34] Therefore, it is important to document the numerical score and the range of the scale, that is, 3 out of 5. The Oucher scale is similar to the FACES, but uses real photographs of children's faces and is available in male and female versions for various ethnic groups.[35] Hester's Poker Chips is another tool to be used with children aged 5 and up. The children are given 4 chips and told that one chip represents a small amount of pain, 2 chips mean more pain, 3 chips mean even more pain, and 4 chips mean the worst pain ever. The children are then asked to put the number of chips in the interviewer's hand that best describes their pain. Any 4 objects of uniform color and size can be used in place of chips.[36] School-age children 7 years and older can generally use a 0 to 10 numerical pain scale, visual analog scale, and verbal report scale similar to those used in adults.

Both preschool and school-age children may attribute their pain to being punished for something they did, and it is important to address this proactively to reassure them that this is not the cause of their pain.

Total pain assessment includes assessing psychological, spiritual, and social components of pain in addition to physical factors (Box 2).

## PEDIATRIC PAIN MANAGEMENT

Pain is a commonly undertreated symptom in pediatrics. One study of children dying from cancer noted that only 27% of children had their pain well controlled. After the establishment of a palliative care program, this same institution discovered that this number had improved to 53%.[37,38] However, this number is still far too low given that pain medications are readily available, and if used correctly have been shown to relieve pain in 90% of adult cancer patients.[39]

The basic principles of pain relief in children are the same as those in adults[27,40,41]:

- Follow the World Health Organization Pain Ladder approach of increasing from simple analgesics to weak opioids, to stronger opioids for increased pain intensity. For mild pain (scores 1–4 out of 10), use acetaminophen, or nonsteroidal anti-inflammatory drugs, if no contraindication. For moderate pain scores of 5 to 7, add a weak opioid such as codeine or tramadol. For severe pain scores of 8 to 10, exchange weak opioid for a strong opioid such as morphine, fentanyl, hydromorphone, or methadone.
- Use round-the-clock dosing or long-acting pain medication for moderate to severe pain with additional pain medication to be used as needed for breakthrough pain.
- Administer pain medication via an oral route if possible.
- Use adjuvant pain medication. These medications, though not primarily indicated for pain relief, can provide pain relief and include anticonvulsants, antidepressants, steroids, muscle relaxers, and so forth.
- Titrate medication upward rapidly using short-acting medication dosed at time intervals based on peak effects (20 minutes for IV route, 60 minutes for oral route) rather than duration of action until pain score is less than 5.
- Reassess pain frequently, and particularly after any dose escalation for worsening pain to ensure adequate relief.
- Anticipate and treat opioid side effects.
- Apply nonpharmacologic adjunctive interventions.
- Treat total pain including psychic, psychological, social, and spiritual aspects.

Common barriers to effective pain management in children occur at the level of the patient, the primary caregiver, the health care provider, and the health care system,

| Box 2 |
| Total pain assessment |

**Psychological**

   Anxiety

   Depression

   Fear

   Sadness

   Anger

   Denial

   Guilt

   Confusion

**Social**

   Loneliness

   Isolation

   Peer-related stress

   Lack of normalcy

   Financial stress

   Family interpersonal dynamics

   Sibling issues

   School milestones

   Social support

**Physical**

   Location

   Quality

   Radiation

   Modifiers

   Intensity

   Interference with activities including sleep, appetite, and play

**Spiritual**

   Meaning of pain and illness

   Meaning of life

   Loss of hope

   Not accepting of situation

   Fear of death

   Attributing pain or illness to being punished

   Lack of closure

and are listed in **Box 3**. Of note, there is no evidence that respiratory depression is more common in children older than 3 months than in adults, occurring at a rate of 0.09%. In addition, there is no evidence that treatment of pain in children with opioids causes addiction. Finally, tolerance to opioids can generally be managed by

---

**Box 3**
**Barriers to effective pain management in children**

Patient Factors

    Fear of stigmatization

    Fear or dislike of side effects, including euphoria

    Dislike of taste of oral medication

    Refusal to report pain, due to fear or guilt

    Nonadherence (especially among older teens and young adults)

    Decision maker most often is not the patient

Healthcare Provider Factors

    Fear of respiratory depression

    Fear of hastening death

    Fear of tolerance and inability to control pain in the future

    Lack of experience

Caregiver Factors

    Fear of stigmatization

    Fear of addiction

    Fear of hastening death

    Denial

    Fear of giving up

    Cultural and religious beliefs

Healthcare System Factors

    Lack of available experts

    Lack of access

    Lack of education provided to pediatric trainees

---

increasing opioid dosages, sometimes to very large, even 100 times average doses, and through opioid rotation. Opioids should not be withheld for fear of tolerance in a patient suffering from pain.[27,41,42]

When prescribing opioids to children, care must be taken to dose according to the child's weight and age. Infants younger than 6 months should be dosed at 30% to 50% of the dose calculated by weight alone. After 6 months of age, weight alone can be used to calculate starting doses of opioids. Adolescents heavier than 50 kg can be dosed using typical adult doses. As in adults, renal and liver function must also be considered and adjusted for according to the degree of organ dysfunction. In addition, the route of administration must be carefully considered. Many children younger than 6 years cannot swallow pills or capsules, leaving only liquid formulations or alternative routes of administration available. Liquid oral morphine is a good option for children with significant pain who cannot swallow tablets. The only long-acting oral liquid opioid available in the United States is methadone. There are extended-release morphine capsules available that technically can be opened and sprinkled into food, but if these are accidentally chewed there is a risk of lethal overdose. Taste is also a consideration when prescribing medication to children, as some will refuse if they dislike the taste. Masking aversive-tasting medication can be accomplished with chocolate or strawberry syrup. Crushable pills can be stirred into pudding or effectively mixed into crème cookie filling. On rare occasions a nasogastric tube is necessary to assist with medication delivery, particularly if the medication is vital to the child's care and it is viewed as the least noxious method of obtaining the medication from the point of view of the child. Some children, especially when ill with mucositis or nausea, refuse or cannot tolerate oral medication. In these instances, transdermal or intravenous routes need to be considered. In general, rectal, subcutaneous, and intramuscular routes of administration of pain medication are avoided in children when possible. Often, and especially if children need intravascular access for other reasons, a percutaneous intravenous catheter or central venous catheter is placed for continuous opioid administration.

Opioid side effects in children mirror those seen in adults. Common side effects include constipation, nausea, somnolence, and pruritus; rare side effects include myoclonus and respiratory depression. Effective pain management may also require the use of palliative disease–directed interventions, such as radiation for metastatic cancer. Rarely a child will require a neurosurgical procedure for placement of an implantable intrathecal pump, or a nerve block to manage refractory pain. In addition, propofol used in subanesthetic doses (0.3 mg/kg/h) has been used for refractory neuropathic cancer pain in children.[41]

### Complementary Therapies

Complementary nonpharmacologic therapies to augment symptom management, especially in the treatment of pain and anxiety, range from simple caregiver maneuvers such as cuddling and providing general social support to more technical interventions such as acupuncture.[41] Psychologists can often provide cognitive behavior techniques, such as hypnosis, guided imagery, biofeedback, and mindfulness-based stress reduction, which have demonstrated efficacy in the treatment of pain and stress.[43,44] Child life specialists can also distract the child with games, toys, and play therapy. Yoga was shown to be effective for reducing anxiety and pain in a small series (N = 20) of pediatric hematology/oncology patients.[45] Massage has been shown reduce anxiety in adult cancer patients and to decrease pain in children.[44,46] Art therapy and music therapy may improve general well-being in terminally ill patients.[46] Acupuncture has been shown to be helpful in the treatment of chemotherapy-induced nausea and vomiting, and pain, in children.[46,47] Accupressure with or without the application of tiny magnets can be offered to young children who are needle-phobic. Transcutaneous electrical nerve stimulation can be used for pain localized in the musculoskeletal system. In addition, heating pads, or sometimes cold packs, can also help to relieve pain.[41] Heated whirlpools can also provide pain relief and general relaxation. Aromatherapy may help with nausea.[48] Finally, improved sleep hygiene can also attenuate pain and anxiety symptoms.

### NONPAIN SYMPTOM ASSESSMENT AND MANAGEMENT
### Nausea and Vomiting

Nausea and vomiting are distressing symptoms resulting from a variety of causes including medication (especially chemotherapy but also opioids), functional or mechanical bowel obstruction, central nervous system pathology, disequilibrium, toxic metabolites, aversive odors or tastes, mucositis, and emotional distress. Vomiting is produced from signals in the vomit center in the medullary reticular formation in the brain on receiving afferent input from the chemoreceptor trigger zone in the fourth ventricle, vagal and sympathetic afferent inputs from the oropharynx and gastrointestinal system, midbrain pressure receptors, labyrinth apparatus, limbic system, and higher cortex.[49] The prevalence of nausea and vomiting in terminally ill children is high, approximately 50%.[38,50]

Assessment of nausea and vomiting can be done through communication with the child and the caregiver, and the use of objective tools. Similar to pain assessment, it is important to understand the terminology used by the child to describe nausea. One available assessment tool is the Pediatric Nausea Assessment Tool (PeNat).[51] The amount of vomiting, the presence of bile or blood, and the ability to tolerate any liquids or solids should be assessed. Physical examination should target central nervous system and abdominal pathology. Once the cause of the vomiting is identified, treatment can be focused on removing triggers (if possible) and alleviating symptoms.

## Constipation

Constipation is a common, uncomfortable, and potentially very painful symptom defined as the difficult passage of hard stool, or frequency of stools less than at least once per 3 days. Common causes of constipation include medication, especially opioids, but also antihistamines and vincristine, and dietary factors (too little fiber or fluid). Constipation is prolonged in up to 50% of terminally ill children, and should be anticipated when prescribing opioids and treated preventively.[38,49,50] Important history elements include number and consistency of stools, pain with defecation, presence of blood, abdominal pain, vomiting, and dietary intake. Physical examination should focus on central nervous system and abdominal pathology. An external rectal examination may be indicated if there is bleeding or if neurologic dysfunction is suspected. Digital rectal examination should be avoided in neutropenic patients. Abdominal radiographs may be indicated if bowel obstruction is suspected. For the prevention of constipation, combination therapy is generally indicated with a stimulant laxative (senna) plus either a stool softener (docusate) or osmotic agent (magnesium, lactulose, polyethylene glycol.) Adding more fiber to the diet may be helpful if liquids are also increased; otherwise they may worsen constipation.

## Dyspnea

Also referred to as breathlessness, dyspnea is a subjective feeling of shortness of breath, which occurs in 30% to 80% of pediatric palliative care patients.[37,38,52] The diseases commonly associated with dyspnea include cystic fibrosis, cancer, congenital heart disease, neuromuscular disease, and renal disease. Causes are numerous and are related to the underlying disease process. The etiology may be at the level of the lungs (infection, secretion, obstruction, bronchospasm, effusion), heart (failure, pulmonary hypertension), and neuromuscular system. Assessment should be aimed at ascertaining the degree of discomfort experienced by the patient, which can be done using a scale such as the Pediatric Dyspnea Scale for younger children[53]or a 0 to 10 scale for older children. Care should be taken to understand the effect of the dyspnea on activities such as walking and talking. Oxygenation status and respiratory rate may not correlate to perception of dyspnea. Physical examination focuses on heart, lungs, fluid status, and neurologic systems. Once the cause of dyspnea is identified, therapy can be aimed at treating the pathology (if indicated by goals of care) and providing comfort measures. Diagnostic tests may be indicated. The mainstay of symptomatic treatment for severe dyspnea is the same as for adults (ie, opioids). Benzodiazepines are indicated for anxiety. A trial of supplemental oxygen is warranted. A trial of steroids for terminal dyspnea due to cancer is also reasonable.

Nonpharmacologic measures include positioning the head of the bed upward for comfort, cool cloths, and a fan blowing toward the child's face.

## Anorexia and Cachexia

Anorexia is a marked decrease or complete absence of appetite. Cachexia is involuntary weight loss. Loss of appetite has been shown to occur in up to 80% of terminal pediatric cancer patients, and is a common in terminal pediatric patients with acquired immunodeficiency syndrome, cardiac disease, lung disease, and complex chronic conditions. Anorexia and cachexia also contribute to increased morbidity and mortality.[38,50] Cachexia is very common in terminal cancer patients and is the result of many factors, including gastrointestinal factors (anorexia, mucositis, nausea, obstruction, malabsorption), catabolic stress (infection, inflammation, cancer), neurohormonal changes, symptoms interfering with food intake such as pain and dyspnea, muscle wasting from inactivity, and psychological factors (aversions, depression). Cachexia is generally not reversible by increasing calorie intake. Assessment of diet, other treatable symptoms, gastrointestinal function, as well as prognosis and goals of care are necessary in developing a care plan. Interventions should be aimed at treating what is potentially reversible, such as pain and depression. Favorite foods and meal-replacement drinks can and should be offered to patients if desired for comfort. Nutritional interventions have not been shown to improve nutritional status, survival time, psychological status, or quality of life in adults with terminal cancer or who are receiving cancer-directed therapies.[54] However, forgoing the provision of artificial nutrition is difficult for many families and health care providers, especially in the face of uncertain remaining time of life. Despite the lack of evidence for it, a trial of artificial nutrition can be offered if desired. Ideally nutrition is given enterally, as the side-effect profile is much more favorable despite the need for a nasogastric or gastrostomy tube. Parenteral nutrition may be the only means for nutritional support if there is concomitant bowel obstruction, severe mucositis, or protracted vomiting. However, side effects include infection, thrombosis, and electrolyte abnormalities. Pharmacologic interventions include appetite stimulants such as megestrol acetate, cannabinoids, and steroids, which have been shown to increase appetite and quality of life though not necessarily weight gain. **Table 3** lists common nonpain symptoms and management. **Table 4** is a formulary for pediatric palliative care.

## PSYCHOSOCIAL ASPECTS OF CARE

Model pediatric palliative care teams are interdisciplinary and their "goal is to promote the healing of the whole child by integrating the developmental, psychosocial and spiritual needs with the medical needs of the patients and their families."[55] As the physician is necessary but not sufficient for the palliative care team, he or she works closely with the psychosocial team to provide a full range of services to the patient and his or her family.[4] Each patient is more complicated than just the symptoms and the diagnosis. He or she presents with a full history, family system, and a unique perspective on life. Each member of the interdisciplinary team is able to offer expertise in psychology, social work, child life, spiritual care, and whatever other therapies the palliative care team has to offer. Each specialty brings a point of view to the entire team that can help in creating an environment of healing and comfort. If the palliative care team is able to recognize all of the needs of the patient and family, then perhaps the patient's suffering and the family's anguish can be lessened.

**Table 3**
**Common nonpain symptoms and management**

| Symptom | First-Line Drug | Second-Line Drug | Nonpharmacologic |
|---|---|---|---|
| Nausea | 5-HT$_3$ antagonist Dexamethasone if due to CNS pressure or edematous bowel obstruction | Add antihistamine Add benzodiazepine | Small low fat meals Aromatherapy Acupressure Hypnosis |
| Constipation | Senna and docusate sodium | Add polyethylene glycol, lactulose, or magnesium agents | Increase fiber and fluids if able. Encourage ambulation/activity as able |
| Dyspnea | Morphine/oxygen | Add benzodiazepine | Increase HOB Music therapy |
| Anorexia/ cachexia | Megestrol acetate | Cannabinoids, cyproheptadine, or steroids | Offer favorite foods or liquid meal replacement. Trial of artificial nutrition |

*Abbreviations:* CNS, central nervous system; HOB, head of bed; HT, hydroxytryptamine.

## Psychological Care

The assessment and treatment of the psychological needs of a child at the end of life are complex at best. Assessment is complicated by the concomitant physical symptoms with which the child may be presenting, and by the need to determine whether the child's symptoms are a normative response or a pathologic one warranting psychiatric diagnosis. Unfortunately, the difficulty in assessing the psychological functioning of children receiving palliative care may result in the failure to notice and appropriately treat psychiatric symptoms, particularly the internalizing symptoms of depression and anxiety.

Terminally ill children present with various physical symptoms, including pain, fatigue, weight loss, sleep disturbance, agitation, and nausea and vomiting, which are difficult for the children, parents, and their treating physicians to discern as being related to depressive or anxiety symptoms or to their medical illness and any interventions they may be receiving.[38] Such physical and emotional symptoms are likely interrelated, and each symptom must be addressed accordingly. However, there is evidence that physicians underestimate the symptoms of depression and anxiety in adolescent cancer patients, as well as in other children with chronic illnesses.[56,57] The focus for physicians may therefore be on the physical symptoms of children at the end of life, and any sadness or anxiety noted may be attributed to a normative response.

Although there is a paucity of epidemiologic studies that examine the prevalence of depression and anxiety in children at the end of life,[58] there is evidence suggesting that these children experience symptoms of distress, nervousness or worry, sadness, fear of being alone, loss of perspective, difficulty talking about feelings, and loss of independence.[59,60] Likewise, children with high-risk malignant disease reported more psychiatric symptoms and decreased quality of life than children with low-risk and moderate-risk malignant disease.[61] To ensure that psychiatric symptoms are appropriately diagnosed and treated, comprehensive assessment is required. Likewise, consideration of individual risk factors is essential, as children with an already limited coping reserve may feel significantly more stressed and overburdened, thus placing them at higher risk for meeting criteria for psychiatric diagnosis. Individual risk factors include preexisting psychopathology, stressful family events, history of substance abuse, prior suicide history, interpersonal isolation or alienation, and pain management issues.[62]

Children with depressive or anxious symptoms must be evaluated to see if they meet criteria for a psychiatric diagnosis of depression or anxiety, and such symptoms must cause significant distress or impairment in social, academic, or other important areas of functioning (eg, activities of daily living). Kersun and Shemesh[58] published a comprehensive article that discusses depression and anxiety in children at the end of life. These investigators note that children receiving palliative care may present with certain types of depressive disorders, including major depressive disorder, dysthymia, and adjustment disorder with depressed mood. In terms of specific anxiety disorders, such children may present with a generalized anxiety disorder, specific phobia, anxiety disorder due to a general medical condition, posttraumatic stress disorder, or adjustment disorder with anxiety. To determine whether a child meets criteria for a psychiatric diagnosis, the use of standardized self-report measures can be used. These measures include items indicating distress, general worry, or a specific anxiety disorder, and have been used successfully in medically ill children (eg, Children's Depression Inventory; Memorial Symptom Assessment Scale; UCLA Posttraumatic Stress Disorder Reaction Index).[63–65] Worrisome information gathered from these measures can then prompt the use of clinician-rated assessment scales or semistructured or structured interviews to determine psychiatric diagnosis.

Once a diagnosis of a psychiatric disorder of depression is established in a child at the end of life, the general treatment approach is to first assess the presence or lack of suicidal ideation, conduct a psychosocial assessment to determine specific areas of treatment focus, and then provide supportive therapy or cognitive behavioral therapy (CBT).[58] Should psychotherapy seem ineffective, a psychotropic medication, specifically a selective serotonin reuptake inhibitor (SSRI), should be tried, as studies are emerging regarding the safety and efficacy of SSRIs in children with medical illnesses. For a psychiatric disorder of anxiety, various cognitive-behavioral interventions are recommended, such as systematic and prolonged exposure to anxiety-producing situations, cognitive restructuring, and increasing available coping resources through teaching specific skills such as relaxation, problem solving, and stress management.[58] The use of benzodiazepine medication has been suggested in the pediatric population, as it addresses neuropathic pain as well as agitation and anxiety. However, benzodiazepines are indicated for short-term use whereas SSRIs are suggested for long-term use. In the cases of both depression and anxiety, the use of psychotropic medications, such as SSRIs, must be done with the utmost caution and with close monitoring because of the increased risk of suicidality, the possibility of bringing about manic episodes should a family history of bipolar disorder be present, impact on liver functioning, and other possible complications.

In addition to considering the psychological functioning of children who are at the end of life, attention should also be paid to the parents and siblings of these children. According to the literature, bereaved parents may be at increased risk for anxiety, guilt, depression, posttraumatic stress, and anger,[66,67] as well as increased parental and marital strain.[68] Likewise, surviving siblings are noted to experience feelings of guilt, anxiety, sleep difficulties, posttraumatic stress symptoms, and higher internalizing and externalizing scores within 2 years of the death of their brother or sister.[69,70] Again, it is essential to assess premorbid psychological functioning and risk factors that may be present among parents and siblings, as the stress related to the experience of anticipatory grief and bereavement can overtax an already frail coping reserve.

**Table 4**
Pediatric palliative care formulary (for infants <6 months, use 30%–50% of opioid dose)

| Drug | Route | Pediatric Dose (mg/kg/dose Unless Otherwise Stated) | Adolescent (>50 kg) Dose (mg/dose) | Comments |
|---|---|---|---|---|
| Nonopioid Pain Medications | | | | |
| Acetaminophen | PO | 15 every 4–6 h | 650–1000 | Max. dose75 mg/kg/d or 4 g/d |
| Ibuprofen (NSAID) | PO | 5–10 every 6–8 h | 400–600 | Maximum dose 3.2 g/d. Inhibits platelet aggregation. |
| Naproxen sodium (NSAID) | PO | 5–7 every 8–12 h | 250–500 BID | Inhibits platelet aggregation. Not for children <2 y. Max. dose 1250 mg/d |
| Opioid Pain Medications | | | | |
| Codeine | PO | 0.5–1.0 every 4–6 h | 30 | 10% of population and newborns cannot convert to active metabolite |
| Tramadol | PO | 1–2 every 4–6 h. Max. 8 mg/kg/d | 50–100. Max. 400 mg/d | Can be compounded to liquid |
| Oxycodone | PO, SL | 0.05–0.2 every 4–6 h | 5–10 | |
| Morphine | PO, SL | 0.2–0.5 every 4–6 h | 5–10 | PCA bolus dose can be 50%–150% every 6–10 min (for children >6 y) |
| | IV/SC infusion | 0.1–0.2 every 2–4 h | 2–4 | |
| | | 0.01–0.03 mg/kg/h | 1–2 mg/h | |
| Fentanyl | IV | 0.5–2 µg/kg every 30 min | 25–75 µg | Caution: rapid IV infusion may cause chest wall rigidity |
| | Infusion | 1 µg/kg/h | 25–100 µg/h | Max. 400 µg per transmucosal dose |
| | Transmucosal | 5–15 µg/kg | | |
| Hydromorphone | PO | 0.03–0.08 every 3–4 h | 1–2 | Not for neonates or young infants |
| | IV/SC infusion | 0.015 every 4–6 h | 1–2 | |
| | | 0.003–0.005 mg/kg/h | 0.3 mg/h | |

| | Route | Dose (mg/kg) | Dose | Comments |
|---|---|---|---|---|
| **Anesthetics** | | | | |
| Lidocaine 2.5% and prilocaine 2.5% (EMLA cream) | Topical to intact skin | 0–3 mo and <5 kg: 1 g and 10 cm² BSA | | Avoid in infants <37 wk GA or <12 mo and receiving methemoglobin-inducing agents |
| For IV punctures and injections | Cover with occlusive dressing | 3–12 mo and >5 kg: 2 g and 20 cm² BSA; 1–6 y and >10 kg: 10 g and 100 cm² BSA; 7–12 y and >20 kg: 20 g and 200 cm² BSA | | Max. time application is 1 h in infants <3 mo and otherwise 4 h |
| Ketamine (low-dose anesthetic agent) | PO; S-ketamine:; Racemic ketamine: IV/SC | Off-label use; 0.25 every 6–8 h; 0.5 every 6–8 h; 0.04–0.15 mg/kg/h to max. 0.3–0.6 mg/kg/h | 10–25 mg every 6–8 h. Can titrate up to 50 mg every 6 h; 2–5 mg/h titrate up every day by 2–4 mg/h to effect | Use injectable form PO. Put in juice to mask taste; This is not commonly used but may be helpful for refractory pain or to reduce total opioid dose |
| **Benzodiazepines** For anxiety, agitation, nausea, muscle spasms, insomnia | | | | May cause respiratory depression especially if on other sedating medication |
| Lorazepam | PO/SL/PR/IV | 0.02–0.05 every 4–12 h | 0.5–4 every 4–12 h | Can cause paradoxic excitation in children <8 y |
| Diazepam | PO; IV/IM | 0.04–0.2 every 6–8 h; 0.04–0.2 every 2–4 h | | Max. dose 0.6 mg/kg within 8-h period |
| **Steroids** | | | | |
| Dexamethasone:  Anti-inflammatory dose | PO/IV/IM | 0.08–0.3 mg/kg/24 h divided every 6–12 h | 0.75–9 mg/24h | Cushinoid side effects |
| Cerebral edema dose | PO/IV | 1–2 mg/kg once, then 1–2 mg/kg/24h divided every 4–6 h | see maximum dose | maximum dose 16 mg/24 h |
| **Tricyclic antidepressants for neuropathic pain** | | | | Can prolong QT interval. Cholinergic side effects |
| Amitriptyline | PO | 0.1 QHS, can increase to 0.5–2 over 2–3 wk | 40–100 mg/d | Use lowest effective dose. Max. 200 mg/d |
| Imipramine | PO | 0.2–0.4 QHS | Max. 1–3 | Titrate up 50% every 2–3 days as needed |

(continued on next page)

**Table 4**
(*continued*)

| Drug | Route | Pediatric Dose (mg/kg/dose Unless Otherwise Stated) | Adolescent (>50 kg) Dose (mg/dose) | Comments |
|---|---|---|---|---|
| Nortriptyline Hydrochloride | PO | 6–12 y: 1–3 mg/kg/24 h divided TID-QID or 10–20 mg/24 h divided TID-QID | 1–3 mg/kg/24 h divided TID-QID or 30–50 mg/kg/24 h divided TID-QID | Do not discontinue abruptly |
| **Anticonvulsants for Neuropathic Pain** | | | | |
| Gabapentin | PO | Day 1: 5 QHS<br>Day 2: 5 BID<br>Day 3: 5 TID; then titrate to effect. Usual dosage range: 8–35 mg/kg/24 h | Day 1: 300 mg QHS<br>Day 2: 300 mg BID<br>Day 3: 300 mg TID; then titrate to effect | Usual dosage range: 1800–2400 mg/24 h<br>Max. dose: 3600 mg/24 h |
| Pregabalin | PO | 75 mg/24 h titrate up by 75 mg/24 h | | Age >10 y. Max. 150–300 mg/24 h |
| **Bisphosphonates** | | | | |
| Alendronate | PO | 0.5–1 every week | 35–70 mg every week | Age >5 y |
| Pamidronate | IV | 1–2 every week | 60–90 mg every week | Age >5 y |
| **Medications for Constipation** | | | | |
| Senna | PO | 1 mo–1 y: 55–109 QHS<br>1–5 y: 109–218 mg QHS | 5–15 y: 218–436 mg QHS | Stimulant laxative.<br>Use prophylactically with patients receiving strong opioids |
| Sennoside | | 1 mo–2 y: 2.2–4.4 mg QHS<br>2–5 y: 4.4–6.6 mg QHS<br>6–12 y: 8.8–13.2 mg QHS | >12 y: 17.6–26.4 mg | Stimulant laxative.<br>Use prophylactically with patients receiving strong opioids |
| Bisacodyl | PO | 3–12 y: 0.3 mg/kg × 1 at bedtime<br><2 y: 5 mg | >12: 5–15 mg. Max. 30 mg/24 h<br>>11 y:10 mg × 1 | Stimulant laxative.<br>Tablets must be swallowed whole and not given within 1 h of antacids or milk |
| | Rectal suppository<br>Rectal enema | 2–11 y: 5–10 mg × 1 | 30 mL × 1 | |

| Drug | Route | Dose | | Notes |
|---|---|---|---|---|
| Docusate sodium | PO | <3 y: 10–40 mg/24 h divided QD-QID; 3–6 y: 20–60 mg/24 h divided QD-QID; 6–12 y: 40–150 mg/24 h divided QD-QID | >12 y: 50–400 mg/24 h divided QD-QID | Stool softener |
| Polyethylene glycol | PO | <20 kg: 0.42 g/kg BID | 17 g mixed in 240 mL QD | Osmotic agent |
| Lactulose | PO | <2 y: 2.5 mL BID; 2–10 y: 2.5–7.5 nL BID; >10 y: 15–30 mL BID | | Osmotic agent |
| Magnesium hydroxide | PO | <2 y: 40 mg divided every 5–24 h; 2–5 y: 400–800 mg divided every 6–12 h; 6–11 y: 800–1200 mg divided every 6–12 h | 1200–2400 mg divided every 6–24 h | Osmotic agent. Not for daily use |
| **Medications for Nausea** | | | | |
| Ondansetron | PO dose based on body surface area / IV | <0.3 m²:1 mg TID; 0.3–0.6 m²: 2 mg TID; 0.6–1 m²: 3 mg TID; >1 m²: 4–8 mg TID; 4–11 y:4 mg TID; 0.15–0.45 every 4 h | >11 y: 8 mg TID Max. dose 32 mg | 5-HT$_3$ antagonist |
| Granisetron | IV/PO | ≥2y: 10–40 mcg per kg/24 h civided every 12–24 h | 1 mg every 12 h | 5-HT$_3$ antagonist. IV max. dose: 3 mg/dose or 9 mg/24 h |
| Prochlorperazine | PO/PR | 0.1–0.5/kg/24 h divided every 6–12 hours >2 y: and >10kg | Immediate release: 5–10 mg/dose TID-QID; Extended release: 10 mg/dose BID or 15 mg/dose QD 25 mg/dose every 12 h | Phenothiazine antiemetic. Do not use IV route in children EPS; give with diphenhydramine |
| | PR | 0.2–0.5 every 8–12 h | | |
| Metoclopramide | IV/IM/PO | 0.1–2 every 2–6 h every 2–6 h | Max 10 mg/dose | Prokinetic agent. Give with diphenhydramine to reduce EPS |

(continued on next page)

**Table 4**
*(continued)*

| Drug | Route | Pediatric Dose (mg/kg/dose Unless Otherwise Stated) | Adolescent (>50 kg) Dose (mg/dose) | Comments |
|------|-------|------------------------------------------------------|-------------------------------------|----------|
| Haloperidol (also treats delirium) | PO/IV/SC | Initial dose 0.025–0.05 per day divided every 8–12 h. Can titrate up over 1 week to 0.15 mg/kg/d | >12 y: 0.5–5 every 4–12 h Max. dose 15 mg/d | Antipsychotic. Lowers the seizure threshold. Not for children <3 y. Can prolong QT interval |
| Chlorpromazine (also treats hiccups) | IV/IM | ≥6 mo: 0.55 every 6–8 h Maximum dose: < 5 y: 40 mg/24 h 5–12 y: 75 mg/24 h | 25–50 mg/dose every 4–6 h | Phenothiazine antipsychotic and antiemetic. Lowers seizure threshold. Risk of EPS. Additive sedative effects with opioids |
| | PO | 0.55 every 4–6 h | 10–25 mg/dose every 4–6 h | |
| Scopolamine (also can decrease oral secretions) | SC/IM/IV | 6 µg/kg every 6–8 h | Max. 300 µg/dose | Anticholinergic side effects. Risk of drug withdrawal after >3 days of use |
| | Transdermal | NA | >12 y: 1.5 mg patch delivers 1 mg every 3 days | |
| Nabilone (also may increase appetite and decrease pain) | PO | <18 kg: 0.5 mg BID 18–36 kg: 1 mg BID >36 kg: 1 mg TID | 1–2 mg every 8–12 h | Synthetic cannabinoid. Has been used in children as young as 10 mo |
| Olanzapine | | Prepubescent: 2.5 mg every day | 5 mg every day Titrate over every 3–4 days to maximum of 20 mg/d | Atypical antipsychotic |
| Droperidol | IV | 0.01–0.07 every 4–6 h | Initial max dose 2.5 mg | Risk of EPS, QT interval prolongation |
| **Antihistamines for Pruritus and Nausea** | | | | |
| Diphenhydramine | PO/IM/IV | 1.25 every 6 h Max. dose 300 mg/24 h | 25–50 mg/dose every 4–8 h Max. dose 400 mg/24 h | Use with caution in infants and young children, and do not use in neonates due to potential CNS effects |

| | | | | |
|---|---|---|---|---|
| Hydroxaz ne | PO | 0.5 every 6–8 h, or alternative dosing by age: <6 y: 50 mg/24 h divided every 6–8 h ≥6 y: 50–100 mg/24 h divided every 6–8 h | 25 mg/dose TID/QID. Max. dose 600 mg/24 h | IV administration is not recommended unless given through central venous catheter |
| **Medication for Somnolence** | | | | |
| Methylphenidate | PO | >6 y: 2.5–5 mg at breakfast and lunchtime | | May increase weekly by 5 mg up to 15 mg/24 h |
| Dextroamphetamine | PO | 6–12 y: 5 mg/24 h divided QD-TID; increase by 5 mg/24 h at weekly intervals to max. dose of 60 mg/24 h | >12 y: 10 mg/24 h divided QD-TID; increase by 10 mg/24 h at weekly intervals to a max. dose of 60 mg/24 h | Do not give with MAO inhibitors or general anesthetics. Not recommended for children <3 y |
| **Medication for Anorexia and Cachexia** | | | | |
| Megestrol acetate | PO | 7.5–10 mg/kg/d divided every 6–24 h | 400–800 mg divided every 6–24 h | Titrate to response. Weight gain may be seen in 2–4 wk |
| Cyproheptadine | PO | 4–8 y:2 mg every 8 h | >13 y: start at 2 mg every 6 h and increase over 3 weeks up to 8 mg every 6 h | |
| Dexamethasone for appetite stimulation | PO | <10 kg: 0.15 every 12 h 10–20 kg: 2 mg every 12 h 21–40 kg: 4 mg every 12 h | >41 kg: 8 mg every 12 h | Not suggested for long-term use |
| Melatonin | PO | 0.5–10 mg QHS | | Consider combining with 5 mL fish oil |

*Abbreviations:* BID, twice a day; BSA, body surface area; CNS, central nervous system; EPS, extrapyramidal side effects; GA, gestational age; IM, intramuscular; IV, intravenous; MAO, monoamine oxidase; NA, not available; NSAID, nonsteroidal anti-inflammatory drug; PCA, patient-controlled analgesia; PO, by mouth; PR, per rectum; QD, every day; QHS, every bedtime; QID, 4 times a day; SC, subcutaneous; SL, sublingual; TID, 3 times a day.

Data from Refs. [41,42,49,50,52,78]

Therefore, psychosocial assessment of the family as a whole is imperative when treating children within the pediatric palliative population, so that appropriate support, interventions, and resources can be offered in a timely manner to maximize the possibility of a healthy psychological adjustment to an otherwise difficult situation.

### Spirituality

Spirituality is a term used to describe everything from religious affiliation to the process by which an individual ascribes meaning to his or her life. Spirituality does not just apply to how one practices a specific religious tradition but rather encompasses the full range of experiences that bring meaning into one's life. For some it may be expressed through the practice of yoga and meditation, for others it may mean going to church every Sunday, while for some spirituality is felt through interpersonal relationships or relationship to nature. Both children and adults have spiritual lives, or ways of understanding how the world works and their place in it.[4,71] When that place is threatened by illness and loss, one's spiritual resources can provide comfort and solace. A parent may say that he or she believes that God will provide a miracle. How this is interpreted by the team can create either an opportunity for healing or a place of divisiveness. The miracle may be reframed; if cure is not possible then perhaps the miracle is the attention paid to the patient's pain and suffering. If, however, the team responds by assuming the family is not coping well, the dynamic in the relationship may change for the worse. Spirituality in palliative care recognizes that children and their families should have a place to express themselves without fear of judgment or retribution from the medical team. A professional spiritual care provider, like a chaplain, can help to bridge the spiritual world and the medical world.

The hopes of the family of the dying or seriously ill family member can often be a complicated jumble of feelings. What can a family hope for when facing their worst nightmare: cure, pain relief, end of the suffering? Often caregivers will hear both the patient and the family question the ultimate reason for their child's illness. Is this a punishment from God? What sin could my baby have committed? From the children one may hear questions about heaven and life after death. Will God take care of me in heaven? Will my parents be okay without me? How the family and the child begin to answer these questions may affect their ability to heal both emotionally and spiritually. For medical caregivers it may be difficult to hear patients and families express religious and spiritual beliefs that are vastly different from their own. Witnessing a child suffer can also cause doubt and frustration on the part of the caregiver's belief system.[71]

In the world of professional chaplaincy the term "ministry of presence" is often used to describe the interventions chaplains and other spiritual care professionals provide to patients and families. To be present implies a gentle approach to the sufferer, to sit and listen without judgment, to affirm belief, and to witness the patient's experience. One need not feel so alone if another is able to sit with you. By listening and being present, the chaplain can identify areas of existential suffering and perhaps help to alleviate some of the anguish simply by naming the spiritual pain. With the help of a chaplain, children can try and make sense of their place in the world and appreciate the meaning that their life has. After a child has died, the chaplain can help the family during the bereavement process as they struggle to come to terms with the death and to make sense of a world in which children die.[71]

### Social

The social worker is an integral part of the interdisciplinary team. The role of the social worker is to focus on the social and psychological health of the patient and family. The initial consultation by the palliative care team should always include an assessment by a social worker. As the family copes with a new diagnosis, they will not necessarily be in a position to identify what they will need medically, financially, or socially. The social worker can work with the family to identify current and future needs, and can help find resources to meet those needs. The social worker will be an ongoing source of support for the patient and family as they cope with the illness and as their needs change during the course of illness. As a nonmedical member of the team, the social worker can help to facilitate communication between the family and the medical staff, and can be a safe person to whom families can express feeling without fear of reprisal from the medical team. Social workers can also help facilitate going to school, transitioning to home or hospice, and can assess the family functioning including sibling adjustment to the child's illness.[72]

## CARE ACROSS SETTINGS

Continuity of care is extremely important in pediatric palliative care. Even if only one member of the health care team can provide care until the child's death regardless of place of care, it may make a positive difference if there is a good relationship between the provider and the child and their family. The loss of a child is often viewed as an extreme tragedy, and possibly the most difficult time the loved ones may ever face in their lives. The continued support of someone who has known the child since the early stages of disease and has remained with the family until the child's death has great potential value. Many families become isolated as they progress through the child's dying process because it becomes too painful or awkward for friends and family to remain engaged. The loss of health care providers at this crucial time further isolates the family.[73]

Traditionally most children die in a hospital setting surrounding by caregivers they have known. This setting may be ideal for some situations and families. Hospitals may be able to provide structured support for the family and to allow a family to have respite from constant caring for the child. In addition, some families are not equipped with the necessary resources to care for their dying child at home, for example because of lack of insurance, space, telephone, and/or social support. However, the hospital setting does have drawbacks. Care is often escalated inappropriately and reflexively in a hospital. For example, in one large study of terminal pediatric cancer patients, 22% died in the pediatric intensive care unit.[37] In addition, multiple family members may not be able to stay the night or be given comfortable sleeping quarters. Vital signs taken every 4 hours prevent comfortable rest for dying patients. Unfortunately, there continues to be a paucity of appropriately trained professionals who can provide palliative and hospice care to children in the home or institutional setting. Flexibility in creating a family-centered care plan for the end of life that meets the expressed goals and wishes of the family and child is paramount.

Hospice care is a comprehensive interdisciplinary type of care developed for terminally ill adult patients. A hospice team generally includes a doctor, a nurse, a social worker, and a spiritual care provider. Often, if a family or child prefers for the child to die at home and a pediatric hospice program is not available, an adult hospice company may be able to offer support. That is, they may be able to provide a nurse's aide, an on-call nurse, intravenous opioids, compounding pharmacies for topical medication delivery, social workers, bereavement support, and spiritual care. However, they often do not have personnel trained in pediatrics, and a pediatric nurse or physician is needed to augment the services with regular home visits.[73]

The home visit is an essential part of allowing a child to die at home. The provider can assess the child's symptoms, surroundings, family members' functioning, and generally the details of the day-to-day routine. The home visitor can assess where and how help may be needed and provided, and can provide anticipatory guidance for the end stages of disease. This visit can also provide a sense of security to the family, reassuring them that they are not being abandoned by their health care team, and it can engender a feeling of trust between provider and patient/family. The decision to allow a child to die at home is a complex one and is largely arrived at through sensitive discussions with the child, the family, and the health care team. Advantages to dying at home include less disruption to family life, better sibling adjustment, the comfort of home for the dying child, increased control by the family, and greater satisfaction with care.[74]

## CARE AT THE END OF LIFE

When it becomes clear that cure is no longer possible, families will want to know what to expect in this last stage of the child's life. Some of the questions they will have include how much time the child has left, what will happen as the active dying process begins, and how the child will die. Unfortunately, the ability to predict with certainty how long any patient has left is poor, with physicians both underestimating and over-estimating the time left.[4] Physicians can inform families what to expect as the child gets sicker and closer to death, and what to expect in the final days and hours. In addition, the team should make sure that the family knows they will not be abandoned by the medical team at any time.

As death becomes imminent, goals may shift toward keeping the child as comfortable as possible. To avoid discomfort, the team must evaluate all of the child's treatments and medications, and revisit the purpose and need for them. Medications that are not contributing to quality of life can be discontinued, with the agreement of the family and child. Similarly, any unnecessary testing or procedures should be stopped. The family will decide whether they want the child to remain at home until death, go to an inpatient hospice, or be admitted to the hospital. Any of those choices is acceptable.[75]

As the child approaches the final weeks of life, parents may notice that he or she is more tired and wants to sleep more or that he or she may not want to get out of bed much. Children may be less interested in things around them and have difficulty concentrating, and may not want as many visitors. The overall rhythm of their daily lives will change with their ability to be up and about. Families can help children by encouraging them to do what they can while respecting the limitations they are developing.[38,59,60] It is important to address the psychological and spiritual symptoms that will arise at this time, as discussed earlier in this article.

Symptom management is obviously of utmost importance. Pain may escalate during this time and pain control needs to be reevaluated frequently. The physician should confer with the child, if possible, and the family to determine their goals for pain control, including whether the child wants pain controlled even at the cost of being sleepy much of the time. Common symptoms at the end of life include pain, anorexia, and dyspnea, and these are reviewed earlier in this article and elsewhere.[38,59,60]

In the final hours of life there are many physical changes that will occur. The skin may become mottled and cool as cardiac output diminishes. Besides, there will be a decrease in urine output and a decrease in level of consciousness. Children may become disoriented and may hallucinate. Parents should be prepared for these changes so that they are not surprised and frightened by them. As the child loses consciousness he or she may not be able to clear secretions well, and may develop the so-called death rattle as secretions pool in the hypopharynx. This process can be very distressing to listen to, even if parents are forewarned, and can be treated with suctioning and/or a scopolamine patch. Parents can continue to help care for their child by repositioning them frequently, performing mouth care, and talking to the child. Even if they are unable to respond, children may hear and feel parents touching them. Children may have involuntary movement and Cheyne-Stokes respirations that can make it look like they are suffering. Families should be reassured that these are a normal part of the dying process and do not indicate that the child is suffering.

When a child is actively dying in the hospital, it is not uncommon for team members to back away from the patient. Whether it is from personal discomfort with death, or not knowing what to say, this may lead to families feeling abandoned. Each member of the team should make an effort to stop by daily to let the family know they are present for them. Often, just listening is enough. Families will remember these acts of kindness.[25,76]

If the child is dying in the hospital, the interdisciplinary team can help prepare the family, including siblings, for what will happen, and can help facilitate the creation of a memory box. This box can include pictures of the child, hand or foot prints, a lock of hair, and anything else the family wants. Most families will want to be with their child after death for a period of time. Many of the tubes and other equipment can be removed, and the family can help bathe the child and dress him or her if they wish. The family can then hold the child or be alone with the child for as long as they wish or need to. Other family members can also come and say goodbye.

The family may have cultural or religious rituals that are important to them. The medical team can ask about this before death so that they can be ready to help families at the time of death. If possible and desired by the family, clergy should be present. Religious rituals should be honored if at all possible.

Even when a family has been anticipating the death of a child for a long time, when the end comes it will be a shock for them. No one can predict how they will react in such a circumstance, and parents respond in all different ways. Some will be loud in their grief; others may appear to be in shock. Whatever form the grief takes, the medical team should be available to support the family through this initial phase of the bereavement process.

## BEREAVEMENT AND GRIEF

Grief refers to the emotional response to loss and mourning, and is the outward expression of that loss. Bereavement includes both grief and mourning and is strongly influenced by culture.[77] The grief process begins before death and is neither orderly nor predictable.[77] Patients grieve the loss of function and the loss of a future. Parents, families, and health care staff can suffer from anticipatory grief while the child is still present. There exist many models and theories on the grieving process, its stages and phases, and how to accomplish the "work" of grieving. Here the authors seek to highlight some special considerations and research pertaining to bereavement that occurs after the death of a child.

The death of a child has a profound impact on the entire family. The parent-child relationship is unique, and a child's death evokes feelings of inadequacy and failure in addition to the typical emotional responses of anger, anxiety, sadness, loneliness, and fear. Grandparents suffer their own loss, and grieve for the loss that their child is suffering as well. Siblings experience a loss of their sibling, a loss of the family unit, and a loss of the caregivers to the grief process.

A bereavement assessment should be included in any inpatient or outpatient intake for a patient nearing the end of life. The assessment should include family composition, past losses, understanding of and attitude toward child's illness and prognosis, cultural practices and beliefs surrounding illness and death, anticipatory grief, and spiritual and other support available. Grief interventions around the time of and following a death include being a presence for the family, identifying and facilitating support systems, involving bereavement specialists, normalizing and individualizing the grief process, providing information, addressing fears, and validating feelings for families and patients.

Assisting families with planning religious or spiritual services and creating a memory box with the family are very concrete tasks that can help families dealing with grief. Providing families with the option to hold and comfort a dying child in the last moments of life[2] and after death can be comforting and can facilitate the grieving process. Often families would prefer to have intravenous lines, endotracheal tubes, and other medical devices removed before or after the child's death; some families are reticent about these requests and appreciate health care providers offering these opportunities.

Families of deceased children have indicated that continued contact with staff after the child's death was meaningful to them; follow-up may be by telephone, mail, and/or in person.[19] Parents also note that certain experiences with the health care staff perceived as painful by the parents can interfere with their long-term grieving process.[19] Specifically, insensitive delivery of bad news, feeling dismissed or patronized, perceived disregard for parents' judgment regarding care of their child, and poor communication of important information were found to disturb family members and complicate grief years later.[19]

## RESOURCES
### For Family

#### Candlelighters for Children with Cancer
Oregon and southwest Washington
   http://www.4kidswithcancer.org/
The mission of Candlelighters for Children with Cancer is to be established as a leader in providing support, education, advocacy, and hope to all children and their families affected by childhood cancer in Oregon and SW Washington.

#### ASK
Central Virginia
   http://askweb.org/
Since its founding, the ASK mission has remained the same: Making Life Better for Children with Cancer. ASK is a 501(c)(3) nonprofit organization that provides financial, spiritual, social, and emotional support directly to more than 1000 children and their families annually.

#### The Compassionate Friends
http://www.compassionatefriends.org/home.aspx
The mission of The Compassionate Friends is to assist families toward the positive resolution of grief following the death of a child of any age, and to provide information to help others be supportive. Today more than 600 chapters serving all 50 states plus Washington DC and Puerto Rico offer friendship, understanding, and hope to bereaved parents, siblings, grandparents, and other family members during the natural grieving process after a child has died. Around the world more than 30 countries have a Compassionate Friends presence, encircling the globe with support so desperately needed when the worst has happened.

*For Health Care Professionals*

*The Initiative for Pediatric Palliative Care, Newton, MA*
http://www.ippcweb.org/index.asp
   The Initiative for Pediatric Palliative Care (IPPC) was launched in 1998 as a research, quality improvement, and education effort aimed at enhancing family-centered care for children living with life-threatening conditions. IPPC's comprehensive, interdisciplinary curriculum, available at www.ippcweb.org, addresses knowledge, attitudes, and skills that health care professionals need to better serve children and families.

*Harvard Medical School Center for Palliative Care; Program in Palliative Care Education and Practice, Boston, MA*
http://www.hms.harvard.edu/pallcare/index.htm
   The Harvard Medical School Center for Palliative Care (HMS CPC) aims to ease suffering and enhance the quality of care for patients and their families dealing with life-threatening illness, through fostering leadership and supporting outstanding educational programs in palliative care. By educating future generations of physicians, nurses, and other health care professionals, the Center serves as a national and international resource for the best practices in palliative care education.
   The Program in Palliative Care Education and Practice—Pediatric Track is designed for physician and nurse educators who wish to enhance their skills in clinical practice, teaching, and program development in palliative care, and who have or seek to develop a leadership role at their institution.

*Children's Hospice and Palliative Care Coalition, Watsonville, CA*
http://www.childrenshospice.org/
   The Children's Hospice and Palliative Care Coalition provides training and support to hospice teams across the state so that when they are caring for a dying child they are able to meet the medical, emotional, and spiritual needs of the child and the family. The CHPCC also works with children's hospitals, home health agencies, hospices, community-based organizations, and the State of California to promote policies and all-inclusive care programs that meet the complex medical, emotional, social, and practical needs of families who are experiencing great loss.

*Children's Hospice International, Alexandria, VA*
http://www.chionline.org/resources/
   CHI's mission is creating public awareness of the needs of children with life-threatening conditions, the issues facing their families, and what children's hospice care can do to meet those needs. CHI seeks to include hospice perspectives in all areas of pediatric care and education, and to include children in existing and developing hospice, palliative, and home care programs. CHI offers education, training, and technical assistance to the health care professionals caring for this special patient population. CHI'S Worldwide Database of Programs Caring for Children with Life-Threatening Conditions and the Families is available at http://www.chionline.org/resources/locate.php

*WHO Pain and Palliative Care Communications Program Resources to Develop and Enhance Pediatric Palliative Care Services*
http://whocancerpain.wisc.edu/?q=node/120

*End-of-Life Nursing Education Consortium, Washington, DC*
http://www.aacn.nche.edu/ELNEC/index.htm

The End-of-Life Nursing Education Consortium (ELNEC) project is a national education initiative to improve palliative care. The project provides undergraduate and graduate nursing faculty, continuing education providers, staff development educators, specialty nurses in pediatrics, oncology, critical care, and geriatrics, and other nurses with training in palliative care so that they can teach this essential information to nursing students and practicing nurses.

### The Children's Project on Palliative/Hospice Services (ChiPPS)
http://www.nhpco.org/i4a/pages/index.cfm?pageid=3409&openpage=3409

ChiPPS is working to concretely enhance the science and practice of pediatric hospice and palliative care, and to increase the availability of state of the art services to families. Several leaders in the field of pediatric palliative care worked collaboratively with the National Hospice and Palliative Care Organization to develop the ChiPPS. The project seeks to make the best-known practices in the field of pediatric palliative care more widely available to care providers.

### REFERENCES

1. Field M, Behrman R, editors. When children die: improving palliative care and end of life care for children and their families. Washington, DC: National Academy Press; 2002.
2. Bartel DA, et al. Working with families of suddenly and critically ill children: physician experiences. Arch Pediatr Adolesc Med 2000;154(11):1127–33.
3. McGrath PA. Development of the World Health Organization Guidelines on cancer pain relief and palliative care in children. J Pain Symptom Manage 1996;12(2):87–92.
4. Himelstein B, et al. Pediatric palliative care. N Engl J Med 2004;350(17):1752–62.
5. Browning DM, Solomon MZ. The Initiative For Pediatric Palliative Care: an interdisciplinary educational approach for healthcare professionals. J Pediatr Nurs 2005;20(5):326–34.
6. Heron M, et al. Annual summary of vital statistics: 2007. Pediatrics 2010;125(1): 4–15.
7. Newacheck PW, Halfon N. Prevalence and impact of disabling chronic conditions in childhood. Am J Public Health 1998;88(4):610–7.
8. Feudtner C, Christakis DA, Connell FA. Pediatric deaths attributable to complex chronic conditions: a population-based Study of Washington State, 1980–1997. Pediatrics 2000;106(1):205–9.
9. ChIPPS Administrative Policy Workgroup of the NHPCO. A call for change: recommendations to improve the care of children living with life-threatening conditions. Alexandria (VA): National Hospice and Palliative Care Organization; 2001. p. 1–37.
10. Atherton JS. Learning and teaching: Piaget's developmental theory. 2010 [cited 2010 July 1, 2010]. Available at: www.learningandteaching.info/learning/piaget. htm.
11. Hinds PS, Drew D, Oakes LL, et al. End-of-life care preferences of pediatric patients with cancer. J Clin Oncol 2005;23(36):9146–54.
12. American Academy of Pediatrics. Committee on Bioethics and Committee on Hospital Care. Palliative care for children. Pediatrics 2000;106(2):351–7.
13. Hays RM, Haynes G, Geyer JR. Communication at the end of life. In: Carter BS, Levetown M, editors. Palliative care for infants, children, and adolescents. Baltimore (MD): The Johns Hopkins University Press; 2004.

14. Levetown M, Committee on Bioethics. Communicating with children and families: from everyday interactions to skill in conveying distressing information. Pediatrics 2008;121(5):e1441–60.
15. Hsiao J, Evan E, Zeltzer L. Parent and child perspectives on physician communication in pediatric palliative care. Palliat Support Care 2007;5(4):355–65.
16. Freyer DR. Care of the dying adolescent: special considerations. Pediatrics 2004; 113(2):381–8.
17. Davies B, Sehring SA, Partridge JC, et al. Barriers to palliative care for children: perceptions of pediatric health care providers. Pediatrics 2008;121(2):282–8.
18. Browning D. To show our humanness—relational and communicative competence in pediatric palliative care. Bioethics Forum 2002;18(3/4):23–8.
19. Contro N, Larson J, Scofield S, et al. Family perspectives on the quality of pediatric palliative care. Arch Pediatr Adolesc Med 2002;156(1):14–9.
20. Kreicbergs U, Valdimarsdóttir U, Onelöv E, et al. Talking about death with children who have severe malignant disease. N Engl J Med 2004;351(12):1175–86.
21. Beale EA, Baile WF, Aaron J. Silence is not golden: communicating with children dying from cancer. J Clin Oncol 2005;23(15):3629–31.
22. Hinds P, Oakes LL, Hicks J, et al. "Trying to be a good parent" as defined by interviews with parents who made phase I, terminal care, and resuscitation decisions for their children. J Clin Oncol 2009;27(35):5979–85.
23. Radwany S, Albanese T, Clough L, et al. End-of-life decision making and emotional burden: placing family meetings in context. Am J Hosp Palliat Care 2009;26(5):376–83.
24. Machare Delgado E, Callahan A, Paganelli G, et al. Multidisciplinary family meetings in the ICU facilitate end-of-life decision making. Am J Hosp Palliat Care 2009;26(4):295–302.
25. Kars M, Grypdonck MH, Beishuizen A, et al. Factors influencing parental readiness to let their child with cancer die. Pediatr Blood Canc 2010;54(7):1000–8.
26. Five wishes: from aging with dignity. 2010. Available at: http://www.agingwithdignity.org/five-wishes.php.
27. Carter B, Levetown M, editors. Palliative care for infants, children and adolescents. Baltimore (MD): The Johns Hopkins University Press; 2004. p. 166.
28. Krechel S, Bildner J. CRIES: a new neonatal postoperative pain measurement score. Initial testing of validity and reliability. Paediatr Anaesth 1995;5:53 61.
29. Ballantyne M, Stevens B, McAllister M, et al. Validation of the premature infant pain profile in the clinical setting. Clin J Pain 1999;15(4):297–303.
30. Lawrence J, Alcock D, McGrath P, et al. The development of a tool to assess neonatal pain. Neonatal Netw 1993;12(6):59–66.
31. Hummel P, et al. Neonatal pain, agitation & sedation scale. 2001.
32. Manworren RC, Hynan LS. Clinical validation of FLACC: preverbal patient pain scale. Pediatr Nurs 2003;29(2):140–6.
33. Gauvain-Piquard A, Rodary C, Rezvani A, et al. The development of the DEGR(R): a scale to assess pain in young children with cancer. Eur J Pain 1999;3(2):165–76.
34. Bieri D, Reeve RA, Champion GD, et al. The faces pain scale for the self-assessment of the severity of pain experienced by children: development, initial validation, and preliminary investigation for ratio scale proportion. Pain 1000; 41(2):139–50.
35. Beyer J. The Oucher: a user's manual and technical report. Evanston (IL): Judson Press; 1984. p. 1–12.
36. Hester NO. Pain in children. Annu Rev Nurs Res 1993;11:105–42.

37. Wolfe J, Hammel JF, Edwards KE, et al. Easing of suffering in children with cancer at the end of life: is care changing? J Clin Oncol 2008;26(10):1717–23.
38. Wolfe J, Grier HE, Klar N, et al. Symptoms and suffering at the end of life in children with cancer. N Engl J Med 2000;342(5):326–33.
39. Zech DF, Grond S, Lynch J, et al. Validation of World Health Organization Guidelines for cancer pain relief: a 10-year prospective study. Pain 1995;63(1):65–76.
40. Clary PL, Lawson P. Pharmacologic pearls for end-of-life care. Am Fam Physician 2009;79(12):1059–65.
41. Friedrichsdorf SJ, Kang TI. The management of pain in children with life-limiting illnesses. Pediatr Clin North Am 2007;54(5):645–72, x.
42. UNIPAC, ed. J.C. Porter Story, S. Levine, and J. Shega. In: Hutton N, Levetown M, Frager G, editors. The hospice and palliative medicine approach to caring for pediatric patients, vol. 8. 3rd edition. Glenveiw (IL): American Academy of Hospice and Palliative Medicine; 2008.
43. Sahler OJ, Frager G, Levetown M, et al. Medical education about end-of-life care in the pediatric setting: principles, challenges, and opportunities. Pediatrics 2000;105(3 Pt 1):575–84.
44. Cassileth BR. Complementary and alternative cancer medicine. J Clin Oncol 1999;17(Suppl 11):44–52.
45. Moody K, Daswani D, Abrahams B, et al. Yoga for pain and anxiety on pediatric hematology-oncology patients: case series and reveiw of the literature. J Soc Integr Oncol 2010;8(3):95–105.
46. Tsao JC, Zeltzer LK. Complementary and alternative medicine approaches for pediatric pain: a review of the state-of-the-science. Evid Based Complement Alternat Med 2005;2(2):149–59.
47. Gottschling S, Reindl TK, Meyer S, et al. Acupuncture to alleviate chemotherapy-induced nausea and vomiting in pediatric oncology—a randomized multicenter crossover pilot trial. Klin Padiatr 2008;220(6):365–70.
48. Ladas EJ, Post-White J, Hawks R, et al. Evidence for symptom management in the child with cancer. J Pediatr Hematol Oncol 2006;28(9):601–15.
49. Waller A, Caroline N, editors. Handbook of palliative care in cancer. Butterworth-Heinemann; 1996.
50. Santucci G, Mack JW. Common gastrointestinal symptoms in pediatric palliative care: nausea, vomiting, constipation, anorexia, cachexia. Pediatr Clin North Am 2007;54(5):673–89, x.
51. Dupuis LL, Taddio A, Kerr EN, et al. Development and validation of the pediatric nausea assessment tool for use in children receiving antineoplastic agents. Pharmacotherapy 2006;26(9):1221–31.
52. Stenekes SJ, Hughes A, Grégoire MC, et al. Frequency and self-management of pain, dyspnea, and cough in cystic fibrosis. J Pain Symptom Manage 2009;38(6):837–48.
53. Khan FI, Reddy RC, Baptist AP. Pediatric dyspnea scale for use in hospitalized patients with asthma. J Allergy Clin Immunol 2009;123(3):660–4.
54. Strasser F, Bruera ED. Update on anorexia and cachexia. Hematol Oncol Clin North Am 2002;16(3):589–617.
55. Desai P, Ng J, Bryant S. Care of children and families in the CICU: a focus on their developmental, psychosocial, and spiritual needs. Crit Care Nurs Q 2002;25(3):88–97.
56. Hedström M, Kreuger A, Ljungman G, et al. Accuracy of assessment of distress, anxiety, and depression by physicians and nurses in adolescents recently diagnosed with cancer. Pediatr Blood Canc 2006;46(7):773–9.

57. Shemesh E, Annunziato RA, Shneider BL, et al. Parents and clinicians underestimate distress and depression in children who had a transplant. Pediatr Transplant 2005;9(5):673–9.

58. Kersun L, Shemesh E. Depression and anxiety in children at the end of life. Pediatr Clin North Am 2007;54(5):691–708, xi.

59. Drake R, Frost J, Collins J. The symptoms of dying children. J Pain Symptom Manage 2003;26(1):594–603.

60. Theunissen J, Hoogerbrugge PM, van Achterberg T, et al. Symptoms in the palliative phase of children with cancer. Pediatr Blood Canc 2007;49(2):160–5.

61. Magal-Vardi O, Laor N, Toren A, et al. Psychiatric morbidity and quality of life in children with malignancies and their parents. J Nerv Ment Dis 2004;192(12):872–5.

62. Kunin H, Patenaude A, Griere H. Suicide risk in pediatric cancer patients: an exploratory study. Psycho Oncol 1995;4:1–7.

63. Kovacs M. Children's depression inventory (CDI). New York: Multi-Health Systems, Inc; 1992.

64. Collins J, Devine TD, Dick GS, et al. The measurement of symptoms in young children with cancer: the validation of the Memorial Symptom Assessment Scale in children aged 7–12. J Pain Symptom Manage 2002;23(1):10–6.

65. Rodriguez N, Steinberg A, Pynoos R. UCLA post traumatic stress disorder reaction index for DSM-IV, child, adolescent and parent versions. Los Angeles (CA); 1998.

66. Hazzard A, Weston J, Gutterres C. After a child's death: Factors related to parental bereavement. J Dev Behav Pediatr 1992;13:24–30.

67. Miles M, Demi A. A comparison of guilt in bereaved parents whose children died by suicide, accident, or chronic disease. Omega 1992;24:203–15.

68. Martinson I, McClowry SG, Davies B, et al. Changes over time: a study of family bereavement following childhood cancer. J Palliat Care 1994;10(1):19–25.

69. Applebaum D, Burns B. Unexpected childhood death: post-traumatic stress disorder in surviving siblings and parents. J Clin Child Psychol 1991;20:114–20.

70. McCown D, Davies B. Patterns of grief in young children following the death of a sibling. Death Stud 1995;19:41–53.

71. Brown AE, Whitney SN, Duffy JD. The physician's role in the assessment and treatment of spiritual distress at the end of life. Palliat Support Care 2006;4(1). 81–6.

72. Doyle D, Hanks GWC, MacDonald N, editors. Oxford textbook of palliative medicine. 3rd edition. New York: Oxford University Press; 2003.

73. Abin A, editor. Supportive care of children with cancer. Baltimore (MD): The Johns Hopkins University Press; 1997.

74. Feudtner C, Feinstein JA, Satchell M, et al. Shifting place of death among children with complex chronic conditions in the United States, 1989–2003. JAMA 2007; 297(24):2725–32.

75. Waggoner J. Shared medical decision making. JAMA 2005;293(9):1058 author reply 1059.

76. Knapp C, Contro N. Family support services in pediatric palliative care. Am J Hosp Palliat Care 2009;26(6):476–82.

77. Davies B, Jin J. Grief and bereavement in pediatric palliative care. In: Ferrell DR, Coyle N, editors. Textbook of palliative nursing. New York: Oxford University Press; 2006. p. 975–89.

78. Custer J, Rau R, editors. The Johns Hopkins Hospital Harriet Lane handbook. 18th edition. Philadelphia: Elsevier Mosby; 2009.

# Index

*Note:* Page numbers of article titles are in **boldface** type.

## A

Abdominal massage, for constipation, 241
Acetaminophen, 201–202, 346
*N*-Acetylcysteine, for COPD, 284
Acupressure
    for nausea and vomiting, 238
    for pain, 341
Acupuncture, for pain, 216, 341
Addiction, to opioids, 204–205
Advance care planning, 185–187
    for COPD, 290
    for dementia, 250–251
    for heart failure, 269
    for kidney failure, 304–306
    for pediatric patients, 335
Agitation, in dementia, 257–258
AIDS. *See* HIV/AIDS.
Albuterol, for COPD, 282
Aldactone, for heart failure, 267
Alendronate, for pain, 348
Allergy, to opioids, 208–209, 211
Alzheimer disease
    clinical presentation of, 248–250
    depression in, 258
    neuropsychiatric symptoms in, 257–258
    treatment of, 253, 255
Amantadine, for pain, 215
American Academy of Hospice and Palliative Medicine, research by, 166
American College of Cardiology, heart failure classification of, 265–266
American Heart Association, heart failure classification of, 265–266
American Pain Society, pain assessment routine of, 197
Amitriptyline, for pain, 214–215, 347
Anal cancer, in HIV/AIDS, 320
Anesthetics, for pediatric patients, 347
Angiotensin receptor blockers, for heart failure, 267
Angiotensin-converting enzyme inhibitors, for heart failure, 267
Anorexia, 225–231
    in cachexia, 229–231
    in HIV/AIDS, 322–323
    in pediatric patients, 343, 351
    treatment of, 351

Prim Care Clin Office Pract 38 (2011) 363–381
doi:10.1016/S0095-4543(11)00033-9
0095-4543/11/$ – see front matter © 2011 Elsevier Inc. All rights reserved.

primarycare.theclinics.com

Anorexia-cachexia syndrome, 230–231
Anticonvulsants, for pain, 214–215, 348
Antidepressants
    for dementia, 259
    for depression, 270
    for pain, 214–215, 347
Antiemetics, 235–237
Antihistamines, for pediatric patients, 350–351
Antipsychotics, for dementia, 258
Antiretroviral Therapy Cohort Collaboration, 313
Anxiety
    in COPD, 279–280, 289
    in HIV/AIDS, 322–323
    in pediatric patients, 344–345
Apnea, sleep, in heart failure, 271
Appetite, loss of. See Anorexia.
Aripiprazole, for dementia, 258
ASK mission, 356
Autonomy, 183–185, 335–336


B

Baclofen, for pain, 214
Barbiturates, for pain, 217
Behavioral disturbances, in dementia, 257–258
Behavioral therapy, for anorexia, 229
Benzodiazepines
    for opioid neurotoxicity, 207
    for pain, 217, 238
    for pediatric patients, 345, 347
Bereavement, 174
    counseling for, in hospice care, 179
    in child's death, 355–356
Beta blockers, for heart failure, 267
Beth Israel Medical Center, Department of Pain Medicine
    and Palliative Care, 243
Billing, for hospice care, 178–179
Bisacodyl, for constipation, 242, 348
Bisoprolol, for heart failure, 267
Bisphosphonates, for bone pain, 215, 348
BODE index, for COPD, 280
Body composition, in cachexia, 230
Body mass index, in COPD, 282, 287–288
Bone pain, 215
Bowel obstruction, 215–216, 236
Brain, lymphoma of, in HIV/AIDS, 319
Breathlessness, in COPD, 289–290
Brief Pain Inventory, 198
Bronchitis Randomized on NAC Cost-Utility Study
    (BRONCUS), 284
Bronchodilators, for COPD, 282–283

Burkitt lymphoma, in HIV/AIDS, 319
Buspirone, for anxiety, 289


C

Cachexia, 229–232, 343, 351
Calcification, coronary artery, in kidney failure, 301
Calciphylaxis/calcific uremic arthropathy, in kidney failure,
   301–302
Cambridge Palliative Assessment Schedule (CAMPAS-R), for nausea and
   vomiting, 233
Cancer
   anorexia in, 225–229
   cachexia in, 229–232
   dementia with, 253
   in HIV/AIDS, 317–320
   pain management in, 187–188, 201–218
   prognostic estimates for, 162–165
Candlelighters for Children with Cancer, 356
Cannabinoids, 216
   for anorexia, 228
   for nausea and vomiting, 236
Capacity, for decision-making, 183–185, 335–336
Carbamazepine
   for dementia, 258
   for pain, 214
Cardiac resynchronization therapy, for heart failure, 268
Cardiopulmonary resuscitation, in dementia, 251
Cardiovascular disease, in kidney failure, 300
Carvedilol, for heart failure, 267
Cascara sagrada, for constipation, 242
Castor oil, for constipation, 242
Celecoxib, 202
Center to Advance Palliative Care, 243
Center to Improve Care of the Dying, 166
Central nervous system, opioid effects on, 205–207
Cerebral edema, 347
Cerebrovascular disease, in kidney failure, 300–301
Certification, of terminal illness, estimation of, 176
Cervical cancer, in HIV/AIDS, 319
Chaplains, 352
Charlson Comorbidity Score, for kidney failure, 304
Children's Hospice and Palliative Care Coalition, 357
Children's Project on Palliative/Hospice Services (ChIPPS), 358
Chlorpromazine
   for nausea and vomiting, 350
   for opioid neurotoxicity, 207
   for pain, 217
Cholinergics, for COPD, 282
Chronic obstructive pulmonary disease, **277–297**
   advanced care planning for, 290

Chronic (*continued*)
  anxiety in, 279–280
  classification of, 277–278
  depression in, 278–279
  exacerbations of, 280–281
  hospice care in, 290–292
  prognosis prediction in, 280–282
  quality of life in, 278
  severity of, assessment of, 277
  treatment of
    associated conditions, 287–289
    end-of-life, 289–292
    oxygen therapy in, 284–285
    pharmacologic, 282–284
    positive pressure ventilation in, 285–286
    pulmonary rehabilitation in, 285
    surgical, 286–287
Citalopram
  for dementia, 258
  for pain, 214
Clinical Practice Guidelines for Quality Palliative Care, 167
Codeine, 202, 346
  dosage of, 210
  metabolism of, 204
Cognitive behavioral therapy
  for anxiety, 289
  for pain, 341
  for pediatric patients, 345
Cognitive dysfunction, pain assessment in, 198–199
Colorectal cancer, in HIV/AIDS, 320
Communication
  in kidney failure, 303–304
  in pediatric palliative care, 330, 332–333
Compassionate Friends, The, 356
Complementary therapy, for pain, 216, 341
Constipation, 238–242
  assessment of, 238–240
  causes of, 238
  definition of, 238
  in pediatric patients, 342, 348–349
  opioid-mediated, 205–206
  pathophysiology of, 238
  prevalence of, 238
  treatment of, 240–242, 348–349
Continuous home care, 177
COPD. *See* Chronic obstructive pulmonary disease.
Coronary artery calcification, in kidney failure, 301
Coronary revascularization, for heart failure, 268
Corticosteroids
  for anorexia, 228
  for COPD, 283

for nausea and vomiting, 235
for neuropathic pain, 213–214
for pediatric patients, 347
Counseling
for cachexia, 232
for constipation, 241–242
for COPD, 285
in hospice care, 179–180
CRIES scale, for pain assessment, 337
Cryptococcosis, in HIV/AIDS, 316
Cultural issues, in pediatric palliative care, 330
Cyclobenzaprine, for pain, 214
Cyproheptadine, for anorexia, 351
Cytokines, in anorexia, 226
Cytomegalovirus infections, in HIV/AIDS, 316


D

Dartmouth Atlas Project, 166–167
Death and dying
idealized good death, 174
Kübler-Ross, Elizabeth on, 174
of pediatric patients, 354–355
valuing of, 174
Death rattle, 355
Decision-making
capacity for, 183–185, 335–336
depression impact on, 290
in COPD, 290
in kidney failure, 303–304
in pain management, 200
in pediatric palliative care, 333–336
in treatment withholding or withdrawal, 186–187
surrogates for, 185–186
Dehydration, in dementia, 251–252
Delirium, pain assessment in, 198–199
Dementia, **247–264**
acute care hospitalization in, 253
acute illnesses in, 253
advanced, 250
Alzheimer, 248–250, 257–258
behavioral problems in, 237–258
cardiopulmonary resuscitation in, 251
chronic diseases with, 253–254
clinical presentation of, 248–250
depression in, 259
feeding in, 251
hydration in, 251–252
Lewy body, 248–250, 253, 255
pain management in, 255–257
prevalence of, 248–250

Dementia (*continued*)
    prognostic estimates for, 162–165
    treatment of, 253, 255
    types of, 248–250
    vascular, 248–249, 253, 255
Department of Veterans Affairs, palliative care in, 167
Depression
    in COPD, 278–279, 288–290
    in dementia, 259
    in heart failure, 270
    in pediatric patients, 344–345
Desipramine, for pain, 214–215
Dexamethasone, 347
    for anorexia, 351
    for nausea and vomiting, 235
    for pain, 214
Dextroamphetamine, for somnolence, 351
Dextromethorphan, for pain, 215
Dialysis
    in elderly persons, 306
    symptom burden in, 302–303
    withdrawal from, 305–306
Dialysis Outcomes and Practice Patterns Study (DOPPS), 302
Diazepam, 347
Dietary counseling
    for constipation, 241–242
    in hospice care, 180
Diffuse large B-cell lymphoma, in HIV/AIDS, 318
Digoxin, for heart failure, 267
Diphenylhydramine, for nausea and vomiting, 237, 350
Diuretics, for heart failure, 267
Docusate, for constipation, 242, 349
Dopamine receptors, in nausea and vomiting, 233
DOPPS (Dialysis Outcomes and Practice Patterns Study), 302
Double effect doctrine, in palliative sedation, 188–189, 217
Douleur Enfant Gustav-Roussy scale, for pain assessment, 337
Dronabinol, 216
    for anorexia, 228
    for nausea and vomiting, 236
Droperidol, for nausea and vomiting, 350
Drug abuse, in HIV/AIDS, 320–321
Duloxetine, for pain, 214–215
Dyspnea
    in COPD, 289–290
    in heart failure, 270
    in pediatric patients, 342–343

E

Eating disorders. *See* Anorexia.
Edmonton Symptom Assessment Scale, 198

for anorexia, 228
for kidney failure, 304
Education
for constipation, 241–242
for COPD, 285
for health care providers, 165–166
Eicosapentaenoic acid, for cachexia, 231–232
Elderly persons, dialysis for, 306
Election statement, for hospice care, 177
Electrolyte imbalance, in kidney failure, 300–301
Emesis. *See also* Nausea and vomiting.
definition of, 232
Emphysema. *See* Chronic obstructive pulmonary disease.
Encephalitis, toxoplasmosis, in HIV/AIDS, 317
Endobronchial valve, for COPD, 287
End-of Life/Palliative Education Resource Center, 243
End-of-Life Nursing Education Consortium, 166, 357–358
Established Populations for Epidemiologic Studies of the
Elderly study, 162–163
Ethical issues, **183–193**
advance care planning, 185–186
in pediatric care, 335–336
pain management, 187–188
physician-assisted suicide and euthanasia, 189
principles of, 183–185
sedation, 188–189
treatment withholding and withdrawal, 186–187
European Association of Palliative Care guidelines, for sedation, 189
EuroQol 5-dimension questionnaire, 278
Euthanasia, 189
Exercise, for COPD, 285
Existential suffering, palliative sedation for, 189
Expectorants, for COPD, 284


**F**

FAACT (Functional Assessment of Anorexia/Cachexia Therapy), 228
Face, Legs, Activity, Cry, and Consolability scale, 198–199, 337
FACES Pain Rating Scale, 198, 337–338
Fatigue, in HIV/AIDS, 322–323
Feeding, in dementia, 251
Fentanyl, 202, 346
metabolism of, 204
side effects of, 205
transdermal administration of, 212–213
Fiber, dietary, for constipation, 242
Fluoxetine, for pain, 214
Food diary, for anorexia, 229
Forced expiratory volume in 1 second, in COPD, 280
Formoterol, for COPD, 282
Frailty, 162–164

Functional assessment, in pain assessment, 199–200
Functional Assessment of Anorexia/Cachexia Therapy (FAACT), 228

**G**

Gabapentin
 for kidney failure, 303
 for pain, 214, 348
Gastrointestinal symptoms, **225–246**
 anorexia. *See* Anorexia.
 cachexia, 229–232, 343, 351
 constipation, 205–206, 238–242, 342, 348–349
 nausea and vomiting. *See* Nausea and vomiting.
Gastrostomy tube feeding, for dementia, 251
Ghrelin, for cachexia, 231
Global Deterioration Scale, for dementia, 250
Global Initiative for Chronic Obstructive Lung Disease (GOLD)
  classification, 277–278
Granisetron, for nausea and vomiting, 349
Grief, in child's death, 355–356
Guaifenesin, for COPD, 284

**H**

HAART therapy, for HIV/AIDS, 311–322
Haloperidol
 for nausea and vomiting, 236–237, 350
 for opioid neurotoxicity, 207
 for pain, 217
Harvard Medical School Center for Palliative Care, 357
Health care proxy document, 185–186
Health Survey Questionnaire, for COPD, 278
Heart failure, **265–276**
 advance care planning for, 269
 classification of, 265–266
 definition of, 266
 internal cardiac defibrillator deactivation in, 271–272
 medication discontinuation in, 271
 prevalence of, 265
 prognostic estimates for, 162–165, 269
 treatment of
  acute decompensated, 268–269
  common symptom management, 270–271
  devices for, 267–268
  hospice, 272–273
  inotropic support in, 272
  medical, 266–267
Heart Failure Society of America, heart failure definition of, 266
Hemodialysis
 in elderly persons, 306
 symptom burden in, 302–303

withdrawal from, 305–306
Hepatitis C, in HIV/AIDS, 321
Hester's Poker Chips, for pain assessment, 338
Hiccups, 227–228
Highly active antiretroviral therapy (HAART), for HIV/AIDS, 311–322
HIV/AIDS, **311–326**
   epidemiology of, 312
   HAART therapy for, 311–322
   hospice care for, 313
   liver disease in, 320–321
   malignancy in, 317–320
   opportunistic infections in, 313–317
   prognostic indicators in, 312–313
   substance abuse in, 320–321
   symptoms of, 322–323
Hodgkin lymphoma, in HIV/AIDS, 320
Home health care programs, 167–168, 177
Hospice care, 168, **173–182**
   benefit limits in, 178
   certification of terminal illness for, 176
   core services in, 179–180
   election statement for, 177
   eligibility for, 175
   for COPD, 290–292
   for heart failure, 272–273
   for HIV/AIDS, 313
   for pediatric patients, 353–354
   history of, 173–174
   payment system for, 177–178
   philosophy of, 173–174
   physician billing for, 178–179
   prognosis in, 175–176
   programs for, 168
   referrals to, 176–177
   regulations for, 175
   team approach to, 175
   treatments covered in, 181
   valuing death in, 174
Hospice Conditions of Participation, 178–179
Hospice of the Bluegrass and Palliative Care Center, 168
Hospitalization, for dementia, 253
Hospitals, palliative care in, 167
Human immunodeficiency virus. See HIV/AIDS.
Hydralazine, for heart failure, 267
Hydration, in dementia, 251–252
Hydrocodone, 202
   dosage of, 210
   metabolism of, 204
Hydromorphone, 202, 210, 346
Hydroxyzine, for nausea and vomiting, 351
Hyoscyamine, for nausea and vomiting, 237

Hyperparathyroidism, in kidney failure, 301–302
Hypersensitivity, to opioids, 208–209, 211


I

Ibuprofen, 346
Illness trajectories, 162–164
Imipramine, for pain, 347
Implantable cardioverter-defibrillators, for heart failure, 267–268, 271–272
Informed consent, 183–185, 188–189
Initiative for Pediatric Palliative Care, 357
Inotropic therapy, for heart failure, 272
Inpatient care
    general, 177–178
    respite, 177
Institute for Healthcare Improvement, 166
Institute of Medicine, end-of-life care recommendations of, 162
Interferons, in anorexia, 226
Interleukins, in anorexia, 226
Internal cardiac defibrillator, for heart failure, 268
International Association of Hospice and Palliative Care, 233, 243
Ipratropium bromide, for COPD, 282


K

Kaposi sarcoma, in HIV/AIDS, 317–318
Karnovsky performance score, 164
Ketamine, 215, 347
Kidney failure, **299–309**
    advance care planning for, 304–306
    causes of death in, 300–302
    decision making in, 303–304
    prognosis of, 299–300
    symptom burden in, 302–303
Kübler-Ross, Elizabeth, on death and dying, 174


L

Lactulose, for constipation, 242, 349
Laryngeal cancer, in HIV/AIDS, 320
Laxatives, 205, 240, 242, 348–349
Left ventricular assist device, for heart failure, 268
Legal issues, in pediatric care, 335–336
Leptin, in anorexia, 226–227
Levonatrodol, for nausea and vomiting, 236
Lewy body dementia
    clinical presentation of, 248–250
    treatment of, 253, 255
Liaison Committee on Medical Education, 165
Lidocaine, 347
Life expectancy, palliative care and, 161–162

Life support, withdrawal of, 186–187
Limb amputation, in kidney failure, 302
Liver disease, in HIV/AIDS, 320–321
Living wills, 185–187
Local coverage determinations, for hospice care, 176
Lorazepam, 347
Lung cancer, in HIV/AIDS, 320
Lung transplantation, for COPD, 287
Lung volume reduction surgery, for COPD, 286–287
Lymphomas, in HIV/AIDS, 318–320


**M**

Magnesium salts, for constipation, 242, 349
Massage
    for constipation, 241
    for pain, 216, 341
Mature minor doctrine, 336
Medicare
    hospice benefits in, 173, 175–179
        for COPD, 291–292
        for HIV/AIDS, 313
    palliative care guidelines of, 168
Medroxyprogesterone acetate, for anorexia, 228
Megestrol acetate, for anorexia, 228, 351
Melatonin
    for anorexia, 351
    for cachexia, 232
Memantine
    for dementia, 258
    for pain, 215
Memorial Delirium-Assessment Scale, 198–199
Memorial Pain Assessment Card, 198
Memorial Symptom Assessment Scale, for anorexia, 228
Meperidine, metabolism of, 204
Metastasis, to bone, 215
Metaxalone, for pain, 214
Methadone, 202, 215
    conversion ratio of, 211–212
    for pediatric patients, 340–341
    mechanism of action of, 203
    metabolism of, 204
Methocarbamol, for pain, 214
Methylcellulose, for constipation, 242
Methylnaltrexone, for constipation, 240–241
Methylphenidate
    for depression, 270
    for somnolence, 351
Metoclopramide
    for anorexia, 228–229
    for nausea and vomiting, 235, 237, 349

Metoprolol, for heart failure, 267
Metropolitan Jewish Hospice and Palliative Care Program, 168
Midazolam, for pain, 217–218
Milrinone, for heart failure, 272
Mini Mental State Examination, 198–199, 250
Ministry of presence, 352
Mirtazapine, for nausea and vomiting, 237
Morphine, 202
    conversion ratio of, 211–212
    dosage of, 210
    for pediatric patients, 340–341, 346
    metabolism of, 204
Mourning, in child's death, 355–356
Mucolytics, for COPD, 284
Muscle relaxants, for pain, 214
Muscle wasting
    in anorexia, 225–228
    in cachexia, 230–232
*Mycobacterium avium* complex infections, in HIV/AIDS, 315–316
*Mycobacterium tuberculosis* infections, in HIV/AIDS, 316


N

Nabilone, 216, 236, 350
Nalmefene, 202
Naloxone, 202, 237
Naltrexone, 202
Naproxen, 346
National Board of Hospice and Palliative Care Nurses, certification from, 166
National Cancer Institute Supportive Care, 243
National Comprehensive Cancer Network Clinical Practice Guidelines, 233
National Consensus Project for Quality Palliative Care, 167
National Emphysema Treatment Trial, 286
National Hospice and Palliative Care Organization, on sedation, 189
National Institutes of Health, research by, 166
National Palliative Care Research Center, 166
Nausea and vomiting, 232–238
    assessment of, 233
    causes of, 233–234
    definition of, 232
    in pediatric patients, 341–342
    opioid-induced, 205–206
    pathophysiology of, 232–233
    prevalence of, 232
    treatment of, 233, 235–238
Neonatal Infant Pain Scale, 337
Neonatal Pain, Agitation and Sedation Scale (N-PASS), 337
Nerve blocks, 341
Neuroleptics, for pain, 217
Neuropathic pain, 213, 215
Neuropeptide Y, in anorexia, 226

Neuropsychiatric symptoms, in dementia, 257–258
Neurotoxicity, of opioids, 205–206
New York Heart Association, heart failure classification of, 266
Nitrates, for heart failure, 267
Nocturnal Oxygen Therapy Trial, for COPD, 284
Noninvasive positive pressure ventilation, for COPD, 285–286
Nonmaleficence, pain management and, 187
Nonsteroidal antiinflammatory drugs, 201–202
Nortriptyline, for pain, 214, 348
Numeric rating scale, for pain assessment, 197–198
Nursing care, in hospice, 179
Nursing education, for palliative care, 166
Nutritional assessment, for anorexia, 229
Nutritional support
    for anorexia, 229
    for cachexia, 232
    for COPD, 287–288
    for dementia, 251
    for pediatric patients, 343


O

Olanzapine
    for dementia, 258
    for nausea and vomiting, 236, 350
    for pain, 217
Ondansetron, for nausea and vomiting, 235, 237, 349
Open Society Institute, Project on Death in America, 165
Opioids, 202–213
    adjuvants for, 213–216
    antagonists for, 202
    chemical classification of, 202
    common pain syndromes and, 213–216
    conversion ratios for, 211–212
    decision pathway for, 209–211
    doses for, 210
    for bowel obstruction, 236
    for COPD, 289–290
    for pain, 238
    for pediatric patients, 338–341, 346
    mechanism of action of, 202
    metabolism of, 203
    mu-receptor agonists, 202–203
    physiologic responses to, 203–205
    psychological response to, 203–205
    rotation of, 211–212
    routes for, 212–213
    side effects of, 205–208, 341
Opportunistic infections, in HIV/AIDS, 313–317
OPTIMIZE-HF model, 269
Osmotic laxatives, for constipation, 242

Osteoporosis, in COPD, 287
Oucher Scale, for pain assessment, 338
Outpatient palliative care clinics, 168
Oxcarbazepine, for pain, 214
Oxycodone, 202, 210, 346
Oxygen therapy, for COPD, 284–285
Oxymorphone, 202, 210


**P**

PACE (Program of All-inclusive Care for the Elderly), 168
Pain
    as vital sign, 197
    characteristics of, 197–198
    concurrent symptoms with, 199
    in cognitively impaired persons, 198–199
    in HIV/AIDS, 322–323
Pain and Palliative Care Communications Program Resources to Develop and
    Enhance Pediatric Palliative Care Services, 357
Pain assessment, 196–200, 255–257, 336–338
Pain Assessment Checklist for Seniors with Limited Ability to Communicate, 255, 257
Pain management, **195–223**
    complementary therapies for, 216
    decision-making process for, 200
    ethical issues in, 187–188
    in dementia, 255–257
    in heart failure, 270
    in kidney failure, 302–303
    in pain crisis, 211
    in pediatric patients, 338–341, 346–347
    palliative sedation in, 188–189, 217–218
    reassessment in, 216–218
    therapeutic plan for, 200–216
Pain Relief Act of 1996, 187
Palliative care
    definition of, 161
    ethical issues in, **183–193,** 335–336
    for chronic obstructive pulmonary disease, **277–297**
    for dementia, 162–165, **247–264**
    for gastrointestinal symptoms, **225–246**
    for heart failure, **265–276**
    for HIV/AIDS, **311–326**
    for kidney failure, **299–309**
    for pediatric patients, **327–361**
    history of, 159–160
    illness trajectories and, 162–164
    in community, 167–168
    in hospice. See Hospice care.
    in hospitals, 167
    need for, 161–162
    nursing education for, 166

overview of, **159–171**
pain management in. *See* Pain management.
physician education for, 165–166
prognostic estimates in, 162–165
research in, 166–167
web resources for, 243
Palliative Prognostic Index, 164
Palliative Prognostic score, 164
Palliative sedation
    ethical issues in, 188–189
    for refractory pain, 217–218
Pamidronate, for pain, 348
Panic attacks, in COPD, 289
Parkinsonism, in Lewy body dementia, 248–250, 253, 255
Paroxetine, for pain, 214
Patient-Generated Subjective Global Assessment, for anorexia, 228
Pediatric Dyspnea Scale, 342
Pediatric Nausea Assessment Tool, 342
Pediatric palliative care, **327–361**
    advanced care planning in, 335
    barriers to, 330
    bereavement and grief management in, 355–356
    communication about, 330, 332–333
    conditions appropriate for, 328
    decision making in, 333–336
    developmental considerations in, 328–331
    epidemiology of, 328–330
    ethical considerations in, 335–336
    formulary for, 346–351
    goals of, 333–335
    in final weeks, 354–355
    information resources for, 356–358
    legal considerations in, 335–336
    pain assessment in, 336–338
    pain management in, 338–341
    psychosocial aspects of, 343–345, 352–353
    settings for, 353–354
    symptom assessment and management in, 341–343
Peritoneal dialysis
    in elderly persons, 306
    symptom burden in, 302–303
    withdrawal from, 305–306
Physical dependence, on opioids, 204
Physical examination, in pain assessment, 200
Physician education, for palliative care, 165–166
Physicians, assisting in suicide and euthanasia, 189
*Pneumocystis jirovecii* infections, in HIV/AIDS, 315
Pneumonia
    in dementia, 253
    in HIV/AIDS, 315
Polycarbophil, for constipation, 242

Polyethylene glycol, for constipation, 242, 349
Positive pressure ventilation, for COPD, 285–286
Pregabalin, for pain, 214–215, 348
Primary central nervous system lymphoma, in HIV/AIDS, 319
Prochlorperazine, for nausea and vomiting, 237, 349
Progestagens, for anorexia, 228
Prognosis estimation, 162–165
    for COPD, 280–282
    for heart failure, 269
    for HIV/AIDS, 312–313
    for hospice care, 175–176
    for kidney failure, 299–300
Program of All-inclusive Care for the Elderly (PACE), 168
Progressive multifocal leukoencephalopathy, in HIV/AIDS, 316–317
Project on Death in America, 165
Prokinetic agents
    for anorexia, 228–229
    for constipation, 242
Promethazine, for nausea and vomiting, 237
Propofol, 217, 341
Prostate cancer, in HIV/AIDS, 320
Proteolysis-inducing factor, in cachexia, 230
Pruritus, opioid-induced, 208
Pseudoaddition, to opioids, 204–205
Pseudoallergy, to opioids, 208–209, 211
Psychosocial issues
    in pediatric patients, 343–345, 352–353
    palliative sedation for, 189
Psychotherapy, for anxiety, 289
Psyllium, for constipation, 242
Pulmonary hypertension, in COPD, 281, 288
Pulmonary rehabilitation, for COPD, 285

Q

Quality of life, with COPD, 278

R

Randomized Aldacton Evaluation Study (RALES), 267
Referrals, for hospice care, 176–177
Refractory symptoms, palliative sedation for, 188–189
Regulations, for hospice care, 175
Rehabilitation, pulmonary, for COPD, 285
Renal failure. See Kidney failure.
Research, in palliative care, 166–167
Resistiveness to care, in dementia, 257–258
Respiratory depression, opioid-induced, 206–208
Respiratory failure, in COPD, 281
Respite care, inpatient, 177
Restraints, for pain, 238
Resuscitation, in dementia, 251

Resynchronization therapy, for heart failure, 268
Retching, versus vomiting, 232
Risperidone, for dementia, 258
Robert Wood Johnson Foundation, palliative care study of, 165


**S**

Salmeterol, for COPD, 282–283
Sarcopenia, in cachexia, 230–232
Saunders, Cicely, as founder of hospice movement, 173–174, 196
Scopolamine, for nausea and vomiting, 237, 350
Seattle Heart Failure Model, 269
Sedation
    ethical issues in, 188–189
    for refractory pain, 217–218
    opioid-induced, 205
Self-bereavement, 174
Self-determination, 183–185
Senna, for constipation, 242, 348
Sensory stimulation, for dementia, 258
Septicemia, in kidney failure, 300–301
Serotonin receptors, in nausea and vomiting, 233
Sertraline, for dementia, 258
Severe Impairment Battery, for dementia, 250
Sleep-disordered breathing, in heart failure, 270–271
Social workers
    in hospice care, 179
    in pediatric care, 352–353
Sodium biphosphate, for constipation, 242
Somnolence, treatment of, 351
Sorbitol, for constipation, 242
Spiritual counseling, 180, 352
St Christopher's Hospice, 173–174
Stimulant laxatives, for constipation, 242
Stool softeners, for constipation, 242
Stroke, in kidney failure, 300
Study to Understand Prognoses and Preference for Outcomes and
    Risks of Treatment (SUPPORT) study, 165, 270
Subcortical ischemic vascular dementia, clinical presentation of, 248–249
Substance abuse, in HIV/AIDS, 320–321
Sudden death, 162
Suicidal ideation, in pediatric patients, 345
Suicide, physician-assisted, 189
SUPPORT (Study to Understand Prognoses and Preference for Outcomes
    and Risks of Treatment) study, 165, 270


**T**

Tapentadol, 202
    dosage of, 210
    mechanism of action of, 203

Team approach
    to hospice care, 174–175, 179–180
    to palliative care, 167
Tegaserod, for constipation, 242
Terminal illness
    certification of, estimation of, 176
    definition of, 175
Test for Severe Impairment, for dementia, 250
Thalidomide, for cachexia, 232
Tiagabine, for pain, 214
Tiotropium, for COPD, 283
Tizanidine, for pain, 214
Tolerance, of opioids, 204
Topiramate, for pain, 214
Total pain concept, 174, 196, 338
Toward a Revolution in COPD Health (TORCH) study, 280–281
Toxoplasmosis, in HIV/AIDS, 317
Tramadol, 202, 346
    dosage of, 210
    mechanism of action of, 203
Transcutaneous electrical nerve stimulation, for pain, 341
Transplantation
    heart, for heart failure, 268
    lung, for COPD, 287
Trazodone, for dementia, 258
Treatment, withholding and withdrawing, 186–187
Tube feeding, for dementia, 251
Tuberculosis, in HIV/AIDS, 316
Tumor necrosis factor, in anorexia, 226


U

United Nations International Covenant on Economic Social and
    Cultural Rights, 187–188
United States Renal Data System database, 300


V

Valvular repair, for heart failure, 268
Vascular dementia
    clinical presentation of, 248–249
    treatment of, 253, 255
Venlafaxine, for pain, 214
Ventilation, positive pressure, for COPD, 285–286
Vomiting. See Nausea and vomiting.


W

Weight loss
    in anorexia, 225–228
    in cachexia, 229–230

in HIV/AIDS, 322–323
Withholding and withdrawing treatment, 186–187
Wong-Baker FACES Pain Rating Scale, 198
World Health Organization
    Pain and Palliative Care Communications Program Resources to Develop
      and Enhance Pediatric Palliative Care Services, 357
    pain management ladder of, 201, 338
    palliative care definition of, 161


Y

Yoga, for pain, 341

# Moving?

## Make sure your subscription moves with you!

To notify us of your new address, find your **Clinics Account Number** (located on your mailing label above your name), and contact customer service at:

**Email: journalscustomerservice-usa@elsevier.com**

**800-654-2452** (subscribers in the U.S. & Canada)
**314-447-8871** (subscribers outside of the U.S. & Canada)

**Fax number: 314-447-8029**

**Elsevier Health Sciences Division**
**Subscription Customer Service**
**3251 Riverport Lane**
**Maryland Heights, MO 63043**

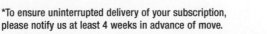

*To ensure uninterrupted delivery of your subscription, please notify us at least 4 weeks in advance of move.

Printed and bound by CPI Group (UK) Ltd, Croydon, CR0 4YY

03/10/2024

01040456-0004